Realize that there is a great wind that blows from heaven and that this wind is Light and Sound. In this stream of Light and Sound, you can dance all the way across the universes. You can turn your consciousness into it, and know that you and the Light are one.

–John-Roger

Being an actor is actually a tough business. It includes intense athletic training and great physical stress. Especially for the last two movies I have done. I recently shot "We Were Soldiers" with Mel Gibson, and "Collateral Damage" with Arnold Schwarzenegger. In preparation, I did vigorous Boot Camp activity for weeks and 680 push-ups a day. My shoulder finally gave out. It just wouldn't heal. And I had to stop working out for a couple of months.

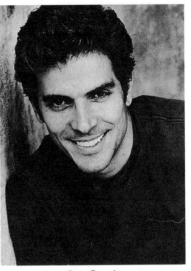

Jsu Garcia

I have been friends with Marc forever, and because many of our acquaintances had been healed by Prolotherapy, I thought I'd give it a shot (no pun intended). After the first set of injections, for a day or so, my shoulder felt like someone had punched it. I was reluctant to be reinjected. Then on a trip with Marc and some friends, while he was injecting them, he said I needed to be injected at least one more time. I agreed, and to my surprise, my shoulder was healed completely within the next couple of days.

Since then, I remain pain-free and am working out like a champ preparing for my next movie.

I entreat you to read this book. It will be an inspiration to you and your friends. Not only will it enlighten you to avoid surgery with a new approach to living pain free, but also will show you the way a doctor is supposed to think and treat his patients. Marc walks the high road and I hope you will follow.

Jsu Garcia

The Collagen Revolution
"Let the Healing Begin"

"Prolotherapy stimulates your body's natural production of collagen and provides relief from chronic pain"

"Be sober and temperate, and you will be healthy."
–Benjamin Franklin

WHAT OTHERS ARE SAYING ABOUT DR. DARROW'S WORK

Dr. Darrow has been a guiding light for my health and wellbeing. It is rare to find a doctor who not only takes the time to care, but also has the wit to find the answers for his patients' problems that other doctors have missed. If you are looking for a pain cure, read this book.

Joe Weider, Muscle and Fitness Guru

This book will help change the way pain medicine is practiced. It will teach your doctor how to heal your pain naturally.

Jack Canfield,
Co-author of Chicken Soup for the Soul®

My career as a bodybuilder was destroyed by an injury. Dr. Darrow's unique therapy that he describes in this book literally saved me. I am pain free again and squatting 700 lbs.

Joe DeAngelis, Mr. Universe, Mr. America

Dr. Darrow's needle feels like an angel dancing on my skin. His treatment gave me my first pain free season in ten years. If you are looking for a doctor who can heal when others fail, read his book.

Johnnie Morton, Jr., Pro Football, Detroit Lions

September 18, 2001
Marc Darrow, M.D., J.D.
Joint Rehabilitation and Sports Medical Center
Los Angeles, CA 90025

Dear Dr. Darrow:

I am so glad to have met you earlier this year. Last year I injured my right shoulder while playing tennis. For months I tried to let it heal by itself, but to no avail. I had pain doing simple tasks such as combing my hair or reaching for my wallet. I finally relented and saw an orthopedist who had it x-rayed. He concluded I had arthritis and there was nothing he could do. I was pretty upset because at age 43 I felt I had many years left to play tennis. That's when I met you. You said you could fix it with a weekly series of Prolotherapy injections. To make a long story short, you were correct. After seven treatments I was back on the court playing pain-free.

However, as you know, that terrific state of affairs didn't last long. Two weeks later I tore two ligaments in my right ankle stepping on a tennis ball while going for a cross-court backhand shot. It blew up like a balloon. After I got an MRI the orthopedist said I would probably need surgery. I told him about you and that I wanted to see what you thought first. We decided to give Prolotherapy a chance. That, combined with an ankle exercise board and heat treatments, and use surgery as a last resort. Well, once again, you worked your magic and two months later I'm back playing tennis with reckless abandon. I don't even need an ankle support. I couldn't be more pleased. I think your book, *The Collagen Revolution: Living Pain Free* should be mandatory reading for anyone who suffers joint pain, no matter what their age. It sure opened my eyes. I plan on playing tennis for another 50 years or so. Thanks for your help Dr. Darrow.

Sincerely,
Bill Strong
Beverly Hills, California

September 22, 2001
Marc Darrow, MD, JD
Joint Rehabilitation and Sports Medical Center
11645 Wilshire Blvd. Suite 120
Los Angeles, California 90025

Dear Marc:

I am writing to give my thanks for the treatment you and your staff have provided me over the past several months. Being a tennis pro is very demanding on my body, and I certainly have my share of aches and pains. I was literally shocked when you told me you could easily heal my knee. It was an injury I had suffered from for years.

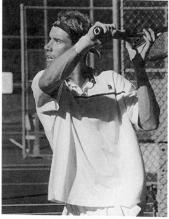

Mark Harradine

Not having had any relief from other practitioners, I was open to just about any kind of treatment whether I had heard of it before or not. Prolotherapy, what the #@*% is that? Needless to say, you were right. After 4 treatments, my knee was completely healed.

As the life of a tennis bum has it, I next injured my wrist. The MRI you took showed nothing more than tendonitis. Hard to believe, it felt like a fracture. Again, after a few sessions of Prolotherapy, the pain is resolving. Sorry, I haven't been a good boy, letting it rest as you suggested. Amazing how the more I beat up my body, the more you love it back to health. You always seem to know I will heal.

God bless you. You are a true healer. I hope your book, The Collagen Revolution: Living Pain Free makes it to every locker room in the world. It will certainly save many of us from long- term pain.

Sincerely,

Mark Harradine

"If I'd known I was gonna live this long,
I'd have taken better care of myself."
–Eubie Blake

The Collagen Revolution

Living Pain Free

by

Dr. Marc Darrow MD, JD

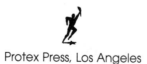

Protex Press, Los Angeles

The Collagen Revolution
Living Pain Free

Marc Darrow, MD, JD

Published by: Protex Press
11645 Wilshire Blvd. Suite 120
Los Angeles, CA 90025, U.S.A.
800-Rehab10 (1-800-734-2210)
310-231-7000
Fax: 310-231-7227
http://www.JointRehab.com
LawDoc@MarcDarrow.com

Printed in the United States of America

Library of Congress Cataloging-in-Publication Data
Marc Darrow, MD, JD
    The Collagen Revolution: Living Pain Free / Marc Darrow, MD, JD.--
1st ed.
    Includes bibliographical references and index.
    ISBN 0-9714503-0-7

    1. Health 2. Medical I. Title.

Book Cover Designer: Nita Ybarra
Book Interior Designer: Pamela Terry

First Edition

Dedication (A Practice)

It is difficult if not impossible, with our lives so full of distractions from our inner worlds, to let those we love really know that we love them. This book is dedicated to all of you whom I love. My work is dedicated to you. My life is dedicated to you.

Michelle— my beautiful wife.

Selma— my loving mother.

Zim— my continuing inspiration from the other side.

Benjy, Jason, Jensen, Jordan and Britt— my sweet children.

Jason, Bill, Frank, Christy, Faith, Shawny, Ben, Joel,

Gary, Stephanie, Gina, Kathy, and Q— my partners in health.

Diane Campbell—without her there could never have been this book.

And that giant of a man who has sculpted me from clay— John-Roger.

Dr. Darrow and David Sloan, Detroit Lions Football Team

About the Author

Dr. Marc Darrow is a Board Certified Physiatrist specializing in Physical Medicine and Rehabilitation.

As medical director of the Joint Rehabilitation & Sports Medical Center in Los Angeles, Dr. Darrow has focused his practice on musculoskeletal injury, pain management, electro-diagnosis (EMG/NCS), and sports medicine and rehabilitation. He works along side Jason Kelberman, D.C. the Director of Chiropractic Services and Bill Bergman, PhD, director of the MedX Department. Together with their staff, they bring healing to patients who have searched far and wide for the answer to their health.

An avid sports enthusiast, Dr. Darrow discovered Prolotherapy after an injury on the golf course (watch out!) caused him to suffer the kind of chronic pain that afflicts millions of Americans.

A skeptical Dr. Darrow became a believer in the therapeutic healing power of Prolotherapy and trigger point injections after only one treatment. Since then he has devoted his practice to Prolotherapy, a little known, natural therapy that is revolutionizing the way we treat pain.

Dr. Darrow lives happily in Los Angeles with his wife and children, and works on his golf swing and tennis serve whenever he finds the time. And a little guitar playing just before bed seems to calm his soul.

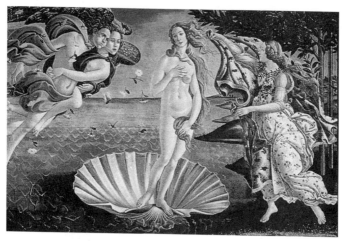

Pearls of the Collagen Revolution

Pearls are formed when something (a grain of sand, a speck of shell) finds itself inside an oyster and creates irritation.

Since the oyster cannot remove the object, it responds by secreting a nacre, commonly called Mother of Pearl (calcium carbonate), to help soothe the irritation.

The nacre covers the object and continues to coat it until the object ceases to irritate. The resulting incrustation, over several years, produces a pearl, one of nature's most precious jewels.

In this book you will discover how Prolotherapy naturally stimulates the body to rejuvenate itself with the proliferation of new collagen.

Disclaimer

This book is designed to provide information about the subject matter covered. It is sold with the understanding that the publisher and author are not engaged in rendering medical or other professional services. If medical or other expert assistance is required, the services of a competent professional should be sought.

It is not the purpose of this manual to reprint all the information that is otherwise available to authors and other creative people but to complement, amplify and supplement other texts. For more information, see the many references.

Healing the human body is not the responsibility of the practitioner without the total commitment of the patient. It is the patient who must make the commitment and leap of faith to be healed. At the same time, every patient is informed that there are no guarantees.

Every effort has been made to make this book as complete and as accurate as possible. However, there may be mistakes both typographical and in content. Therefore, this text should be used only as a general guide and not as the ultimate source of information about healing your pain.

The purpose of this manual is to educate and entertain. The author and Protex Publishing shall have neither liability nor responsibility to any person or entity with respect to any loss or damage caused or alleged to be caused directly or indirectly by the information contained in this book. In medicine there are no guarantees.

If you do not wish to be bound by the above, you may return this book to the publisher for a full refund.

Prolotherapy – The rehabilitation of an incompetent structure as a ligament or tendon, by the induced proliferation of new cells.

Rehabilitation – To restore or bring to a condition of good health, ability to work, or productive activity.

Rejuvenation – To restore to youthful vigor; make young again.

– Webster's New Collegiate Dictionary

"Although the world is full of suffering, it is also full of the overcoming of it."

-Helen Keller

Table of Contents

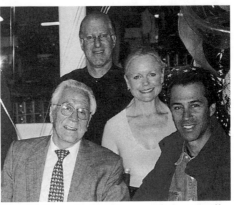

Joe Weider with Dr. Darrow, Robert Reiff (Photographer for Weider Publications), and Janet Miller

Foreword by Joe Weider

I consider myself an evangelist of health. I have spent my life with a single purpose: to bring joy to my fellow man. My focus has been to educate the public on the many wonders and paths to excellent health.

Through my own experience, I found that exercise, good diet, and high-minded thinking are all important to maintain a state of well-being. In my process, I have developed among other enterprises, a food supplement company, an exercise equipment line, and seven magazines that focus on health and fitness.

Because of my early success, I have always taken pride in giving talented individuals a stepping-stone to their success.

Part of my good fortune was my referral by my friend and doctor, Leroy Perry, DC, to a creative healer, Marc Darrow, MD.

Like many of the current heroes of modern medicine, Marc walks to the beat of a different drummer. His strong spiritual ties have led him to a field that is yet unmapped. He doesn't need devices of the high-tech age to diagnose or treat. He uses his hands and intuition just like his mentors of years past.

Instead of copping out to the surgical quick fix of mainline medicine, Dr. Darrow stimulates the body to naturally heal and rejuvenate itself.

The aphorism, "Physician Heal Thyself" applies in his case since the magical treatment that he administers to his patients, was first used on his own body and saved his sports life after years of gymnastics and other sports injuries.

Prolotherapy is the technique that has changed my life and the lives of a multitude of Dr. Darrow's patients. I first learned about it from associates of mine who had experienced miracle pain cures after 2-3 sessions.

It made no sense to me, and in fact seemed like a fairy tale. I had been treated without relief by many of "the best" practitioners, including surgeons and podiatrists, for chronic foot and toe pain. They told me the ligaments in my toes had become stretched from years of athletics such as repetitive toe raises and mountain climbing. Nevertheless, after three to four weeks of Prolotherapy, much of the pain that I had experienced for years, disappeared. As I write this, my foot feels 80% better!

I not only recommend Prolotherapy to those of you who suffer, but I expect you to buy this book for your friends, families, and doctors, and educate them about this therapy. There is new hope for the elimination of your chronic pain.

Joe Weider, Muscle and Fitness Guru

"Every human being is the author of his own health or disease."

–Sivananda

1

My Medical Path

Prolotherapy and Healing

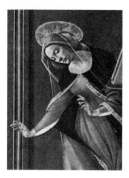

I am about to introduce you to a revolutionary therapy that is radically changing the face of orthopedic medicine and the treatment of chronic pain.

It is called Prolotherapy and I believe it to be a "miracle cure." A miracle, because the results with my patients astound me. Injuries and chronic pain that previously continued for years even with treatment, can now be healed.

If you, or a loved one, suffer from chronic pain, and have found little or only temporary relief through conventional treatments, I have good news for you. It is possible for you to live your life pain free.

That's right, *you do not have to suffer pain any more,* even if you have been led to believe that your pain is *"untreatable"*, or that surgery is the only answer.

This is important, so I'm going to say it again. You can **live your life pain free**.

Think about that for a minute. What would your life be like if you no longer had to endure the chronic pain that plagues you?

Imagine, you could walk, run, lift your child, garden, hike, or just resume your daily activities, no longer afflicted with the pain you thought was your lot to bear.

Sounds pretty sweet, doesn't it? Almost too good to be true? Many of you have probably tried everything already: physical therapy, drugs, surgery, acupuncture; the list goes on.

Maybe you had temporary relief, a lessening of pain, a little more range of motion, but still, chronic pain persists.

You have probably been told that your pain is inevitable; a part of the aging process, the result of injury, arthritis, or repetitive stress.

You have probably heard that there is no real cure for chronic pain or arthritis, that the best you can do is manage it or live with it.

You've probably lived with your pain for so long, that you've given up hope of ever finding true relief, let alone a cure.

I know, because I myself was once a skeptic. And, with good reason.

You see my interest in the treatment of pain and musculoskeletal injuries is not just professional. It's personal.

I too have suffered from chronic pain nearly all of my adult life. And I know how frustrating the experience can be.

I was born into a family of doctors. My grandfather, 3 brother-in-laws and several uncles were all doctors. Their devotion to their patients and the practice of medicine was an inspiration. From a young age I felt the calling.

In fact, growing up in a typical Jewish family that stressed academic achievement and social standing, it was almost preordained that I would become a doctor or a lawyer.

Because I have a typical type A personality, driven to succeed and highly competitive, I went one better. I became both: a doctor and a lawyer. And, I threw in another degree, just for fun, Masters of Business Taxation. I am nothing, if not driven.

That drive has served me well, most of my life. My parents expected a lot from me and I did not disappoint them. I excelled academically, skipped twice in grammar school and graduated from high school at the age of 16 and college at the age of 20. After graduating from Northwestern University, I fled from my Chicago traditions to the wilds of Berkeley, California. I practiced law for fifteen years while the medical calling pestered me until I entered medical school in Hawaii at the age of forty-one. The dean of admissions, Dr. Linman, told me he was going to save my soul. He would deliver me from the despised legal profession to the lofty medical profession.

In fact, Dr. Linman helped establish a program for students without intense science backround: The Liberal Arts Doctor of Medicine Program. A spot in the medical school class 2 years ahead was saved for me if I could successfully complete premed. When I asked what successfully complete meant, Dr. Linman said he didn't know, but that I better get straight A's. Out of the fear of not being accepted, I did excel, but only received a 3.94 out of 4 grade point average. One professor gave me a B and told me that no one had gotten 100% on his exams. Therefore, I must have broken into his computer. He threatened to report me. I'm so glad I'm finally done with school.

I was interviewed for medical school by Gary Watabayashi. After answering a few of Gary's questions, I took what I thought was a big risk, and told him about my mentor, John-Roger. He suddenly put down his pad of paper and began staring into my eyes. This process lasted for quite some time. I can still see his beautiful face and am very moved as I write this. He then broke his gaze and told me my teacher had sent me to him and that I had been admitted to medical school. He stood up and I followed, then he embraced me. I was shocked, feeling my knees tremble and go weak. Gary told me to relax and sit down. He then told me his journey of being a Zen master who had taken a "menial" job in the world. He said that one of his jobs was to get me admitted to medical school. Apparently, no one knew his past. He gave me 2 books on Zen and told me to read them before I returned to Hawaii to start school so that we could discuss them. Unfortunately, we never had that conversation; I was busy with school and before we could meet, Gary died.

The same drive that fueled my academic life translated into a love of sports. I was a fierce competitor. I was one of the top gymnasts in the state of Illinois. I lifted weights till my arms became black and blue. Every sport I did, including golf and tennis was done with the precision of a gymnast. I still am not fulfilled unless I drive the ball 300 yards or ace my opponent with a rocket-speed tennis serve.

By the time I was in my 20's I had racked up my share of injuries. In gymnastics I had fallen from a bar to the hard floor with my legs piked to my face. A great target for my tail bone. And then there was a high-speed water skiing fall in Tahiti. Back and neck pain persisted for years. My right shoulder was later wrenched by a weight-lifting injury. After a year of shoulder pain, guided by my orthopedic surgeon preceptor in medical school, a "simple" arthroscopic surgery was performed on my shoulder.

After all, surgery is what you do when everything else fails, right?

That is what western medicine teaches us and it was what I had been trained to believe. So after a failure with physical therapy and two cortisone injections into the shoulder, I opted for surgery as a quick fix. I was told I would be back to sports in three weeks.

After the surgery, in a story that is sadly all too familiar, my shoulder was much worse. It blew up like a balloon full of fluid. When I walked, it sloshed. It took a year after the surgery to return my shoulder to the baseline pain I had experienced before surgery. On top of the chronic neck and back pain, my right wrist, which had suffered years of abuse from the constant wear and tear of gymnastics, tennis, and golf was bothering me and I had a wicked case of tennis elbow that occasionally flared. Pain was my constant companion.

Like many of my patients, I learned to live with the pain. I "knew" there would never be a cure. In fact, I sometimes worried that I would be crippled as the pain kept extending to different areas. Many of the injuries I suffered in my teens and 20's that I thought were healed were revisiting me, one by one.

Then a light turned on. During my fourth year of residency in Physical Medicine and Rehabilitation (PM&R) at UCLA, a PM&R doctor gave a lecture on Prolotherapy. I immediately liked Andrew Kochan, MD because he was more down to earth than other doctors that had taught me. He was a bit radical in his approach, showing how traditional medicine failed those in pain. His subject was the miracle of Prolotherapy. He said it helped 80-90% of his patients. What didn't make sense was why none of us had heard about it. I spent time in Andrew's office watching his technique. It never occurred to me that this therapy would change my life.

Then, while playing golf, I missed the ball and hit the ground with my club at about 100 miles per hour. My right wrist was forcefully hyper-extended backwards. The pain was excruciating. Mind you, my wrist was often sore, but this injury brought pain to a whole new level for me.

The pain was so intense I could barely write. Nothing helped. It still felt like a freshly injured wound months after the injury. Therapy did not help and the pain would not go away. I had to give up all sports except running. Needless to say, I was miserable.

Dr. Kochan invited me to a medical convention for the American Association of Orthopedic Medicine. During a workshop on Prolotherapy, I happened to complain to one of the lecturers that my wrist was probably worse than the one he was describing. He quickly told me that he could fix my wrist with Prolotherapy.

I did not believe him. After all, chronic pain and sports medicine was my specialty and almost no one knew what it was. And then, when he explained to me that he would inject my wrist with dextrose and lidocaine, and that this would heal my injury, I had to hide my skepticism. Inject me with sugar water? He had to be kidding! And, honestly, I was not interested in a shot in my wrist. It hurt enough already!

Up until that point, although I had watched Prolotherapy and heard patients rave about it, I never thought I would let anyone inject me. My theory about shots was it was better to give than receive. But this doctor was persuasive, and I was desperate. A match made in heaven.

He explained that Prolotherapy worked by causing inflammation at a trigger or tender point where the tissue had been irritated or injured. The injection stimulates the body's natural healing process. Like the oyster that protects itself from the irritating grain of sand by producing a protective pearl, the human body has it's own defense mechanism which promotes healing. It is called inflammation. That's right, inflammation.

But wait, inflammation is what causes the pain in the first place. That is why we take anti-inflammatories to reduce inflammation and pain, right?

Well, sort of. You see, inflammation is your body's siren call. It's nature's way of letting you know that something has gone wrong.

The problem with anti-inflammatory pills is that they work by relieving the symptom, but do nothing to cure the problem. Kind of like winning the battle, but losing the war. While the anti-inflammatory reduces inflammation, it also shuts down the body's natural healing process.

Since I had reached the point where I would try almost anything to fix my wrist and I knew that sugar water would not harm me I agreed to try Prolotherapy. What doesn't kill me makes me stronger, right?

So I received my first injection. I found the injection to be almost painless. However, my wrist was really stiff for about twenty-four hours afterwards. Although he told me this was to be to expected, the skeptic in me was working overtime. I thought that not only is this not going to work, but it made my wrist worse. Then something truly amazing occurred. After about 24 hours my wrist felt about 50 percent better. How could this happen after months of pain with no improvement? I then proceeded to inject the wrist myself over the course of the next several weeks.

And it was after that that the miraculous occurred. My wrist was almost completely healed. A mere shadow of the injury remained. I could hardly believe it myself. But it was true. My sports life was regained. Needless to say I became a believer. Like C. Everrett Koop, MD, our previous surgeon general, who was also healed by Prolotherapy, and began to practice it because he was so impressed by the resuts, I too became a practitioner of Prolotherapy.

After my own healing, I started to perform this procedure on any of my patients I could convince to try it. Many had heard of and had trigger point injections, but few had heard of Prolotherapy. The strange thing that I later discovered is that when a doctor performs trigger point injections, he is also doing Prolotherapy.

I had also cured my tennis elbow and long standing shoulder pain with my own injections. On several occasions, Dr. Kochan, and Dr. Bjorn Eek, an orthopedic surgeon, have injected every vertebrae from my neck to sacrum. Recently, I have been able to play hours of tennis without neck or back pain. Previous to Prolo, one set of tennis would have had me limping for a couple of days.

Although I am grateful for what Prolo has done for me, one of my deepest satisfactions is keeping my patients from unnecessary surgery. It is rare that a patient undergoes surgery after Prolotherapy. The healings continue in my office. To such an extent, that I am often emotionally moved by the surprise and joy of my patients. You will be reading some of their stories in the pages that follow.

Please know that I am grateful to be a doctor. Next to being a husband and father, my love of medicine gives me my greatest joy. May the information in this book help change your life and the lives of your friends and family as it has changed my life.

*"The optimist already sees the scar over the wound;
the pessimist still sees the wound underneath the scar."*

– *Ernest Schroder*

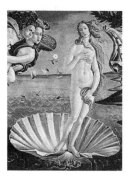

2

The Collagen Revolution

Living Pain Free

ollagen is a thing of beauty. It is one of our body's most precious resources. Collagen, quite literally, is the glue that holds our bodies together. In fact, when you boil collagen down, you are left with glue.

As you begin to appreciate the role collagen plays in healing your body, you will see why I call this approach to curing chronic pain 'The Collagen Revolution'. And you will understand why I believe collagen to be, like the pearl, one of nature's most precious jewels. And like the oyster, the body can be irritated or stimulated to produce or proliferate collagen with Prolotherapy.

> Collagen "is a major structural protein, forming molecular cables that strengthen the tendons and vast, resilient sheets that support the skin and internal organs." [1]

Collagen is a type of protein. It is in fact our body's most abundant protein. *Collagen represents approximately 30% of all the protein found in the body.*

Our bodies use protein to do all sorts of things both *"functional"* (i.e. to circulate blood, aid digestion) and *"structural"* (build ligaments, tendons, joint capsules, and muscle). Ligaments, tendons, cartilage, muscle, bones, skin, and teeth are composed of collagen as well as other substances.

Collagen is found in a number of tissues in various forms, but is most abundant in the soft tissues in and around our joints, particularly our tendons, ligaments and cartilage. In fact, collagen is the major component of all of our connective tissue—70-90% by weight.

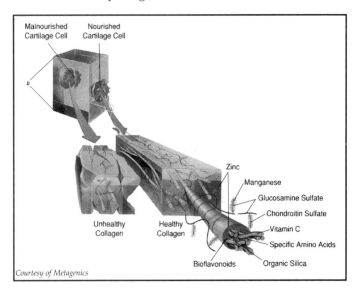

Courtesy of Metagenics

Most of you are probably familiar with collagen because of its cosmetic benefits. Skin, our body's largest organ, is held together by collagen. Young skin has plenty of natural collagen that makes it smooth, full and wrinkle-free. As we age the quality and quantity of collagen in our skin diminishes and breaks down. Years of sun exposure, facial movement, and gravity aggravate that: wrinkles and creases appear; the cheeks are not as full; and the upper lip usually thins out.

And just as the collagen in our face deteriorates, so does the collagen all over our body. It is noticeable in the skin, but it is not visually seen in the other hidden parts of the body. However, in parts of the body other than skin, this breakdown may show itself by causing pain. As the collagen stretches, dries with age, breaks down with arthritis, or becomes injured, we notice more and more aches and pains. Why this happens more in some individuals than others is speculation at this time. There are many theories including but not limited to poor genetic makeup, blood type with its specific dietary requirements, viral or bacterial load, pathological conditions, acidity in the body, and food allergies to name a few.

The cosmetic industry, recognizing the role that collagen plays in the appearance of youthful skin, devotes millions of dollars in research trying to discover the best ways to deliver collagen in a cream for the skin. They spent millions advertising collagen as the fountain of youth, and a gullible public spent billions of dollars on various creams and potions which promised to enhance the collagen in the skin.

Unfortunately you can't bind collagen to your skin topically. The collagen molecule is too large to penetrate the skin. Applying these creams and compounds did nothing to actually increase or enhance the production of collagen in your skin. But when there is a will, there is a way. And many people in our youth-obsessed culture will try anything to insure that there is no way they will ever look their age.

The FDA approved the injection of collagen for cosmetic purposes in 1981. Ever since, collagen injections have been one of the top ten cosmetic procedures performed in the United States [2]. Millions of men and women receive collagen injections to smooth out their furrows and wrinkles in order to appear younger. "Cosmetic surgeons use a form of collagen derived from cows (injectable bovine collagen). The bovine collagen is purified to create a product similar to human collagen[3]." It is then injected just beneath the skin. Some people are allergic to bovine collagen and experience side effects such as rash, hives, joint and muscle pain, and headaches.

Most people who have collagen injection are happy with the results. Unfortunately, the results are not usually permanent because the body eventually metabolizes the injected material. Depending upon the individual, the effects can last anywhere from only a few weeks, to a couple of years to, in extremely rare cases, indefinitely [4]. The average time the injection lasts is three to six months [5].

One of the most promising new procedures in the fields of cosmetic surgery and dermatology is use of a laser using

Intense Pulsed Light, (known by various trademark names: IPL Photorejuvenation, FotoFacial, Photoderm and Multilight). Considered a breakthrough because it cosmetically treated a number of conditions such as age spots, sun damage, broken capillaries and rosacea, with very little downtime, excitement grew as studies revealed that its therapeutic effects were even more impressive.

While improving the appearance of the skin, the intense pulsed light was also *rejuvenating the skin by stimulating the growth of new dermal collagen*. In a recent study "five patients underwent four sessions of dermal remodeling with an intense pulsed light source. All patients received a pretreatment biopsy and a second biopsy 6 months after the final treatment…All patients showed histologic evidence of new upper papillary dermal collagen formation.[6]"

As one of my patients happily put it, " It's cosmetic Prolotherapy! New collagen not only cures my aches and pains, it makes me pretty from the inside out!"

Just as collagen can rejuvenate damaged skin to make you look better, *collagen can rejuvenate your soft tissues to make you feel better*. Prolotherapy promotes the growth of collagen, which in turn alleviates chronic pain. That in a nutshell is the "Collagen Revolution".

It is significant to note a crucial difference between the cosmetic use of collagen and Prolotherapy for pain:

Prolotherapy is NOT the injection of cow's collagen. Prolotherapy consists of generally innocuous compounds like dextrose and Lidocaine being injected into your body, prompting an inflammatory response which we allow to run it's course so that *your body naturally produces it's own collagen and heals*.

Prolotherapy is the proliferation of new cells, which rehabilitate an incompetent structure.

Collagen: a component of ligaments, tendons, cartilage, muscle, joint capsule, and the outer covering of muscle called fascia. All of the soft tissue of the body is composed of collagen.[9]

Ligaments are sheets or bands of connective tissues made out of collagen that provide stability to the joints of the body by connecting two or more bones together. When ligaments become weak or damaged, healing is often slow and the injury may not fully recover, primarily because the blood supply to ligaments is limited. Ligaments also contain many nerve endings that can exacerbate the pain a person feels when ligaments are injured or attenuated.[9]

Tendons are fibrous connective tissue made out of collagen, which connect muscles to bones. Like ligaments, when tendons become damaged or attenuated they may cause pain.[9]

In healthy ligaments or tendons, the collagen fibers are flexible, but do not stretch very far. They have elasticity. Injuries can tear these fibers or they may become frayed or even torn by repetitive motion. When stretched beyond their normal limits, pain is perceived. Inflammation produces pain, which is a sign the body's healing process is happening. "If the healing process is completely successful, the ligaments are returned to their normal length and strength, and you can return to your normal activities. If the healing process does not completely work, the ligaments will heal stretched.[10]" "This "stretched out" ligament, often called *ligament relaxation*, or *ligament laxity* will produce pain and discomfort, especially with movement because the connection of the ligament or tendon to the bone may be inflamed and the the joint may move beyond its normal range of motion. In the same way muscle fascia or joint capsular tissue may be stretched or strained.

"The abnormal motion allowed by the strained ligament will produce painful ensations...which include feelings of 'numbness and tingling' and a phenomena of referred pain. Referred pain is created by the ligament laxity around a joint but is felt at some distance from the injured joint. These painful points that refer elsewhere are called trigger points, and will be dealt with later. The abnormal joint movement also creates many protective actions by adjacent tissues. Muscles will contract in spasm in an attempt to pull the joint back to the correct location or stabilize it to protect it from further damage. We then feel the muscle spasms which are related to ligamentous laxity.[10]" Orthopedic surgeons often reduce vertebral instability by fusing the vertebrae with bone and/or metal fixation. But there is often an easier and more conservative way to achieve the same stabilization. And this is the outcome of Prolotherapy.

Unfortunately, this is where chronic problems begin, because the conventional medical practice with its emphasis on pain relief, treats the symptom, *pain*, and not the problem, *laxity*. Most likely, a patient will be told to take anti-inflammatories, which is often precisely the wrong thing to do, because as we should know by now, inflammation is the first part in the body's healing process. By blocking inflammation, we never allow complete healing, and instead, aggravate the situation. Nonsteroidal anti-inflammatories (NSAIDS) and cortisone (an anti-inflammatory steroid) give immediate relief with the added bonus of a long term injury with chronic pain.

Inflammation and the healing process

The above illustration shows the inflammatory response with collagen production during the healing of an injury.

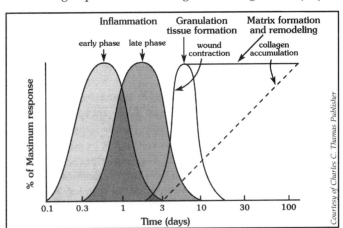

If we allow the inflammation process to run it's cycle without interference, we see that inflammation leads to granular tissue formation which results in new collagen tissue being created. The new collagen forms new threads, which attach themselves to the damaged tissue. Because new collagen fibers are short, they lose water and shrink, and as they attach themselves to the old ligament, muscle, joint capsule, or tendon, these tissues actually contract and become more anatomically sound. This process is much like the scab on a wound or scar that tightens up and shrinks once healing occurs. The difference is that with Prolotherapy, biopsies have shown brand new beautiful tissue without evidence of scarring. In essence, the tissue is healed, rejuvenated and made stronger than before.

A closer look at Collagen

The collagen in our bodies, especially in the tissue around and near our joints, is prone to breakdown. We subject our joints to wear and tear whether through repetitive movement, injury, accident or any other number of reasons. Because the connective tissue around our joints and cartilage has poor blood circulation, conventional treatment maintained that any injury to connective tissue was often irreparable.

In a 1983 study of Prolotherapy's effectiveness, Y. King Liu injected 5 percent sodium morrhuate solution into the medial collateral ligaments of rabbits. He found that after five injections, the ligament mass increased by 44 percent, the thickness by 27 percent, and the strength of the ligament bone junction increased by 28 percent.[7]

Liu's study confirmed the results of an earlier study done by George Hackett, (widely considered to be the father of

> When properly nourished and stimulated by provoking the body's natural healing process with Prolotherapy and Trigger Point injections, the cells reproduce and rejuvenate. This results in the growth of new collagen, which not only heals the pain, but makes the ligaments, tendons and surrounding tissue even stronger than before.

Prolotherapy). In 1955 [12]Hackett and Henderson reported two years experimentation on the effects of the proliferant Sylnasol when injected into rabbit tendons.

In 48 hours, histological tissue examinations revealed an early inflammatory reaction surrounding the nerves and blood vessels with lymphocytic infiltration throughout the area between the two tendons and between the tendons and it's sheath.

Microphotographs of sections represent the effect of proliferating action on the tissues in the formation of permanent bone and fibrous tissue.

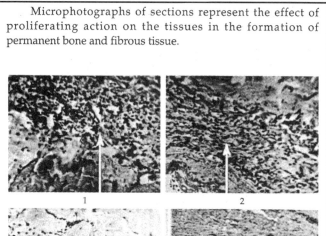

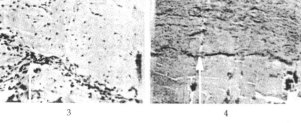

Fig. 29 (1-2-3-4). Microphotographs of sections from rabbit tendons following the injection of the proliferant, Sylnasol (G. D. Searle & Co.), within the fibrous strands. The same technic was used as that which is used clinically.

1) Arrow points to moderate infiltration of lymphocytes 48 hours after injection of proliferating solution. Note absence of necrosis in surrounding tissue.

2) Beginning fibroplastic organization present in adjacent tissues. Arrow points to capillary proliferation with moderate infiltration of lymphocytes. Two weeks after injection.

3) Fibrous tissue now present. Lymphocytic infiltration minimal. One month after injection. Arrow points to few fibroblasts.

4) Fibrosis now present, lymphocytes absent and sheath thickened and fibrosed nine months after initial injection. Arrow points to junction of tendon and its sheath. Nine months after initial injections.

Photographs and x-rays reveal the gross production of permanent bone and fibrous tissue.

Courtesy of Charles C. Thamas Publisher

Two weeks after the injection, fibrous tissue was present; lymphocytic infiltration had diminished, although some was still present, which indicated that the proliferation of new white fibrous tissue was still being stimulated.

One month after injection, fibrous tissue was present, and lymphocytic and fibroblastic activity was greatly diminished.

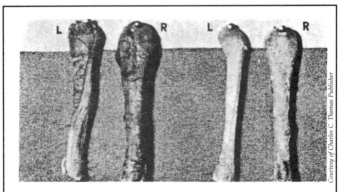

9 months   12 months

Fig. 30. Photograph of rabbit tendons at nine and 12 months after three injections of proliferating solution into the right tendons. Left, controls; right, proliferated. The tendons on the right reveal an increase in diameter of 40 per cent, which is estimated to double the strength of the tendon. The upper portion reveals the attachment of the ligament to the bone which has increased 30 per cent in diameter. The proliferating solution stimulates the production of new fibrous connective tissue cells which become organized into permanent non-elastic fibrous tissue.

And as you can see from the illustration above, one year after three injections of the proliferant solution, the diameter of the tendons increased dramatically, which is estimated to double the strength of the tendon.[12]

The Collagen Triple Helix

Collagen is composed of three chains, wound together in a tight triple helix that forms long ropes and tough sheets that are used for structural support in mature animals, and as pathways for cellular movement during development. All contain a long stretch of a triple helix connected to different types of ends.

VITAMIN C & COLLAGEN

Modifying normal proline amino acids after the collagen chain is built creates Hydroxyproline, which is critical for collagen stability. The reaction requires vitamin C to assist in the addition of oxygen. Unfortunately, we cannot make vitamin C within our bodies, and if we don't get enough in our diet, the results can be disastrous. An example is the rampant cases of scurvy that plagued early sailors, deprived of Vitamin C. Their gums bled easily, teeth would loosen, and spontaneous hemorrhages would occur over any part of the body. Vitamin C deficiency slows the production of hydroxyproline and stops the construction of new collagen. [8]

The purpose of Prolotherapy and Trigger Point Injections is to stimulate growth of new collagen. By doing so, musculoskeletal injuries are healed, and chronic pain is finally eliminated.

We will discuss the importance of nutrition and supplements in the nourishment of soft tissues more thoroughly in a later chapter.

Prolotherapy and Trigger Point Injections share things in common with other alternative therapies such as acupuncture and homeopathic remedies, which are also ignored by conventional medicine and not taught in most medical schools. However these therapies are widely gaining acceptance by the general public based on a track record of results.

Using needles and trigger points in Prolotherapy to stimulate the circulation of blood to bring nutrients to the area is similar to some of the principles used in Acupuncture. But Prolotherapy is like "acupuncture plus". Acupuncture plus homeopathy, because by introducing a natural substance into the body we are provoking a reaction that triggers the body's natural healing response, much like the principle of homeopathic medicine. And what's more impressive is that Prolotherapy not only promotes the growth of new collagen, thus healing damaged tissue, but in the process of doing so, it rejuvinates the ligaments, muscle fascia, joint capsular tissue, and tendons.

Just like collagen injections firm up your face to make you look younger, Prolotherapy injections promote collagen growth which firms up your ligaments and tendons and makes you feel younger!

Welcome to the Collagen Revolution !

Let the healing begin...

---

[1] Goodsell, David S. "Collagen." Protein Data Bank: Molecule of the Month. http://www.rcsb.org/pdb/molecules/pdb4_1.html.

[2] "Collagen and Liquid Silicone Injections." FDA Backgrounder: Current & Useful Information from the Food & Drug Administration. August 1991. http://www.fda.gov/opacom/backgrounders/collagen.html

[3] Ebody.com. "Collagen Treatment." Plastic Surgery. http://www.ebody.com/plastic_surgery/collagen_ treatment.html.

[4] Plastic Surgery Information Service. "Injectable Fillers in Plastic Surgery." Surgical Procedures. American Society of Plastic Surgeons, Illinois. 1996 http://www.plasticsurgery.org/surgery/inject.htm.

[5] "Collagen Replacement Treatments." Topdocs.com: The Internet's Cosmetic Yellow Pages. Topdocs, Inc. 2000. http://www.topdocs.com/collagen.htm.

[6] New collagen formation after dermal remodeling with an intense pulsed light source. Goldberg, DJ. , J Cutan Laser Ther 2000;2:59-61

[7] Liu Y, Tipton C, Matthes R, Bedford T, Maynard J, Walmer H. An in situ study of the influence of a sclerosing solution in rabbit medial collateral ligaments and its junction strength. Connect Tissue Res. 1983;11:95-102.

[8] H.M. Berman, J. Westbrook, Z. Feng, G. Gilliland, T.N. Bhat, H. Weissig, I.N. Shindyalov, P.E. Bourne: The Protein Data Bank. Nucleic Acids Research, 28 pp. 235-242 (2000) <http://www.rcsb.org/pdb/molecules/pdb4_3.html> David S. Goodsell

[9] In Alternative Medicine, the Definitive Guide, chapter co-written by Marc Darrow, MD, JD, and copyrighted and compiled by The Burton Goldberg Group.

[10] Prolotherapy or the Injection Treatment of Ligamentous Laxity: American Association of Orthopaedic Medicine; Michelle Fecteau, D.O. and Tom Ravin, M.D. http://www.aaomed.org

[11] Ligament & Tendon Relaxation Treated Prolotherapy by George Hackett & Gus Hemwall 1993 Charles C. Thomas Publisher

[12] Ligament & Tendon Relaxation Treated Prolotherapy by George Hackett & Gus Hemwall 1993 Charles C. Thomas Publisher

"It is more important to cure people than to make diagnoses."

– August Bier

3

Pain, Friend or Foe?

*M*ost of us have been led to believe that pain is our adversary, something to be avoided, eradicated, eliminated; the sooner the better. We are a quick fix society. The drug companies understand this. They spend millions in advertising, to make billions in profit, by promising quick "relief" from pain.

Some of these drugs are quite effective in the short term. Most of them reduce inflammation, which reduces pain. If you're one of the lucky ones, your strain, sprain, or injury is transient, temporary or superficial and easily healed.

However, I suspect that if you're reading this book, you are one of the millions in this country who suffer from chronic pain.

Dramatic Increase in Chronic pain

Chronic Pain - pain that continues a month or more beyond the expected recovery period for an illness or injury, or pain that persists for months or years. It may be constant, or come and go.

The amount of chronic musculoskeletal pain has risen dramatically the second half of the nineteenth century. According to data from the National Center for Health Statistics, musculoskeletal system surgeries are the second leading type of surgeries performed in the United States annually.

Chronic pain is an affliction that disables, to some degree, about 86 million Americans. It is estimated that chronic pain costs U.S. businesses and industry, about $90 billion dollars annually.

Myofascial pain syndrome is one of the most common disorders seen in chronic pain clinics. Myofascial pain syndrome occurs due to damage or injury in the soft connective tissues in our bodies. When the soft tissue does not heal properly, **"trigger-points"**— develop.

> **Myofascial Pain Syndrome is a common painful muscle, tendon, ligament, or joint capsule disorder characterized by Trigger or Tender Points.**
>
> **Trigger or tender points are hyperirritable bundles of muscle fiber, ligament, or tendinous soft tissue that produce both local and referred pain when pressed.**

Trigger or tender points have been associated with all sorts of soft tissue injuries that result in patients complaining of headache, neck pain, low back pain, knee pain and various other musculoskeletal disorders. Patients with active trigger points typically complain of pain—which may be characterized as either sharp or dull, localized muscle swelling or weakness, as well as generalized fatigue & malaise. Trigger points were noted in 30% of patients at a University who presented with pain as the chief complaint.

A recent Newsweek article stated that "Twenty million American's suffer from Arthritis, suffering joint pain that ranges from the annoying to the crippling…and account for seven million doctors visits each year. Dr. John Klippel, medical director of the Arthritis Foundation, expects that figure to rise to about 30 million by 2020. This year American surgeons will perform as many as 267,000 total knee replacements (more than double the figure from 1990) and 168,000 artificial hip implants, up by a third from a decade ago."

Taking an anti-inflammatory for pain?
Better think twice.

In 1974, Ibuprofen hit the market. "It was such a hit that within two years the company had churned out 1.7 billion tablets..." In my opinion, the moment inflammation became the enemy is the moment chronic pain started becoming a billion dollar business for drug companies.

Today, over 100 million prescriptions for pain relievers are written every year and 15 *tons* of aspirin are consumed each day. Unfortunately, these drugs only mask the problem and come with their own risks of addiction and unpleasant side effects.

Anti-inflammatory drugs are classified as "non-steroidal anti-inflammatory drugs" or "NSAID's."

If you suffer from myofascial pain, joint pain, arthritis, sprained or strained ligaments, almost any kind of pain, most likely your doctor will prescribe one of the non-steroidal anti-inflammatory drugs, or NSAID's.

These drugs will reduce the inflammation, which in the short term reduces the pain. However, in the long term they set you up for more pain and a long term chronic injury.

In addition to the potential side effects NSAID's can cause which include "gastrointestinal upset and bleeding, kidney and liver damage...the worst side effect of NSAID's is hardly ever mentioned in conventional medicine. *What you aren't told is that these drugs have been shown to increase the destruction of cartilage lining the ends of the bone.*"

That's right, the drugs you are being prescribed, the NSAID's, are actually destroying your cartilage and setting you up for chronic pain. NSAID's do nothing to treat the underlying source.

"In a study of 186 arthritis patients, doctors in Norway studied the x-rays of 294 arthritic hips. Fifty-eight of the patients were taking the NSAID Indocin, and 128 were not taking NSAID's. Those on Indocin had far more rapid hip destruction than the non-medicated group.[7]

Anti-inflammatory drugs like taken for pain-related problems account for one-third of all the side effects reported by the FDA. More than 100,000 people are hospitalized each year for gastrointestinal complications resulting from the use of anti-inflammatory medicines, and over *16,000 deaths* can be attributed to these complications.

> **PLEASE DON'T BE FOOLED. IT IS THE PATIENTS WHO DO NOT HAVE STOMACH DISCOMFORT THAT DIE FROM GASTROINTESTINAL BLEEDING. THOSE WHO EXPERIENCE STOMACH DISCOMFORT USUALLY STOP THE NSAID BEFORE THEY START BLEEDING!!!!!**

In other words, the fact that you tolerate NSAIDS does not protect you from their side effects.

Two new anti arthritis drugs which were heavily adverised and marketed on TV directly to consumers, Celebrex and Vioxx recently caused concern when "a leading cardiologist reported that the two drugs could pose a small but disturbing additional risk of heart attack...[5]" In my office, more than one alarmed patient had to stop the use of Celebrex because of stomach discomfort, nausea, and dizziness.

The Newsweek article goes on to note that "for drug companies, arthritis has been a boon: a nonfatal, incurable disease that may require patients to take pain-relief medication every day for decades. Since their introduction in 1999— Celebrex and Vioxx have captured more than 60% of the $6.6 billion arthritis drug market – a figure that doesn't even include products like acetaminophen, which are used to treat other conditions as well.[5]"

NSAIDs or (Non-steroidal anti-inflammatory drugs)

Aspirin
Ibuprofen (*Advil,Bayer,Motrin*)
Carprofen (*Rimadyl*)
Celecoxib (*Celebrex a Cox.2 inhibitor*)

Choline Magnesium Trisalicylate *(Trilisate)*
Choline Salicylate *(Anthropan)*
Diclofenac *(Volaren)*
Diflunisal *(Dolobid)*
Etodolac *(Lodine)*
Fenoprofen calcium *(Nalfon)*
Indomethacin *(Indocin)*
Ketoprofen *(Orudis)*
Ketorolac tromethamine *(Toradol)*
Magnesium salicylate *(Doans, Magan, Mobidin…)*
Meclofenamate sodium *(Meclomen)*
Mefenamic acid *(Ponstel)*
Naproxen *(Naprosyn)*
Naproxen sodium *(Aleve, Anaprox)*
Piroxicam *(Feldene)*
Sodium Salicylate
Tolmetin *(Tolectin)*

Corticosteroids

Cortisone & Prednisone *(most commonly used steroids)*

Potential Side Effects of Aspirin & NSAID's*

- Gastritis, esophagitis, bleeding ulcers
- Renal (kidney) insufficiency
- Liver abnormalities
- Fluid retention
- Platelet inhibition
  (and therefore possible prolonged bleeding)
- Tinnitus (ringing in the ears)
- Exacerbation of asthma

Potential Complications of Steroid Use[10]*

- Growth retardation in children
- Cataracts
- Osteoporosis
- Aseptic necrosis of the femoral head
- Proximal myopathy
- Delayed wound healing
- Decreased resistance to bacterial and yeast infections
- Buffalo hump

- Skin striae
- Mood disturbances
- Psychosis
- Adrenal suppression
- Cushing's syndrome
- Increased blood pressure
- Glucose intolerance
- Restlessness, nervousness, insomnia
- Increased appetite
- Weight gain
- Hirsutism (increased body hair)
- Gastrointestinal bleeding

*These medications are not as benign as many people, *including doctors*, think and should not be taken long term for the management of chronic pain.

NEVER TAKE TWO OR MORE OF THESE MEDICATIONS AT THE SAME TIME WITHOUT THE ADVICE OF YOUR DOCTOR!!!!

Partners Against Pain commissioned a survey of more than 1,000 people to identify the scope of pain management, including access and barriers to treatment within the United States. According to the National Institutes of Health, pain costs Americans more than $100 billion each year in health care costs and lost productivity. (November 2000)

"Pain is a serious public health problem for patients and the physicians who care for them. When inadequately treated, pain interferes with patients' quality of life," stated Kathleen Foley, M.D., professor and neurologist at Memorial Sloan-Kettering Cancer Center and Partners Against Pain advisor.

"Many of the surveyed patients believe their family is tired of hearing about their pain-related problems, such as quality of life issues, and feel that their family doesn't understand how their pain affects their life.

Patients reported generally receiving treatment first with non-prescription medications such as aspirin, acetaminophen, nonsteroidal anti-inflammatories (NSAIDS), and physical therapy according to their needs. The range of prescription pain treatments includes NSAIDs, Cox 2 inhibitors, low dose anti-depressants, anti-convulsants and opioid analgesics (NARCOTICS).

SURVEY FACT SHEET [11]

■ At least one member of almost half of America's 44 million households (43%) suffers from chronic pain due to a specific illness or medical condition.

■ Among the survey respondents, 48% experienced pain related to skeletal problems, which include; back pain, as well as problems with the knees, neck, shoulder/arm, ankle/foot, joints, bones, hips and bursitis; and other sources, such as arthritis (28%), headaches (16 %), nerve problems (10%), surgical/post-operative (4%) and traumatic injury (2%).

■ 80% of patients surveyed thought that their pain was a normal part of their medical condition and something with which they must live.

■ For one third of sufferers, their chronic pain is so severe and debilitating, they feel they can't function as normal people and sometimes is so bad they wish to die.

■ Some 40% of sufferers are uncomfortable discussing their pain and 37% say it can be isolating, leaving them feeling alone.

■ One-third of sufferers do not believe people understand how much pain they are in and one-quarter say their family is tired of hearing about their pain, do not understand how it affects them and feel inadequate as a spouse/partner because of it.

- 56% of patients suffering from severe pain feel that their pain interferes with sleeping. They also report that pain affects their overall mood (51%), ability to drive (30%), to have sexual relations (28%), and to feed themselves (7%).

- Those not completely happy with their physician cited unsuccessful treatment (62%) as the main reason for dissatisfaction. Survey respondents expressed their dissatisfaction through comments such as "has not helped me" and "not doing as much as he/she could."

- Patients in chronic pain are so dissatisfied with the efficacy of their prescription and over-the-counter (OTC) pain control medications, that 78% are willing to try new treatments and 43 %would spend all their money on treatment if they knew it would work.

- Two thirds (66%) of the surveyed pain patients said their OTC pain medication is not completely or very effective and of those that rely on prescription drugs, 52% said they also are not completely effective or not very effective.

- Many patients have been suffering for years, with more than half of sufferers (62%) having experienced pain for at least five years. Even for those patients who say their pain is under control, it often has taken a long time to happen.

- On average, chronic pain patients have seen three physicians for their pain and have taken 3.7 different kinds of prescription medications as part of their pain treatment.

In my practice, many patients have seen up to a dozen or more practitioners without lasting relief. I am often their last hope. And the work that is done at my clinic is often their medical salvation.

TYPES OF PAIN

Transient Pain – lasts only a short time, though it may be severe.

Acute Pain – new onset: it doesn't imply the severity of the pain. It complicates injuries and diseases of all kinds. Common kinds of acute pain are low back pain and headache, which can last for several days or more.

Persistent Pain – unrelenting with time, requires long term use of analgesics. Most typical persistent pain is low back pain, but any pain that has not relented after conventional therapies used is generally described as persistent.

Chronic Pain – Pain generally lasting 3 months or more. Patients are disabled by their pain and often suffer severe depression and anxiety, and, often drug abuse.

Unfortunately, it may be the doctor that becomes the enabler of the patient's drug habit. Since most doctors do not know how to heal their patient's pain, they simply sedate the patient.

Personally, I am against the chronic daily use of narcotics. Patients become tolerant to them and live in a depressed state of conciousness. They often give up on life. Studies show that treatment at a multidisciplinary practice is the fastest way to reduce pain.

Melzack and Wall's Gate Control Theory

In 1965, Drs. Ronald Melzack and Patrick Wall introduced the *Gate Control Theory* of pain. They determined that "thoughts and emotions in human beings play an important role in determining (1) whether pain impulses reach the brain and (2) if they do, how the brain will interpret them. They hypothesized that certain higher order functions of the brain, such as those relating to thoughts and emotions, could open or close a mechanism that operates like a gate in the nervous system. When the "gate" is open, pain signals flow freely to the brain. When closed, it is as if the pain impulse has insufficient change for the toll taker. For example, powerful emotions such as anger, frustration or anxiety were thought to activate parts of the brain that served to swing the gate fully open. Alternatively, more pleasant feelings or states of mind resulted in swinging the gate fully or partly closed.[10]

It is thought that a noxious stimulus such as the needle of acupuncture, trigger point therapy, or Prolotherapy can shut the pain gate. This is done by sending the stimulus to the spinal cord or brain where the pain generators are up-regulated and in a sense letting them know that their job is finished. There is no longer a need to protect the nervous system by causing pain and its sequelae of physical limitations. A simple form of this is obtaining relief by rubbing an area that has been injured.

"Most physicians and patients see pain as a symptom of an underlying disease," says Jeffrey Lackner, Psy.D., director of the Behavioral Medicine Clinic at the Pain Management Center at the University at Buffalo. In a study appearing in the journal Spine last November, Lackner described how a person's perceptions can influence the physical experience of pain. [11] I am certainly a believer in this phenomenon and therefore one of the first things I do with a new patient is work to convince them that they are healthy. I take away the diagnosis that they have been branded with and move them to a state of healing. The rest is usually simple.

"Patients who develop chronic problems appraise and process pain stimuli differently than do healthy controls. These patients attend selectively to pain cues, mislabel bodily sensations, inaccurately predict the probability of painful events, and have distorted memories for pain episodes," says Lackner. Specialists in researching and treating chronic pain believe it involves the complex interplay of biology, psychology and learning.

"With chronic pain, frequently there is no physical cause. For example, less than 25 percent of disability from low-back pain can be traced to a physical dysfunction," says Lackner. Most researchers agree that psychological factors, such as attention to and fear of pain and how the pain is interpreted, can cause a gate to open or close. It is thought that when nerve signals reach the brain, they are processed in the context of a person's mood, emotions, beliefs and thought patterns. [11]

According to the official definition set down by the International Association for the Study of Pain, pain is a two-fold experience: both **physical** and **emotional**.

For me, it just makes sense that when treating a patient, it is more important to focus on the totality of the patient's life. I must consider their emotional, spiritual and physical needs as we proceed together down the path towards healing. I'm less interested in their diagnosis, and more interested in their prognosis. And the prognosis we have some ability to manipulate.

> The Collagen Revolution requires us to change our attitudes and belief about pain and the role it plays in our ultimate recovery.

Pain, a tough friend

Pain is a friend, smart and vigilant, ready to point with relative precision at any problem that indicates something is not right with our bodies. We need to listen. Often the voice that speaks is more than that of the body itself.

After a long period of "mourning" because I could not play golf secondary to an elbow injury from playing too much golf, I was told in a dream that the injury was in essence a gift. At first I didn't understand. Then I got it; I was out of sync with my work and family because I was escaping to the golf course at every possible moment. And I was secretly distraught because I was not tending adequately to my responsibilities. "Golf was so relaxing."

When I realized that because of the injury I was actually much happier overall, it made me think about the positives of pain. This is not always easy to do in dire straits. At the same time we must use everything to our advantage. And it does no good to feel sorry for yourself. Believe me, I've tried without success. I look at every person's pain as a message. I'm certainly not the judge of what the message is, but I present the options to my patients. All messages in one way or another force us to look inside. Pain is possibly the greatest messenger.

The pain signal is our body's first line of defense. Without such warning, a person with a broken leg might attempt to walk and permanently ruin the leg.

Pains might be sharp, dull, aching, burning, lingering, or imaginary; or possess countless other attributes or combinations thereof. But whether real or imagined, pain is always a clue to a genuine problem of some sort, whether small or serious, physical or psychological, and often it is a combination of the two.

Understandably, people do not like to feel pain and would like to prevent it at all costs. They want immediate relief and getting rid of the inflammation often provides that relief.

Why you may win the battle, but lose the war

The basic truth is that immediate relief does not equal long-lasting relief. Interfering with the body's healing process by stopping inflammation to reduce pain causes long term suffering down the road.

Inflammation does indeed cause pain. But remember pain is your friend. It is the body's siren alerting you that you have injured yourself. Getting rid of inflammation provides some immediate relief from pain. It sets you up to win the battle, but lose the war.

> By stopping inflammation we shut down the body's natural healing which inhibits the growth of new tissue.

Inflammation and the pain that accompanies it are actually your allies in healing.

Prolotherapy & Natural Healing

1. During inflammation the blood vessels in the area of injury expand, causing the swelling that is experienced.

2. This expansion enables more blood to flow into the injured area. The blood carries with it white blood cells and other immune cells, such as macrophages, whose

job it is to destroy and remove bacteria, foreign bodies, and dead tissue.

3. The expanded blood cells press on sensory nerves, and produces the pain that you feel.

4. Once finished, these cells are replaced by fibroblasts, which are cells whose job it is to repair the damaged area by laying down new collagen to strengthen connective tissues.

5. Once new collagen formation occurs, pain is greatly reduced, if not entirely eliminated, and the damaged tissue is rejuvenated and stronger than before.

Like the pearl that is sometimes perfectly round and other times imperfect in shape, some healing is not as complete. This is when Prolotherapy should be used. Prolotherapy, by injecting a natural irritant into the trigger point of pain, provokes an inflammatory reaction. Most commonly, the irritant is as basic as dextrose, which is sugar water. The dextrose is combined with Lidocaine to numb the area. Dextrose works by osmosis. It draws water into itself, drying out the tissue and thus causing the inflammation.

Prolotherapy simply triggers the body to once again begin the healing process when the body could not do it itself. And this time, we allow it to complete the process by not interfering with anti-inflammatory medication.

"Why wasn't my body able to completely heal itself on its own?"

Ligaments, and tendons, the soft tissue culprits behind chronic pain, tend to have poor healing abilities because of the poor blood supply to these areas. The healing rate for ligaments and tendons takes more time than that of muscle and bone. The body's reconstructive processes stop a few weeks after injury. In some instances this does not allow enough time for the ligaments to complete their healing.

Healing takes time. When inflammation is allowed to run it's course, without interference, your body's natural healing process has a much better chance to complete itself.

If it's instant gratification you want, anti-inflammatories are an option, but only short term. They are likely to do more harm then good, and can lock you into a cycle of chronic pain.

Over the past 50 years more than one million patients have been successfully treated with Prolotherapy— but most doctors still don't even know about it.

Pharmaceutical companies aren't interested in promoting Prolotherapy because there's no money in it for them. The fluids used in the injections contain common and inexpensive ingredients.

And since drug companies can't obtain patents or lock up exclusive manufacturing rights to these substances, they will not be spending dollars to advertise it. Without such advertisement, doctors simply will not get the message.

I have successfully used Prolotherapy to treat almost every part of the musculoskeletal system from head to toe. And I have transformed my patient's lives in the process, just as my life has been transformed.

Becoming your own Advocate

Fortunately, the electronic media revolution, culminating in the phenomenal explosion of the Internet —has made it easier than ever to gather information. (See our Resource Guide).

Much of this knowledge is available to the public at large, and a little "preventive research" can lead to great personal gains for anyone wishing to optimize their medical support structure.

When faced with chronic pain and injuries that diminish the quality of your life you must insist upon the most progressive, up-to-date, and proven-to-be-effective treatment.

That choice is Prolotherapy. It is safe, highly effective, and yields benefits well beyond the palliation of pain.

It actually rejuvenates and heals. It is the Collagen Revolution.

[1] American Chronic Pain Association;
http://www.theacpa.org

[2] Gerwin RD: The Clinical Assessment of Myofascial Pain.
In Turk DC, Melzack R (eds) Handbook of Pain Assessment.
New York, Guilford Press,1992;p.61

[3] Lewis S. Nelson, MD, Robert S. Hoffman MD;Intrathecal
Injection;Universal Complication of Trigger Point Injection
Therapy.N.Y. University Medical Center/Bellevue Hospital
Center & N.Y. City Poison Control Center;presented in ab-
stract form at N.American congress of clinical Toxicology.
Rochester 1995

[4] Skootsky SA,Jaeger B.,Oye RK;Prevalence of Myofascial
pain in general internal medical practice.West J Med
1989;151:157-160

[5] Newsweek September 3, 2001p. 40-46;
newsweekmsnbc.com

[6] Fishman, Scott, M.D. The War On Pain. New York, Harper
Collins Publishers, 2000.

[7] http://www.health-today.net/arthritis.htm

[8] Chino, Alan F. and Davis, Corinne D. Validate Your Pain!:
Exposing the Chronic Pain Cover-Up. p.135 Florida: Health
Access Press, 2000.

[9]Contemporary diagnosis and Management of Pain;Second
ed.;Donlin M. Long, MD copyright by Handbooks in Health
Care Co., a division of Associates of medical marketing;p.36

[10] Validate your Pain;Allan F.Chino,Ph.D.,Corrine Dille
Davis,MD Health Access Press;p.132; 136;184

[11]http://www.newswise.com/articles/2000/11/PAIN.PPH
.html University at Buffalo 4-Apr-00

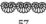

"The wish for healing has ever been the half of health."
– Seneca

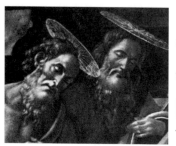

4

What is Prolotherapy?

The Way to Proliferate Collagen!!!

*P*rolotherapy works by rejuvenating the body's connective tissue and support structures to correct problems associated with damaged muscles, tendons, ligaments, and joints.

> Prolotherapy, is a safe, highly effective yet relatively unknown therapy used to heal chronic pain and musculoskeletal injuries. Prolotherapy stimulates the growth, or "proliferation", of new collagen tissue that rejuvenates and rehabilitates the damaged ligaments, tendons, muscle fascia, and joint capsules responsible for most chronic pain.

With an injection of natural substances into precisely targeted areas of the body, known as **"trigger points"**, the doctor activates the body's natural healing process which stimulates the growth of new collagen and in turn strengthens and repairs weak or damaged soft tissue structures.

A simple and cost-effective alternative to drugs and surgery, Prolotherapy is an effective cure for many pain syndromes, including degenerative arthritis, low back and neck pain, joint pain, carpal tunnel syndrome, fibromylagia, migraine headaches, and torn ligaments and cartilage.

Unlike conventional medical treatments with their emphasis on surgery and drugs, Prolotherapy stimulates the body's own healing processes to effect a natural and long-lasting cure.

A Brief History of Prolotherapy

Although Prolotherapy is a relatively new therapy, first used by Dr. George S. Hackett, in 1939, it is actually based on medical theory dating as far back as ancient Greece.

Hippocrates, the father of Western medicine who lived in the 5th century, B.C., used a cauteric technique much like Prolotherapy, to treat the pain and heal the dislocated shoulders of Javelin throwers in ancient Greece. It is said that he would place a heated metal probe into a shoulder that had dislocated, in order to contract the lax collagen. By the 16th Century A.D., the French surgeon Pare't was using "sclerotherapy" to promote healing.[1]

Like the pioneers before him, Dr. Hackett's therapy in 1939 involved the injection of an irritating compound to activate the body's natural mechanisms.

But unlike Pare't's technique, Dr. Hackett's did not involve the formation of scar tissue, thus the evolution from "sclero-" (meaning "scar") to "prolo-" (short for "proliferation") therapy.

> Prolotherapy prompts the production or "proliferation" of new collagen tissue, which in turn results in rejuvenation and rehabilitation of damaged tissue.

Prolotherapy gained more recognition in 1955, when a progressive physician, Gustav A. Hemwall, M.D., attended a presentation by Dr. Hackett at the national meeting of The American Medical Association.

Thoroughly impressed by Dr. Hackett's new therapy, Dr. Hemwall soon became its leading practitioner.

His first attempts with Prolotherapy yielded astounding results. Patients with chronic pain that he had been treated unsuccessfully for years, were suddenly healing and living nearly pain free after only a few sessions.

"Many intelligent people never move beyond the boundaries of their self-imposed limitations"
–John C. Maxwell

Unfortunately for the history of this revolutionary therapy, and for the millions of pain-sufferers who might have benefited from its proliferation, (no pun intended), Prolotherapy experienced a major setback in 1959 due to one careless physician—and the over-zealous reaction of the traditional medical establishment.

The case involved a fatality, caused when a reckless physician broke every established rule of the procedure and injected the wrong solution into the wrong part of the patient's body. Just as other promising therapies have been set back for political reasons, Prolotherapy was soundly attacked by a group of physicians representing their own interest, in this case, Neurosurgery.

Their assault on Prolotherapy arrived in the guise of a feature article in the August 8, 1959 edition of The Journal of The American Medical Association.[2]

Although Dr. Richard Schneider admitted in the article that the offending physician had grievously erred in his procedure, he proceeded to jump to the unfair and erroneous conclusion that "… this technique… appears to be neither sound nor without extreme danger."

While this setback undoubtedly impeded the acceptance of Prolotherapy as a mainstream treatment, fortunately for us, there remained a number of fair minded and forward thinking doctors who recognized the remarkable promise of Prolotherapy, and were not detered.

I am certain that as the word spreads about the amazing results achieved by Prolotherapy in treating chronic pain and musculoskeletal injury, wider acceptance for Prolotherapy in the medical community will follow. After all it took 12 years and two lawsuits against the AMA until the medical profession was forced to stop maligning chiropractors, and now, chiropractic is accepted as conventional treatment by most insurance companies.

ACUPUNCTURE, TRIGGER POINTS & PROLOTHERAPY: Similarities and Differences

Acupuncture, although used for at least 5000 years in China, was not well known or widely accepted as a therapeutic treatment in the Western medical community, until recently.

Acupuncture is based on Eastern philosophical premise that all matter is permeated with energy—called **Chi**—which flows in patterns in the body called meridians. An obstruction of these patterns interferes with basic vitality by disrupting the energy flow. This is analogous to cholesterol plaques clogging the precious flow of blood through our circulatory system. The needles used in acupuncture are inserted into the skin at precisely mapped meridian points which affect the flow of the Chi, redirecting or restoring it until the energy flow patterns are balanced and health is restored. Without surprise, most acupuncture points have been mapped to be the exact same points as trigger points. And again, without surprise, there is a technique to heat acupuncture needles and use them as Hippocrates did for guess what: Prolotherapy.

Trigger Point Therapy also uses needles to eliminate irregularities in the body's normal functioning, in this case the taut bands of pathological muscle tissue are known as *trigger points*. However, tendons, ligaments and joint capsules may also refer pain to areas distant from the actual trigger point. Tender points, which are points that are sore with pressure or palpation of the doctor's hand, may also be treated with trigger point injections or Prolotherapy. Unlike the dry needle of acupuncture, the trigger point or Prolotherapy needles deliver fluid to the target area to be treated. By puncturing the tissue, trauma to the area is caused, resulting in a rush of white blood cells to the area that provokes a reaction and stimulates the healing process. Frequently, in trigger point therapy the physician will use a local anesthetic solution such as lidocaine to relieve the pain as well.

Trapezius m.
Origin
Insertion

Palpable
hard bands

Courtesy of Charles C. Thomas Publisher

Fig. 1.7 Tight "cords" or "bands" in the upper back and neck are frequently reported by patients. These localized areas of muscle spasm are accompanied by tender sites at the origin and insertion of the muscles affected.

Acupuncture needles act as "magnetic" attractants to steer the Chi energy into proper channels. However, acupuncture needles can also be used in a pecking fashion and reach the same end as trigger point therapy or Prolotherapy. The deep tissue injection of the trigger point attacks the problem directly, causing physical changes and subsequent pain reduction in the tissue provoked by the needle.

Since acupuncture works on the energy flowing through the entire body, it is effective on all parts including the organs. At present, trigger point is used primarily for myofascial pain and dysfunction.

Prolotherapy takes trigger point theory a step further, by adding an irritant solution, like dextrose or phenol to the injection process. This irritant solution helps speed up the proliferation of new collagen tissue.

It is highly effective for rejuvination of joints, muscles, tendons and ligaments. Acupuncture, trigger point therapy, and Prolotherapy are basically variations of the same therapeutic process, all originating from ancient medical arts, best known in China and Greece.

Diverse though they are, all three therapies use needles and all have been very successful, often exceeding or succeeding where traditional treatments have failed. Simple but sophisticated, based on theories of healing dating back several centuries, Prolotherapy has been honed over the last five decades into an incredibly successful, natural therapy, proven to correct many of the deeper, structure-related problems such as chronic pain and myofascial pain Yet despite the overwhelming evidence of its effectiveness, it has yet to achieve full acceptance by the medical community. Perhaps it is because, as Dr. William Faber, Director of the Milwaukee Pain Clinic and a leading authority in the field of Prolotherapy, points out, "… the substances used in Prolotherapy are not patented and therefore would not provide the huge profits that pharmaceutical therapies receive." Nevertheless, the big companies have nothing patented in the field of trigger point therapy or acupuncture, both of which are accepted today. Could it be that there is a resistance to Prolotherapy because it would substantially reduce the number of surgeries? If this is the case, it is a sad comment on our dollar driven medical system. Without all of the unnecessary surgeries, would hospitals go out of business?

> Years of research and study have confirmed that Prolotherapy is less risky, less expensive and more effective than surgery in the proper cases; that it aids in the prevention of future injuries, and that it provides a lasting boost to a person's energy and endurance.

Prolotherapy also requires specialized training, sometimes with long needles, and only 200 or so physicians have made the commitment to master the procedure. But based on the public demand, this is about to change.

As the general public becomes more and more sophisticated in making decisions that affect their health and well-

TRIGGER POINTS OF PAIN AND NEEDLES IN POSITION FOR CONFIRMATION OF THE DIAGNOSIS AND FOR TREATMENT OF LIGAMENT RELAXATION OF THE LUMBOSACRAL AND PELVIC JOINTS. TRIGGER POINTS OF LIGAMENTS

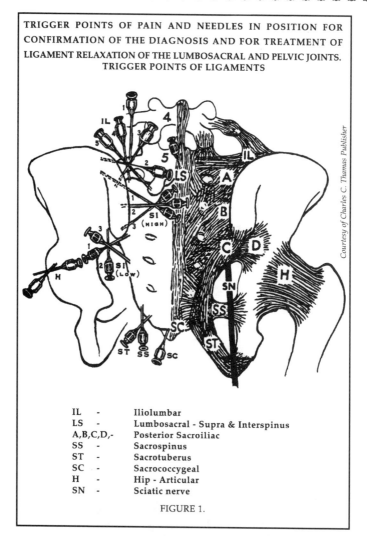

Courtesy of Charles C. Thomas Publisher

IL	-	Iliolumbar
LS	-	Lumbosacral - Supra & Interspinus
A,B,C,D,-		Posterior Sacroiliac
SS	-	Sacrospinus
ST	-	Sacrotuberus
SC	-	Sacrococcygeal
H	-	Hip - Articular
SN	-	Sciatic nerve

FIGURE 1.

being, and show a more willing acceptance of so called "alternative" medicine, the miraculous benefits of Prolotherapy will soon replace the drugs and surgeries that are being show not to help the patient.

As we avail ourselves to the internet, the information revolution will help establish Prolotherapy among enlightened doctors and their patients as a mainstream, frontline therapy, providing better, faster and more permanent relief to the millions who suffer from pain.

Although all of these treatments cause tissue injury, inflammation, and probable proliferation of collagen, insurance companies usually do not pay for Prolotherapy. Medicare states that there isn't enough scientific evidence to support its use. Why don't they look at the studies? The answer is unclear.

> When a doctor performs trigger point therapy, he unknowingly is doing Prolotherapy. When a doctor performs Prolotherapy, he is also doing trigger point therapy. Although a more irritating solution may be used with Prolotherapy than traditional trigger point therapy, in perhaps 20-30% of patients, there is instant and lasting relief. This shows the trigger point effect of the treatment, not the proliferative effect, which if it were to occur, would take weeks to months.

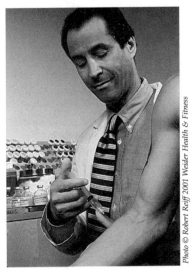

Photo © Robert Reiff 2001 Weider Health & Fitness

Dr. Darrow injects an elbow

How Prolotherapy Works

The term **"Prolotherapy"** is short for "proliferation therapy"—referring to the proliferation (i.e. "rapid production") of collagen. Doctors use Prolotherapy to treat a number of different types of pain, which will be reviewed later in this book.

> Like homeopathy, Prolotherapy heals the body by prompting the body to heal itself.

Prolotherapy consists of a series of injections—not of collagen—but of innocuous substances that stimulate the production of collagen by your body, via its natural repair mechanisms.

Collagen is a naturally occurring protein in the body. It is a necessary element for the formation of new muscle fascia, joint capsular tissue, tendons and ligaments, the semi-elastic tissue that supports our skeletal infrastructure. Most people know it only as the precious rejuvenating ingredient used extensively in the health and beauty industry.

> **The beauty of Prolotherapy is that, unlike the cosmetic use of collagen which requires injecting bovine collagen into the skin to rejuvenate and restore a more youthful appearance, it stimulates your body to produce it's own collagen. This rejuvenates and rebuilds your body's infrastructure, and allows you to move once again with youthful vigor.**

The injections used in Prolotherapy consist of a variety of different compounds. The compounds have been tested and refined throughout years of trial and research.

Although they all work safely, and on similar principles, they work their wonders in slightly different ways. Your physician will determine what works best for you.

Solutions Commonly Used in Prolotherapy

1. Irritants – Phenol, quaicol, tannic acid, sodium morrhuate (arachadonic acid), dextrose, pumice, zinc sulfate, glucose, glycerin

2. Anesthetics – Lidocaine, Procaine, Bupivacaine

The injections stimulate the production of collagen at the source of the injection, often commonly referred to as a **"trigger point."**

The injections at the trigger points cause an irritation, that stimulates the body's natural process for repairing damaged tissue—by causing an influx of **fibroblasts**, the healing cells which create collagen.

The collagen thus produced works to increase the formation of fresh muscle fascia, joint capsule, ligament, and tendon tissue, which increases support for joints weakened by arthritis, injury or degeneration. The increased support eliminates stress on the muscles, bones and nerves, and thus alleviates the pain which inevitably accompanies such pathology.

Although simple in principle, Prolotherapy is actually quite sophisticated in both theory and application, thanks to the enthusiastic involvement of dedicated physicians who have researched and improved the techniques over the last half-century.

With successful case studies now numbering in the tens if not hundreds of thousands, Prolotherapy has been proven to be safe and highly effective. Connective tissues are repaired and strengthened. Joints are pulled back into proper alignment as the collagen reinforces the muscles, tendons and ligaments, then shrinks to tighten them, all part of the natural healing process. Rather than just alleviating the symptoms like pharmaceutical pain-killers do, Prolotherapy fixes the very structure of the body, effecting a hopefully permanent cure.

And unlike old-fashioned surgical treatments that cause greater trauma to the body, Prolotherapy's "kinder and gentler" approach restores and improves the body, rather than diminishing it.

**"Before the art of medicine
comes the art of belief."**

–Depak Chopra

What exactly is injected during Prolotherapy?

There are a number of different types of injections which have proven to be successful in Prolotherapy. Although they work in different ways, motivating the body to heal itself through a variety of natural responses, the end result is the same: to cure pain by building new tissue and stabilizing the joints.

All of the solutions used in Prolotherapy are designed to have a "double-edged" effect: a combination of **anesthetic** and **proliferant** qualities.

The anesthetic agent alleviates the **"pain trigger"** while at the same time the proliferant agent begins to strengthen the ligaments and tendons at the **trigger or tender point**.

Some prolotherapists use mild **chemical irritants**, such as phenol, guaiacol or tannic acid, to trigger the healing process. These substances attach themselves to the walls of the cells wherever they are injected, causing irritation that stimulates the body's reactive healing process. Others prefer to use **chemotactic agents**, primarily morrhuate sodium, a fatty acid derived from cod liver oil. Most closely aligned to the compound **Sylnasol** used by Dr. Hackett in his pioneering efforts, these proliferants attract immune cells directly to the injected area.

The dramatic sounding **"osmotic shock agents"** are actually simple compounds like dextrose and glycerine.

These are the most commonly used ingredients in the arsenal of Prolotherapy. Extremely safe and water-soluble, they are easily excreted from the body after having their initial desired effect. They work by causing cells to lose water, which leads to inflammation and the subsequent stimulation of the healing response.

Particulates such as pumice flour are microscopic particles that attract macrophages, tiny organisms which gobble them up, in turn secreting polypetide growth factors that result in collagen production.

Besides these general differences, the specific combinations of chemicals and substances used are as varied as the "schools" of Prolotherapy using them.

Some practitioners add **co-factors**, such as the anti-oxidant mineral manganese, or a combination of glucosamine sulfate and confroitin sulfate which is believed to aid in the repair of arthritic joints, or other co-factors believed to increase the efficacy of the compounds they are used with.

Despite the enormous success of the compounds used today, the most exciting advances in Prolotherapy may be just around the corner, in the form of **Growth Factors** or **Growth Hormones**. In addition, **Fetal Stem Cells** have been injected.

Growth factors cut to the chase, so to speak, acting directly on the cells and joints of the body to stimulate the proliferation of fibroblasts and regeneration of collagen and cartilage.

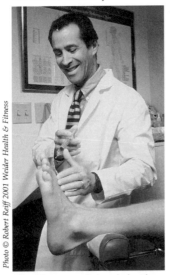

Photo © Robert Reiff 2001 Weider Health & Fitness

Dr. Darrow giving injection

The most important variable of all, however, as in all medical practices, is *the ability and experience of the therapist one chooses.* Besides being a licensed medical doctor, it is important that the prolotherapist also be in tune with the underlying premise of homeopathy. It is not our duty to cure, but rather to entice the body into curing itself.

Prolotherapy takes trigger-point therapy one step further by injecting an irritant into the trigger-point which increases the proliferation of fibroblasts that produce new collagen.

"Is not the body the soul's house?
Then why should we not take care
of the house that it fall not into ruins?"

–Philo

The Natural Healing Cascade

In order to fully appreciate how Prolotherapy works, it is essential to understand the natural healing process that it mimics, known in the world of medicine as "the natural healing cascade."

This process is complex, but has been extensively studied by the medical community and is readily understood, even by the layman.

When an injury occurs to a muscle, joint, tendon or ligament, or loss of fluid in the body through aging or illness causes a weakening of these tissues, it becomes inflamed, or irritated. This irritation provokes a defensive immune response and sequestering of fibroblasts into the damaged area. These rejuvinative cells produce the miraculous healing: collagen.

Absorbed into and around the damaged tissue, the collagen builds up and fortifies these structures. It then shrinks and stabilizes. After proliferative therapy, a ligament can become 50% thicker and 200-400% stronger.

It is interesting to consider that **inflammation** is the inciting factor that actually stimulates the entire healing process.

In his massive and scholarly tome, "Prolo Your Sports Injury Away," Dr. Ross Hauser suggests a very intriguing theory about inflammation and sports injuries. Sports injuries are commonly "treated" with an injection of **steroids**—which are administered specifically for their **anti-inflammatory effect**.

Hauser wonders if **recurring sports injuries** aren't in fact **caused** by this routine use of steroid injections — which by their very nature would interfere with the body's ability to produce fibroblasts and therefore to produce the collagen it sorely needs to repair and strengthen its damaged tissue.

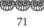

If this indeed proves to be true, then the decision to choose Prolotherapy over corticosteroid injections could mean the crucial difference to an athlete—the difference between a *record-breaking* career and or a *career-breaking* decision.

A BRIEF HISTORY OF TRIGGER POINT THERAPY

Trigger point therapy is a fairly modern science, which developed as a result of decades of observation and studies into the nature of pain by researchers around the world. Various techniques of therapy blossomed with each new revelation, evolving from deep massage to the needle therapies *(i.e.—acupuncture, trigger point, or Prolotherapy)* used today.

Trigger point therapy is an extension of the principles of acupuncture. Both of these therapies, although rooted in non-traditional (by Western standards) medicine, have eventually been accepted by the medical establishment, including most insurers.

The German physician Froriep took the first recorded step in the trigger point arena in 1843. He coined the phrase "muskelschwiele" *(muscle callouses)* to identify the hard cords found in muscle tissue in cases of rheumatic pain. Other physicians adopted his ideas and continued studying the problem of muscle pain based on Froriep's assumption. But by the end of the century, one of his countrymen debunked the theory on the grounds that no real "callouses" of deposited material were found in these tender muscles.[7]

Although German physicians held the lead for many years to come[8][9][10], Swedish and British researchers conducted their own studies and offered their own contributions, with the same mixed results.

Many of these pioneers stumbled onto important nuggets of information and—even when they were wrong—ended up advancing the science by uncovering possibilities that were eventually eliminated.

The cryptic and elusive nature of the pathology, and an incomplete understanding of the intricate structures of the human physiology hampered early researchers and clinicians. Today, much progress has been made thanks to advanced scientific technologies like Magnetic Resonance Imaging and ultrasonic devices.

American researchers in the 1930s were among the first to describe instances of referred pain[11] [12], and a major breakthrough was achieved in 1939 when British researchers Kellgren and Lewis proved that the previously held but not widely accepted notion of referred pain was indeed rooted in fact.[13] But even their observations were limited by the then rudimentary understanding of the complexities of the spine and nervous system.

Other brilliant researchers came forth with major findings shortly thereafter. Polish physician Gutstein, writing first in German, and later in English (as Gutstein-Good), after relocating to Great Britain, advanced the concept of trigger points, which he called "myalgic spots," as well as the importance of analyzing the patient's pain reaction, later called the "jump sign." Contributing over a dozen papers between 1938 and 1957, his observations on trigger points were highly astute, and steered his colleagues in the proper direction.[14] [15] [16]

Hans Kraus introduced a great advancement in the treatment of muscle pain in 1937 when he pioneered the use of vapocoolant spray to treat muscle pain and relieve trigger points.[17] In 1970, Kraus published a book on the beneficial effects of exercise on patients with back pain.[18]

Janet G. Travell, M.D., reached prominence as the personal physician to Presidents John F. Kennedy and Lyndon Baines Johnson, two of the brightest men ever to occupy the Oval Office. David Simons, M.D. was a U.S. Air Force Flight Surgeon conducting experiments in the nascent field of Aerospace Medical Research when he and Travell met at the School of Aerospace Medicine.

Together they produced one of the most comprehensive reference manuals in the history of pain medicine, "Myofascial Pain and Dysfunction: The Trigger Point Manual," an exhaustive presentation covering every practical aspect of Trigger Point Therapy. It included descriptions of techniques and ingredients to maps of all the known trigger point reference patterns.[19]

A CLOSER LOOK AT TRIGGER POINTS

A normal healthy body contains an intricate framework of bones and cartilage supported in perfect harmony by a network of semi-elastic tissues, mainly tendons and ligaments.[20] Dysfunction in these tissues causes a wide variety of problems.

When the tendons or ligaments, which anchor the structure, are weakened or damaged, the stress and friction created by the misalignment of joints results in chronic pain. Similar stresses can be caused by the action of dysfunctional muscles, tendons, or ligaments containing problem areas known as **"trigger points"** or **"tender points"**— hyperirritable, painful soft tissue areas. Normal healthy soft tissue does not contain trigger or tender points.

The source of muscle pain is called the **active trigger point**.[21] In some cases, the pain occurs directly in the active trigger point that caused it. This is called a **primary trigger point**. Pain can also manifest in distant areas away from the active trigger point. Such pain is called **referred pain**. Cases of referred pain may involve either secondary or satellite trigger points.

A **secondary trigger point** is a hyperirritable spot in a muscle or fascia that became active because the muscle (in which it manifests) has an antagonistic or a synergistic relationship with the muscle actually triggering the pain. That is, it works with, or against, the muscle which hosts the primary trigger point.

A **satellite trigger point** is simply one that receives pain because it is located in a zone of reference linked directly to the active trigger point, an area known as the **essential pain zone.** There are also areas known as **spillover pain zones** that receive pain signals that spill out beyond the normal boundaries of the essential pain zone where it originates.

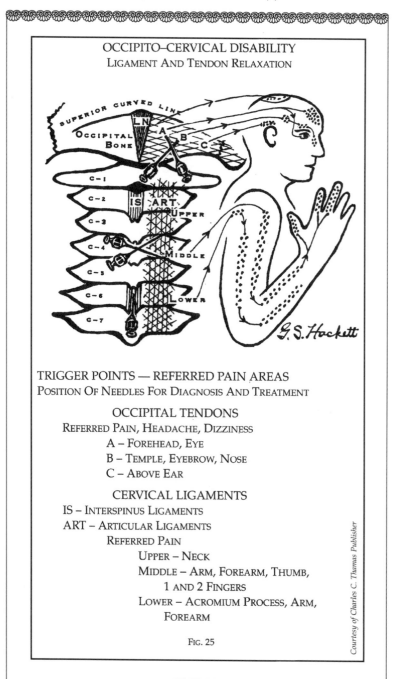

OCCIPITO–CERVICAL DISABILITY
LIGAMENT AND TENDON RELAXATION

TRIGGER POINTS — REFERRED PAIN AREAS
POSITION OF NEEDLES FOR DIAGNOSIS AND TREATMENT

OCCIPITAL TENDONS
REFERRED PAIN, HEADACHE, DIZZINESS
A – FOREHEAD, EYE
B – TEMPLE, EYEBROW, NOSE
C – ABOVE EAR

CERVICAL LIGAMENTS
IS – INTERSPINUS LIGAMENTS
ART – ARTICULAR LIGAMENTS
REFERRED PAIN
UPPER – NECK
MIDDLE – ARM, FOREARM, THUMB,
1 AND 2 FINGERS
LOWER – ACROMIUM PROCESS, ARM,
FOREARM

FIG. 25

Besides the pain caused by active trigger points, there are symptoms other than pain that are caused by **latent trigger points.** Some common latent symptoms include weakness, stiffness or restriction of movement. Both active and latent trigger points cause dysfunction—but only active ones cause pain.[22]

> **Myofascial pain – Pain associated with damage or injury to the soft connective tissues in our body**

Myofasciitis is a general term used to describe pain or other dysfunctions in the network of muscles, tendons, and ligaments and other soft connective tissue that holds our bodies together. Myofascial pain may start abruptly or gradually. Abrupt onset is usually the result of trauma to the muscle, such as a sudden overload or over-extension, while a gradual onset is due to chronic overload, virus, or other disease, or psychogenic stress.[23]

Through an understanding of the various symptoms of pain, such as whether it occurs at rest or during activity, what muscles it is related to, whether it is primary or referred, and countless other factors, the doctor can isolate the problem and treat it with a technique known as **trigger point therapy.** It is an underlying premise of this treatise, that Prolotherapy may be much more effective than simple trigger point therapy.

Diagnostic procedures include testing for taut bands of muscle fiber, twitch response, and applied pressure to check for referred pain triggers. There is evidence to suggest that trigger points are caused by impaired circulation and/or an increased metabolic demand.[24]

Skeletal muscle tissue accounts for about 40% of our body weight, and includes nearly 700 individual muscles.[25] When active trigger points are present, passive or active stretching of the muscle produces pain.[26] And this pain can occur with the slightest activity or even at rest. Biofeedback has proven that muscles are in a state of contraction and activity even when we believe we are at rest.

When myofascial pain is related to a single muscle trauma, or exhibits a stable pattern over any length of time, it is usually easy to diagnose and treat.

In cases where pain appears in multiple muscles, spreads to other areas, or there is evidence of increasing fibrosis or other contributing factors, pain can be very difficult to diagnose and treat. Once the proper diagnosis is ascertained, however, various treatments are available to deal with the problem effectively.

Knowledge of the referred pain pattern characteristic of each muscle is often the most important single source of information used in diagnosing pain. The patient's examination begins with observation of their posture, movements, body structure and symmetry. It progresses with specialized screening movements to isolate the problem areas and identify trigger points.

> <u>Referred (Trigger-Point) Pain</u> – **Pain that arises in a trigger-point, but is felt at a distance, often entirely remote from its source. The pattern of referred pain is reproducibly related to its site of origin.** *The distribution of referred trigger-point pain rarely coincides with the entire distribution of peripheral nerve or dermatomal segment.* [35]

Once a diagnosis is made, an appropriate treatment can be effected. Simple problems might respond to non-invasive treatments like the "**stretch and spray**" technique pioneered by Hans Kraus to relieve simple musculoskeletal pain.[27] Described by Travell-Simons[28] as the "workhorse" of myofascial syndrome, stretch and spray treatment inactivates myofascial trigger points quickly and with little discomfort to the patient. A single-muscle syndrome of recent onset frequently responds with full pain-free function with just two or three sweeps of ethyl chloride or fluori-methane spray while the muscle is being passively stretched.

More complex problems, or seemingly simple ones that do not respond to stretch and spray therapy, need more intensive treatment with the addition of needle therapy.

REFERRED PAIN AND SCIATICA–
ILIOLUMBAR, POSTERIOR SACROILIAC,
SACROSPINUS AND SACROTUBERUS
LIGAMENTS .
(LUMBOSACRAL AND SACROILIAC JOINT
INSTABILITY.)

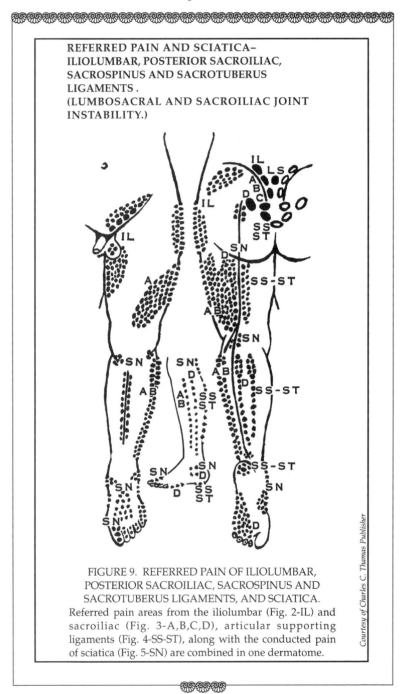

FIGURE 9. REFERRED PAIN OF ILIOLUMBAR,
POSTERIOR SACROILIAC, SACROSPINUS AND
SACROTUBERUS LIGAMENTS, AND SCIATICA.
Referred pain areas from the iliolumbar (Fig. 2-IL) and
sacroiliac (Fig. 3-A,B,C,D), articular supporting
ligaments (Fig. 4-SS-ST), along with the conducted pain
of sciatica (Fig. 5-SN) are combined in one dermatome.

Courtesy of Charles C. Thomas Publisher

"Injection and stretch" or "trigger point injection therapy" is highly effective, but a bit more complicated, involving the actual injection of a dry needle or a solution into the problem area.

It is advisable to immediately follow up injection therapy with "spray and stretch" treatment, especially if there is residual pain or restriction of movement in the treated area. Hot packs are also used following the injections, to relieve post-injection soreness.

Injection has proven to be an effective treatment in various cases, whether a dry needle is used[29] or various solutions, including procaine or other anesthetics, isotonic saline,[30] and occasionally steroids.[31]

Physiatrists are Doctors specializing in Physical Medicine and Rehabilitation. They typically have the most experience in administering trigger point injections because of intense training in their 4-year Physical Medicine and Rehabilitation residency program that occurs after medical school. They are skilled at using their hands to find and identify trigger points, as well as the subtler art of distinguishing true trigger points from simple tender areas that might have been caused by contusions.

Once a **Physiatrist** identifies a problem area, he or she will proceed with a series of pinches, pokes or other touch techniques known to elicit twitches or other specific responses from the body, thus refining the search for the root of the problem, honing in on the trigger or tender point and targeting the precise area which needs to be treated.

A great debt is owed to Doctors Janet G. Travell and David G. Simons, who mapped out the human body and contributed a comprehensive guidebook to the paths of pain in the body.[32]

Often, just as in acupuncture, a **dry needle** is sufficient to provoke a healing response. Unlike acupuncture, however, trigger point therapy involves a deep tissue invasion by the needle with injection of fluid, and more concentrated manipulation by the practitioner.

Although dry needling is highly effective, it is too painful for many patients to endure comfortably. Most Prolotherapists administer the injections with an anesthetic. In addition in my practice I also use an anesthetic jet (see photo on page 132) which is administered prior to injection so that the "pinch" of the needle is not felt.

Procaine is widely used in cases where an anesthetic solution is desired. It is cheap, non-irritating, easy to sterilize, and has minimal systemic toxicity combined with reasonable duration of activity. Another big advantage of adding Procaine to the treatment is its vasodilating effect. Since lack of circulation is a leading cause of trigger point activation, the Procaine helps considerably in this area.[33]

Lidocaine is a favorite alternative to procaine, for its longer-lasting effects, which is why it has found favor in dentistry and other fields of minor surgery where pain reduction is an important part of the equation.

Besides the pain-relieving properties of these fluid injections, there is a strong but unproven assumption that they may also wash out any nerve-sensitizing substances contributing to the trigger point, which further reduces the problem.

> **Prolotherapy and Trigger-Point therapy are essentially the same thing. Both Prolotherapy and Trigger-Point injections can reduce or eliminate pain and result in the growth of new cells to support weakened ligaments and tendons.**

Although generally safe and effective, there are cases where trigger point injection therapy just will not do the trick. Some of the more common reasons include cases involving stress due to psychological factors, chronic infection, skeletal asymmetry, nutritional deficiencies, metabolic problems, allergy, or disease. In many cases involving skeletal misalignment, or myofascial pain Prolotherapy may offer the only effective cure.

[1] Techniques of Prolotherapy, K.Dean Reeves, M.D. Chapter 7, p.57.

[2] "Fatality After Injection of Sclerosing Agent to Precipitate Fibro-osseous Proliferation." Journal of the AMA, Aug. 8, 1959. Richard Schneider, M.D.

[3] Faber, W., Walker, M. Pain Pain Go Away, Ishi Press Intl, Menlo Park, CA 1998.

[4] "Prolo Your Sports Injury Away" by Ross A. Hauser, M.D. and Marion A. Hauser, M.S., R.D., Beulah Land Press, 2001.

[5] Froriep, R: Ein Beitrag zur Pathologie und Therapie des Rheumatismus, Weimar, 1843.

[6] Virchow, R: Ueber Parenchymatose Entzundung, Arch Path Anat Chap. 4, p. 269-70, 1852.

[7] Strauss, H: Uber die Sogenannte "Rheumatische Muskelschwiele," Klin Wochenschr, 35:89-91, 121-123, 1898.

[8] Schade, H, Z Gestamte Exp Med, 7:275-374, 1919, Muensch Med Wochenschr, 68:95-99, 1921.

[9] Glogowski, G, Wallraff, J, Z Orthrop 80:237-268, 1951.

[10] Miehlke, Schulze, Eger, Z Rheumaforsch, 19:310-330, 1960.

[11] Hunter, C, Myalgia of the Abdominal Wall, Con Med Assoc, 28:157-161, 1933.

[12] Edeiken, J., Wolferth, C.C., Persistent Pain in the Shoulder Region Following Myocardial Infarction, American Journal of Medical Science, 191:201-210, 1936.

[13] Kellgren, J.H., Lewis, T, Observations Relating to Referred Pain Visceromotor Reflexes and Other Associated Phenomena, Clinical Science, 1:47-71, 1939.)

[14] Gutstein, M, Diagnosis and Treatment of Muscular Rheumatism, British Journal of Physical Medicine 1:302-321, 1938

[15] Gutstein, M, Common Rheumatism and Physiotherapy, British Journal of Physical Medicine 3:46-50, 1940.

[16] Gutstein-Good, M, Idiopathic Myalgia Simulating Visceral and Other Diseases, Lancet 2:326-8, 1940.

[17] Kraus, H, The Use of Surface Anesthesia for the Treatment of Painful Motion, JAMA, 116:2582-2587, 1941.

[18] Kraus, H, Clinical Treatment of Back and Neck Pain, McGraw-Hill, New York, 1970.

[19] Myofascial Pain and Dysfunction: The Trigger Point Manual, Janet G. Travell, M.D., David Simons, M.D., Illustrations by Barbara D. Cummings, Williams & Wilkins, Baltimore, MD 1983.

[20] Bardeen, C.R. The Musculature, Section 5, p. 355, Morris's Human Anatomy, Ed. by C.M. Jackson, Blakiston's Son & Co., Philadelphia, PA, 1921.

[21] Janet G. Travell, M.D. and David G. Simons, M.D., Myofascial Pain and Dysfunction: The Trigger Point Manual, p.1-4, Williams & Wilkins, 1983.

[22] Janet G. Travell, M.D. and David G. Simons, M.D., Myofascial Pain and Dysfunction: The Trigger Point Manual, Chapter 2, p.13, Williams & Wilkins, 1983.

[23] Janet G. Travell, M.D. and David G. Simons, M.D., Myofascial Pain and Dysfunction: The Trigger Point Manual, Chapter 3, p.53, Williams & Wilkins, 1983.

[24] Janet G. Travell, M.D. and David G. Simons, M.D., Myofascial Pain and Dysfunction: The Trigger Point Manual, Chapter 2, p.34, Williams & Wilkins, 1983.

[25] Bardeen, C.R. The Musculature, Section 5, p. 355, Morris's Human Anatomy, Ed. by C.M. Jackson, Blakiston's Son & Co., Philadelphia, PA, 1921.

[26] Macdonald, AJR, Abnormally Tender Muscle Regions and Associated Painful Movements, Pain, 8:197-205, 1980.

[27] Modell, Travell, Kraus, et al, Relief of Pain by Ethyl Chloride Spray, New York State Journal of Medicine, 48:2050-59, 1948.

[28] Janet G. Travell, M.D. and David G. Simons, M.D., Myofascial Pain and Dysfunction: The Trigger Point Manual, Williams & Wilkins, 1983.

[29] Lewit, K, The Needle Effect in the Relief of Myofascial Pain, Pain 6:83-90, 1979.

[30] Frost, Jessen, Siggaard-Andersen, A Control, Double-Blind Comparison of Mepivacaine Versus Saline Injection for Myofascial Pain, Lancet, 1:499-501, 1980.

[31] Zohn, Mennell, Musculosketal Pain: Diagnosis and Physical Treatment, p.126-9, Little, Brown & Co., Boston, 1976.

[32] Janet G. Travell, M.D. and David G. Simons, M.D., Myofascial Pain and Dysfunction: The Trigger Point Manual, Chapter 2, p.34, Williams & Wilkins, 1983.

[33] Good, M.G., The Role of Skeletal Muscles in the Pathogenesis of Diseases, Acta Med Scand 138:285-292, 1950.

[34] George Stuart Hackett, MD., Gustav A. Hemwall, MD, and Gerald A. Montgomery, MD., Ligament and Tendon Relaxation Treated by Prolotherapy, Charles C. Thomas 1993

[35] Janet G. Travell, M.D. and David G. Simons, M.D., Myofascial Pain and Dysfunction: The Trigger Point Manual,p.3; Williams & Wilkins, 1983

"When you get sick and tired of being tired and sick —you'll change"

–John-Roger

"The practice of forgiveness is our most important contribution to the healing of the world."

–Marianne Williamson

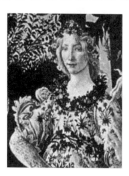

5

Back Pain

Surgery doesn't cut it

*T*he New England Medical Journal reports that back pain is the second most common medical complaint reported in the U.S. today.[1] After the common cold, it is the second leading cause of work absenteeism, averaging 100 million lost work days per year.[2,3] According to the National Safety Council, the total annual cost of back injury disabilities in the United States is between $30 billion and $60 billion annually.[4]

60 to 90 percent of adults experience an acute episode of low back pain at least once in their lifetime.[5] Preventing low back injuries- the single most frequent injury requiring days off from work- was the focus of the 1998 Labor Day CheckList, issued by the American College of Occupational and Environmental Medicine (ACOEM). The U.S. Bureau of Labor Statistics (BLS) in 1996 recorded a total of 490,608 back injuries that resulted in time away from work.[6] The same study showed men outnumber women almost two to one in sustaining back injuries requiring time off the job. Operators, fabricators, and laborers experienced close to 42 percent of injuries, followed by those in service professions, who had 20 percent.[7]

Although symptoms are usually acute and self-limited, low back pain often recurs,[8] and in 5-10% of patients, low back pain becomes chronic.[9,10] Back symptoms are the most common cause of disability for persons under age 45.[11]

80% of Americans will suffer some type of back pain in their lives.[12] For 85% of back pain sufferers, the primary site of back pain is the lower back.[13]

51% of the nearly 30 million musculosketal impairments reported in 1988 were back-related.[14] A 1988 National Health Interview Survey[15] found that one of every eight Americans suffer from back/spine impairments, most prevalently among 45-64 year-olds. Not surprisingly, this demographic represents people young enough to be active, but old enough to start letting themselves go, buying into the mindset that physical deterioration of the body is an inevitable part of the aging process.

> **"Those who think they have not the time for bodily exercise will sooner or later have time for illness."**
> **-Edward Stanley**

Epidemiologic evidence suggests that several modifiable risk factors, including smoking, obesity, and certain psychological profiles, predispose subjects to develop low back pain.[16] Studies have shown that smokers have a 1.5-2.5-fold increased risk of back pain compared to nonsmokers.[17][18][19] A biologic basis for this risk is suggested by a recent study of identical twins discordant for smoking, showing that smoking increases degenerative changes of the spine.[20]

Prospective and cross-sectional studies have also associated obesity with back pain.[21][22]

Psychological risk factors, including depression, anxiety, and perceived high occupational stress, have also been associated with the development of low back pain.[23][24]

A study conducted at Ohio State University provided the first-ever link between stress and back pain.[25] The study, published in the December 1, 2000 issue of the journal Spine, found that people with certain personality types may increase their risk of back injury if they experience workplace stress. According to study co-author William Marras, professor of industrial, welding, and systems engineering, "The results take a first step toward explaining why people with certain personality types — namely, introverted people and those who dislike performing repetitive tasks — are more likely to report back pain on the job. The criticism just rolled right off the extroverts, but introverts changed the way they used their muscles, so that lifting became much more mechanically stressful."

When stressed, introverts began employing muscles in their abdomen or sides — muscles that weren't necessary for lifting. As a result, different forces on the spine increased as introverts lifted the box. The same held true for intuitors.

For introverts, spinal compression increased by almost 14 percent, while sideways forces on the spine increased by about 27 percent. For intuitors, spinal compression increased by almost 11 percent, and sideways forces by about 25 percent.

In another study[26] involving the psychological roots of pain, Stanford researchers completed a rigorous comparison of the MRI and discography results of 96 patients with known risk factors for disc degeneration, with surprising results. People whose discs had high intensity zones were only slightly more likely to experience back pain during normal activity than those without obvious disc problems. Additionally, high intensity zones were found in 25 percent of people who — despite their known degenerative disc disease — had no corresponding symptoms of low back pain.

The Stanford team concluded that the presence of the high intensity zones — and thus torn discs — doesn't automatically mean that the patient is experiencing pain during everyday activities, or that they will feel pain during a discography.

> **This suggests that not every disc tear is painful, and not all low back pain results from a damaged disc. This concept is one most importance.** *It means that if you have back pain and have a disc problem, having surgery to remove the disc may not end your pain.* **Most back pain is from a sprain of the sacroiliac and iliolumbar ligaments. Prolotherapy can heal this.**

A better predictor of pain, they found, is an abnormal result on psychometric testing. Basically... that the amount of discomfort that people have... is, in many patients, most closely related to psychological and social issues," said Dr. Eugene Carragee. "People with poor coping skills... are more

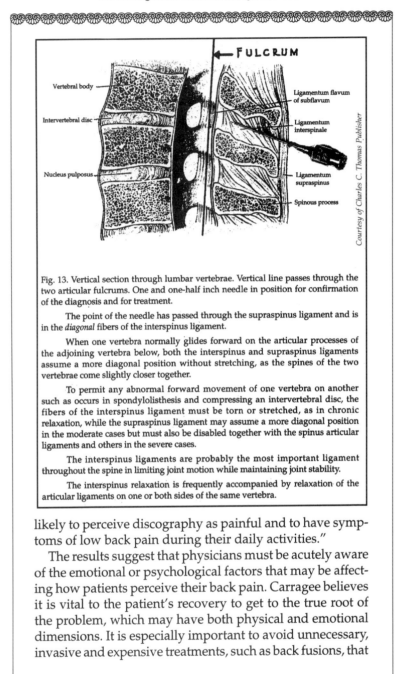

Fig. 13. Vertical section through lumbar vertebrae. Vertical line passes through the two articular fulcrums. One and one-half inch needle in position for confirmation of the diagnosis and for treatment.

The point of the needle has passed through the supraspinus ligament and is in the *diagonal* fibers of the interspinus ligament.

When one vertebra normally glides forward on the articular processes of the adjoining vertebra below, both the interspinus and supraspinus ligaments assume a more diagonal position without stretching, as the spines of the two vertebrae come slightly closer together.

To permit any abnormal forward movement of one vertebra on another such as occurs in spondylolisthesis and compressing an intervertebral disc, the fibers of the interspinus ligament must be torn or stretched, as in chronic relaxation, while the supraspinus ligament may assume a more diagonal position in the moderate cases but must also be disabled together with the spinus articular ligaments and others in the severe cases.

The interspinus ligaments are probably the most important ligament throughout the spine in limiting joint motion while maintaining joint stability.

The interspinus relaxation is frequently accompanied by relaxation of the articular ligaments on one or both sides of the same vertebra.

likely to perceive discography as painful and to have symptoms of low back pain during their daily activities."

The results suggest that physicians must be acutely aware of the emotional or psychological factors that may be affecting how patients perceive their back pain. Carragee believes it is vital to the patient's recovery to get to the true root of the problem, which may have both physical and emotional dimensions. It is especially important to avoid unnecessary, invasive and expensive treatments, such as back fusions, that reinforce the perception that the patient has a grave disease of the spine, he said.[28] Currently a standard treatment for severe, persistently painful, vertebral disc tears, as many as 30,000 back fusions are performed annually in the United States, Carragee estimates, although they are often not very successful at relieving the patient's pain.

> Over 250,000 back surgeries are performed in the U.S. annually, and the number of back surgeries is linearly related to the number of back surgeons in the region.

But it isn't only adults or workers who suffer from serious back problems. Adolescent athletes — gymnasts in particular — are prone to back injuries because they're often competing at high levels and putting stress on immature bones, said Dr. Vesna Martich Kriss, M.D., an associate professor of radiology and pediatrics at the University of Kentucky College of Medicine, Lexington. In a study at the University of Kentucky, of 69 children complaining of low back pain, 21 were identified as having back lesions by bone scan, or single photon emission computed tomography (SPECT), while X-ray detected problems in only 8 children.[29]

"Back pain is common in adults, and the majority of the time, it's nothing serious," said Dr. Kriss, M.D., "But when children complain, doctors and parents should be concerned. Even if an initial X-ray doesn't show anything, parents shouldn't stop there if pain persists... sometimes a fracture after a trauma doesn't show up in an X-ray for a week or two. A second X-ray may be necessary if the child continues to complain, and occasionally, a bone scan may be necessary to get to the root of the problem."[30]

Pregnant women are yet another high risk group for back pain, due to increased stress on muscles bearing the increased forward weight of the torso.[31] In the words of study co-author Jon R. Davids, MD, a member of the American Academy of Orthopedic Surgeons, "When pregnant women walk, their muscles must work harder to accomplish the same gait pattern they normally can without the added weight."

"Pregnant women who are not physically fit are at greatest risk of overuse injury," said lead author Theresa Foti, PhD, Motion Analysis Laboratory, Shriners Hospital for Children, Greenville, S.C.

"Despite major anatomical changes associated with pregnancy, the appearance of women's gait changed very little," said Dr. Foti. "However, measures indicating increased muscular effort at the hips and ankles were found. This suggests an increased use of muscles to compensate for increases in body mass and weight distribution during pregnancy to keep walking speed, stride length, cadence and joint angles relatively unchanged."

Dr. Davids said that it is this extra work by these muscles that potentially contributes to low back pain, hip and pelvic pain, leg cramps and other lower extremity musculoskeletal conditions associated with pregnancy.

"Women who are physically fit before pregnancy are less likely to get these problems during pregnancy," he said. "Pregnant women also should consider engaging in some type of exercise and conditioning program approved by their physician."

SPINAL CORD INJURY

Spinal Cord Injuries (SCI) represent the most dreaded and debilitating type of back injury. In their most severe form the result is crippling paralysis.

There are two classifications for SCI's. In a complete injury, nerve damage obstructs every signal coming from the brain to the body parts below the injury. In an incomplete injury, some residual motor and sensory function remains below the level of SCI.[32]

Approximately 450,000 people in the United States have sustained traumatic spinal cord injuries, with more than 10,000 new cases of SCI emerging in the U.S. every year. Males account for 82 percent of all SCI's and females for 18 percent.[33]

Motor vehicle accidents are the leading cause of SCI (44 percent), followed by acts of violence (24 percent), falls

(22 percent), sports injuries (8 percent), and other causes (2 percent).

Currently, there is no cure for spinal cord injuries. However, ongoing research to test surgical and drug therapies is progressing more rapidly than ever before. Injury progression prevention drug treatments, decompression surgery, nerve cell transplantation, nerve regeneration, and complex drug therapies are all being examined as a means to overcome the effects of spinal cord injury.

Overall, 85 percent of SCI patients who survive the first 24 hours following injury are alive 10 years later.

SYMPTOMS OF SPINAL CORD INJURY

The rings of bone that make up the spinal column are known as vertebrae. Grouped according to their location on the spinal column are the Cervical, Thoracic, Lumbar and Sacral vertebrae.

The seven vertebrae in the neck are the Cervical Vertebrae. Severe SCI at cervical levels usually causes a loss of independent breathing and loss of function to the arms and legs, thereby resulting in quadriplegia which is now termed tetraplegia.

The twelve vertebrae in the chest are called the Thoracic Vertebrae. Thoracic level injuries usually affect the chest and the legs and result in paraplegia.

The five vertebrae in the lower back are known as the Lumbar Vertebrae. Lumbar level injury typically results in loss of control of the legs, bladder, bowel and sexual functions.

The Sacral Vertebrae are the five vertebrae that run from the pelvis to the end of the spinal column. Sacral level injuries generally damage the nerves emanating from the distal spinal cord conus and typically cause lower motor neuron flaccid paralysis type lesions involving some loss of function in the legs and difficulty with bowel, bladder and sexual control.

PREVENTION: THE BEST MEDICINE

TIPS TO SPARE YOUR BACK

Although there is some evidence that exercise (flexion, extension, aerobic, or fitness) protects against the development of low back pain, the effect is modest and of unknown duration, and the interventions have not been demonstrated in typical clinical settings. Thus, there is insufficient evidence to recommend for or against counseling patients to exercise specifically to prevent low back pain. There is however, medical exercise equipment that has been widely studied to relieve back pain. It is a computerized dynomometer named MedX. Dr. William Bergman, PhD, an exercise physiologist trained by Arthur Jones, the inventor of MedX, (also the creator of Nautilus exercise equipment), directs our MedX department in Los Angeles.

Given some evidence that mechanical supports may increase the risk of low back pain, recommendations can be made against their use except in the context of comprehensive programs where their use can be carefully monitored to avoid injury.

Occupational back injury is routinely caused by heavy lifting and repetitive motion activities.[35] Persons in occupations that require repetitive lifting and heavy industry,[36] are especially at risk. Based on national data, occupational groups with the highest estimated prevalence of low back pain (10.1-10.5%) include mechanics and repairers of vehicles, engines and heavy equipment; operators of extractive, mining, and material-moving equipment; and people in construction trades and other construction occupations.[37]

The most commonly prescribed strategies[38] to prevent low back pain and injury are:

(a) back flexion, back extension, and general fitness exercises

(b) improved back mechanic and ergonomic techniques

(c) mechanical back supports (back belts or corsets); and

(d) risk factor modification[39]

HOW TO HAVE A HEALTHY BACK:[40 41 42 43]

- Keep lifted objects close to your body at waist level.

- Evenly balance loads with both arms.

- Don't strain your muscles by attempting to lift too much weight. Get help if the load is too bulky or heavy for you, or split it into smaller/lighter loads.

- Take rest breaks to change position and stretch.

- Avoid twisting, bending and reaching while lifting— rotate entire body instead.

- Bend with the knees, not the back.

- Alternate between standing and sitting tasks.

- During long periods of standing, rest one foot on a low support. When sitting, rest both feet flat on floor.

- Use a chair with good back support.

- When driving, move seat forward to keep knees level with hips.

- Keep both hands on wheel. Use a lumbar support for lower back.

- When working or exercising, wear comfortable, low-heeled, non-slip, non-skid, cushioned shoes.

- Learn relaxation techniques to manage stress on and off the job.

- Exercise regularly to keep back/abdominal muscles strong and flexible.

- Maintain your proper weight.

- Drink plenty of water for good hydration.

- Avoid smoking, which reduces blood/fluid flow to spine.

- Get plenty of sleep on a firm mattress.

Lower Back Pain

Lower back pain is one of the most widely reported types of pain in the United States today. It is the most common cause of industrial disability, and the leading cause of physical disability payments taxing our Social Security system.[44]

Studies suggest that the prevalence of lower back pain in the adult population of the United States is at least 60% and its incidence, about 30%. Astonishing as it may sound, 10-12% of the population is seeking health care for low back pain at any given moment.

Because the structures of the lower back are very complicated, and the specific symptoms of lower back pain are highly varied, lower back pain is one of the most difficult to diagnose and treat.

While some forms of back pain are transient—such as simple bruises caused by light trauma, which require at most an analgesic treatment to ease the pain until it heals naturally,—persistent or chronic lower back pain usually develops over an extended period of time, due to interacting causative factors involving the vertebrae and their supporting tissues. Although these two types of "extended pain" are similar in many respects, researchers have distinguished them according to a few basic guidelines.

Generally, pain is described as **"persistent"** if it does not heal promptly, based on statistical standards; or, if it recurs regularly, in defiance of any treatments provided. **"Chronic"** is the term usually reserved for pain lasting longer than three months, which, in both cause and effect, often involves psychological as well as physical factors, or combinations of the two.

As with all types of pain, there are many possible factors causing or contributing to both types of extended lower back pain. The two main causes are **spondylosis**, or **degenerative disk disease**, and **muscular or ligamentous inflammation**. *In fact, damage to ligaments is estimated to be responsible for up to 70% of all cases of lower back pain.*[45] In my clinic, I would estimate these causes to be a high as 95% of back pain.

The chronic lower back pain patient typically experiences some type of trauma to the lower back that causes injury to the interspinous and supraspinous ligaments.

This may causes some forward slippage of the fifth lumbar vertebra onto the sacrum, which in turn causes excessive pressure on the vertebra disk. Fissures may occur at the annulus fibrosis, and this begins the degenerative disk problem.[46]

Ligaments are designed to handle a normal amount of stress that will stretch them to their natural limit, and will return to their normal length once the stress is removed. If additional (traumatic) stress is applied— stretching the ligament beyond its natural range of extension—the ligament will not return to its normal length, but will instead remain permanently overstretched, diminishing its power. Such a condition is called **ligament laxity**. Ligament laxity in the lower back, as elsewhere in the body, may be caused by a major traumatic injury, repeated minor injuries to the same area, or simple normal aging. Unlike muscle tissue, ligaments have a very limited circulatory system that means a poor supply of blood to replenish them. This is why ligaments do not heal well on their own, and why Prolotherapy is needed in these types of injuries to stimulate circulation and to promote new cell growth.

With its overburdened matrix of ligaments, muscle, nerves, and small, interlocking bones, the spine is an area that benefits greatly from Prolotherapy.

The **sacrum** at the base of the spine is the "keystone" bone, on which all of the most vital structures of the body rest. Besides the lower vertebrae and the rest of the spinal column that it supports, it bears the weight of the entire torso with all its major organs.

And since the core of the central nervous system is housed in the spinal cord, and the nerves affect not only the legs and other extremities, but also the glands and the organs, the importance of keeping this area healthy and properly aligned becomes readily apparent. It also explains why so much of the pain reported to physicians is rooted in the lower back.

TRIGGER POINTS OF PAIN AND NEEDLES IN POSITION FOR
CONFIRMATION OF THE DIAGNOSIS AND FOR TREATMENT OF
LIGAMENT RELAXATION OF THE LUMBOSACRAL AND PELVIC JOINTS.
TRIGGER POINTS OF LIGAMENTS

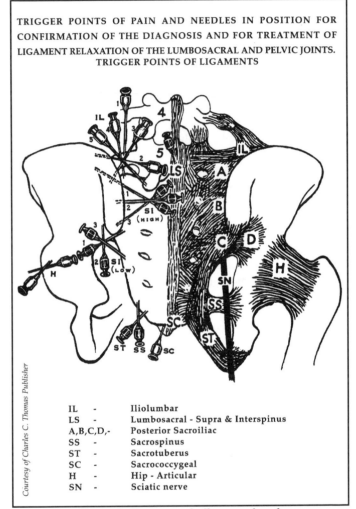

Courtesy of Charles C. Thomas Publisher

IL	-	Iliolumbar
LS	-	Lumbosacral - Supra & Interspinus
A,B,C,D,-		Posterior Sacroiliac
SS	-	Sacrospinus
ST	-	Sacrotuberus
SC	-	Sacrococcygeal
H	-	Hip - Articular
SN	-	Sciatic nerve

Descriptions and diagnosis of common low back pain include:

Lumbrosacral strain or sprain indicates a soft tissue injury of the lower back, equivalent to a sprained ankle.

Discogenic syndrome is used to describe pain originating in the lumbar disk, due to tears in the annulus, release of chemical mediators, or micromotion.

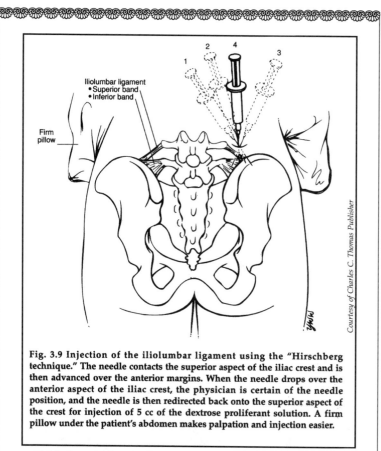

Courtesy of Charles C. Thomas Publisher

Fig. 3.9 Injection of the iliolumbar ligament using the "Hirschberg technique." The needle contacts the superior aspect of the iliac crest and is then advanced over the anterior margins. When the needle drops over the anterior aspect of the iliac crest, the physician is certain of the needle position, and the needle is then redirected back onto the superior aspect of the crest for injection of 5 cc of the dextrose proliferant solution. A firm pillow under the patient's abdomen makes palpation and injection easier.

Disk herniation indicates a displacement of the nucleus pulposus from the intervertebral space into the spinal canal or foramen, or outside the foramen. This can "pinch" a nerve root and cause sciatica.

Facet syndrome describes pain originating in the zygapophyseal or "facet" joints between the vertebrae, characteristically localized in the back, aggravated by movement and alleviated by rest.

Spondylolisthesis is the slipping forward of one vertebral segment onto another. **Retrolisthesis** describes the inverse: the slipping backward of one vertebra onto another.

Spondylolysis indicates a defect in the structure of the pars interarticularis, while **spondylosis** is a catch-all phrase describing the changes that occur as a result of degenerative disk disease, such as desiccation of the disk, narrowing of the interspace, inflammation, spurring or degeneration of the bone, and ligament hypertrophy.

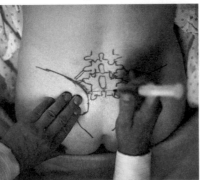

Photo ©1999 K.L. Pomeroy, MD.

Sacroiliac join injection

Spinal stenosis is used to describe the narrowing, in part or in whole, of the spinal canal, either through spondylosis or a congenital defect.

Spinal instability is a very general term used when a more precise diagnosis eludes the physician. Specifically, it refers to excess motion of the vertebrae, and can be shown on flexion and extension x-rays. If instability is severe, it can cause spinal cord injury and paralysis.

Perhaps the most distressing is **"failed back syndrome"** — an official-sounding term to describe the pain of those poor patients whose surgical attempts have failed to correct their problem.

> **The most common cause of failed back syndrome is poor judgement on the part of the physician. Surgery prescribed as a last resort, with a hope and a prayer that it might alleviate the pain.**

Unfortunately, often times surgery does little to help, and in fact can make things worse. Frequently surgery results in post-operative scarring, which often exacerbates the initial problem or causes new pain syndromes.

Subsequent "corrective" surgery can help in some cases, particularly if the damage done by the first operation involves clearly observable physical complications like nerve root compression, massive scarring, bone spurring or foraminal compression.

Unfortunately, the rate of success for second surgical operations in the case of "failed back syndrome" is no greater than it was for the initial operation, and declines with further attempts. In the words of a surgeon involved in such procedures, "In our extensive experience, satisfactory outcome is achieved about 60% of the time." Evidence indicates that many patients suffering from residual pain after multiple operations can benefit from an intensive rehabilitation program.

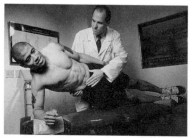

Dr. Kelberman with Johnnie Morton Jr.

Photos © Robert Reiff 2001 Weider Health & Fitness

Chiropractic care, although dreaded by the medical community, is desired more than any other therapy by the public. An excellent chiropractic methodology is called Applied Kinesiology (AK). The reason that it is often the best form of care post-surgically is that it does not involve "cracking" the vertebrae (although I must admit, I love to have my neck and back adjusted). Jason Kelberman, D.C., is the director of chiropractic at our clinic and practices many forms of chiropractic, with a specialty on AK.

A synergistic form of back strengthening for the muscles of the back and

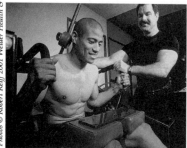

Dr. Bill Bergman Ph.D with Johnnie Morton Jr. on Med-X back machine

neck is MedX computerized exercise equipment. It was developed by Arthur Jones who also developed Nautilus. Bill Bergman, PhD is our director of the MedX department. Bill actually trained with Arthur in the early days of MedX and is the most experienced practitioner in the world, having helped over 8000 patients back to health.

With a combination of chiropractic care, Prolotherapy, MedX, and an intensive rehabilitation program that focuses on stretching, elimination of local inflammatory changes, spinal muscle strengthening, and general reconditioning, most patients improve by increasing function and mobility, and decreasing pain.

Prolotherapy to the Rescue

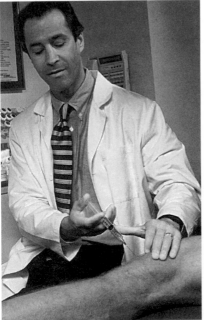

Photo © Robert Reiff 2001 Weider Health & Fitness

Dr. Darrow injects a knee

A study[47] published in1987—by which time the procedures of Prolotherapy were fairly well established—offered dramatic support to proponents of the still basically unknown technique. In the first double-blind study on the effects of the treatment, two groups of carefully screened patients—with at least a one year history of back problems that hadn't responded to other non-surgical treatments—were injected with either a true prolotherapy proliferant (a dextrose-glycerine-phenol solution originally developed to treat varicose veins), or with a saline-based placebo.

The test subjects had been thoroughly pre-screened, with full clinical evaluations, x-rays and lab tests, and the 82 patients accepted had arrived with painful conditions. 60% were currently using non-steroidal anti-inflammatory drugs. A half-dozen were experiencing such intense pain that they were taking narcotics for relief. A whopping 91% had difficulty sitting still for any length of time, and 65% had difficulty sleeping due to their pain. 17% had difficulty walking, sexual activity was down in 21%, and 4% were completely bed-ridden.

Six months after the treatment, 35 of the 40 people who'd received the actual Prolotherapy treatment had experienced at least a 50% reduction in pain—a success rate of 88%. And 15 of them were comletely pain free—compared to only 4 in the control group.

Other "pain score" indicators backed up the results of this data, confirming the success of the therapy. One thing was eminently clear:

Prolotherapy worked for the treatment of chronic low back pain.

---

[1] Frymoyer JW. Back pain and sciatica. N Engl J Med 1988; 318:291-300.)

[2] McElligott J, Miscovich SJ, Fielding LP. Low back injury in industry: the value of a recovery program. Conn Med 1989; 53:711-715.

[3] Batti, MC, Bigos SJ. Industrial back pain complaints: a broader perspective. Orthop Clin North Am 1991;22:273-282.

[4]http://www.spinenet.com/articles.patient/backstats.html, National Safety Council.

[5]http://www.newswise.com/articles/1998/8/BCKINJRY.A CO.html, American College of Occupational & Environmental Medicine, Aug.12, 1998.

[6]http://www.newswise.com/articles/1998/8/BCKINJRY.A CO.html, American College of Occupational & Environmental Medicine, Aug.12, 1998.

[7]http://www.newswise.com/articles/1998/8/BCKINJRY.A CO.html, American College of Occupational & Environmental Medicine, Aug.12, 1998.

[8] Mitchell LV, Lawler FH, Bowen D, et al. Effectiveness and cost-effectiveness of employer-issued back belts in areas of high risk for back injury. J Occup Med 1994;36:90-94.

[9] 1. Liebenson CS. Pathogenesis of chronic back pain. J Manipulative Physiol Ther 1992;15:299-308.

[10] Nachemson AL. Prevention of chronic back pain: the orthopaedic challenge for the 80's. Bull Hosp Joint Dis Orthop Inst 1984;44:1-15.

[11] Dwyer AP. Backache and its prevention. Clin Orthop 1987;222:35-43.

[12] http://www.spinenet.com/articles.patient/back stats.html, American Academy of Orthopaedic Surgeons.

[13] http://www.spinenet.com/articles.patient/back stats.html, AAORS.

[14] http://www.spinenet.com/articles.patient/back stats.html, AAOS, Musculoskeletal Conditions in the U.S., Feb 1992.

[15] http://www.spinenet.com/articles.patient/back stats.html, AAOS, Musculoskeletal Conditions in the U.S., Feb 1992.

[16] Andersson GB. Factors important in the genesis and prevention of occupational back pain and disability. J Manipulative Physiol Ther1992;15:43-46.

[17] Deyo RA, Bass JE. Lifestyle and low-back pain; the influence of smoking and obesity. Spine 1989;14: 501-506.

[18] Boshuizen HC, Verbeek JH, Broersen JP, et al. Do smokers get more back pain? Spine 1993;18:35-40.

[19] Cox JM, Trier KK. Exercise and smoking habits in patients with and without low back and leg pain. J Manipulative Physiol Ther 1987;10:239-245.

[20] Batti, MC, Videman T, Gill K, et al. Smoking and lumbar intervertebral disk degeneration: an MRI study of identical twins. Spine 1991;16:1015-1021.

[21] Deyo RA, Bass JE. Lifestyle and low-back pain; the influence of smoking and obesity. Spine 1989;14: 501-506.

[22] Gyntelberg F. One year incidence of low back pain among male residents of Copenhagen aged 40-59. Dan Med Bull 1974;21:30-36.

[23] Frymoyer JW, Rosen JC, Clements J, et al. Psychologic factors in low-back-pain disability. Clin Orthop 1985;195: 178-184.

[24] Pope MH, Rosen JC, Wilder DG, et al. The relation between biomechanical and psychological factors in patients with low-back pain. Spine1980;5:173-178.

[25] Marras, W, Heaney, C, Davis, K, Maronitis, A, Allread, G, Job Stress May Lead to Back Injury for Some People, Spine, 12-1-00.

[26] Carragee,E, Paragioudakis, S, Khurana, S, Stanford University Medical Center, State of Mind Contributes to Low Back Pain, Spine, Dec. 2000.

[27] Carragee,E, Paragioudakis, S, Khurana, S, Stanford University Medical Center, State of Mind Contributes to Low Back Pain, Spine, Dec. 2000.

[28] Carragee,E, Paragioudakis, S, Khurana, S, Stanford University Medical Center, State of Mind Contributes to Low Back Pain, Spine, Dec. 2000.

[29] Kriss, V.M.,Szafranski, B, Rwankole, P, Kentucky Medical Center, Back Pain in Children May Signal Something Serious, Nov. 29,1999.

[30] Kriss, V.M., Szafranski, B, Rwankole, P, Kentucky Medical Center, Back Pain in Children May Signal Something Serious, Nov. 29,1999.

[31] Foti, T, Bagley, A, Davids, J.R., Pregnant Women's Back Pain, Calf Muscle Cramps, The Journal of Bone and Joint Surgery, May 12, 2000.

[32] Christopher Reeve Paralysis Foundation, http://www.crpf.com/

[33] National Spinal Cord Injury Statistical Center, University of Alabama, Birmingham, http://www.sci.rehabm.uab.edu/shared/faq.data.html

[34] Lahad A, Malter AD, Berg AO, et al.The effectiveness of four interventions for the prevention of low back pain. JAMA 1994;272:1286- 1291. Copyright 1994, American Medical Association.

[35] Venning PJ, Walter SD, Stitt LW. Personal and job-related factors as determinants of incidence of back injuries among nursing personnel. J Occup Med 1987;29:820-825.

[36] Behrens V, Seligman P, Cameron L, et al. The prevalence of back pain, hand discomfort, and dermatitis in the US working population. Am J Public Health 1994;84:1780-1785.

[37] Behrens V, Seligman P, Cameron L, et al. The prevalence of back pain, hand discomfort, and dermatitis in the US working population. Am J Public Health 1994;84:1780-1785.

[38] Nordin M, Weiser S, Halpern N. Education: the prevention and treatment of low back disorders. In: Frymoyer JW, ed. The adult spine and practice. New York: Raven Press; 1991:1641-1654.

[39] Deyo RA, Loeser JD, Bigos SJ. Herniated lumbar intervertebral disk. Ann Intern Med 1990;112:598-603.

[40] Liles DH. Using NIOSH lift guide decreases risk of back injuries. Occup Health Safety 1985;54:57-60.

[41] Haag AB. Ergonomic standards, guidelines, and strategies for prevention of back injury. Occup Med 1992;7:155-165.

[42] Harvey BL. Self-care practices to prevent low back pain. Am Assoc Occup Health Nurs J 1988;36:211-217.

[43] Graveling RA. The prevention of back pain from manual handling. Ann Occup Hyg 1991;35:427-432.

[44] Contemporary Diagnosis and Management of Pain, Donlin M. Long, M.D., p.58, Handbooks in Healthcare, Newtown, PA, 2001.

[45] The Mystery of Low Back Pain, Gillies and Griesdale, p.55, The Canadian Journal of Continuing Medical Education, September, 1997.

[46] Prolo Your Sports Injuries Away! Ross Hauser, M.d. and Marion Hauser, M.S., R.D., Chapter 17, p.226, Jean-Paul Ouellette, M.D., Beulah Land Press, 2001.

[47] A New Approach to the Treatment of Chronic Low Back Pain, Ongley, Klein, Dorman, Eek, Hubert, The Lancet, p.143, July 18, 1987.

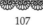

"To wish to be well is a part of becoming well."

–Seneca

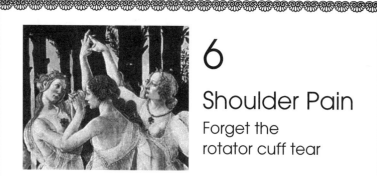

6

Shoulder Pain
Forget the
rotator cuff tear

*T*he shoulder is in reality several joints combined by an intricate arrangement of muscles and tendons that provide a great deal of flexibility and stability, and allow a wide range of motion to the arm.[1]

The **rotator cuff** is a group of four shoulder muscles that surround the top of the upper arm bone, known as the **humerus**, and hold it in the shoulder joint. These muscles are responsible for moving the arm in various directions, and unlike the massive deltoid muscle of the upper arm, are smaller and generally more vulnerable to injury. The 4 muscles and tendons of the rotator cuff are the supraspinatus, infraspinatus, teres minor, and subscapularis. The 4 tendons merge like a glove around the shoulder, but the part that is most commonly inflamed or torn is the supraspinatus.

> **Almost all of my body builders complain of anterior shoulder pain that is caused from wide bench presses. Although they often have fear of impending rotator cuff surgery, it is usually nothing more than a stretch injury easily healed by Prolotherapy.**

Because they are subjected to a wide range of motions, shoulders often suffer from problems of instability or impingement of soft tissue, resulting in pain. The pain may be constant, or may occur only when the shoulder is moved.

In any case, any shoulder pain that persists more than a few days should be diagnosed and treated as necessary.

Diagnosis of shoulder pain

More than 4 million people in the U.S. seek medical care each year for shoulder problems. [2]

As with all problems in the body, a proper diagnosis of shoulder pain is essential to determine the root cause of the problem and the proper method of treatment. Because many shoulder conditions are caused by specific activities, a medical history is an invaluable tool. A physical examination should include screening for physical abnormalities- swelling, deformity, muscle weakness, and tender areas—and observing the range of shoulder motion—how far and in which directions the arm can be moved.

Although X-rays may be helpful in defining problems, more elusive ones may require computerized tomography (CT scan), which provides a more detailed view of the shoulder area. Electrodiagnostic studies such as the electromyogram (EMG) and nerve conduction study can indicate nerve damage versus local injury in the tissue. Magnetic Resonance Imaging (MRI) and ultrasound are other safe and effective diagnostic tools, providing images of the soft tissues without using radiation.[3] An arthrogram is an x-ray study or MRI in which dye is injected into the joint for added contrast.

Arthroscopy is an invasive surgical procedure, which is commonly used by traditional orthopaedists, but generally disdained by progressive therapists, due to its damaging effects on the tissues of the body. It involves the insertion of a sizable metal instrument into the area, and practitioners who favor it are often proponents of further invasive procedures involving cutting and removal of bone, cartilage and muscle, inflicting permanent damage on their patients.

Most shoulder problems involve the soft tissues— muscles, ligaments, and tendons—rather than the bones. These soft tissue injuries are precisely the kinds of injury that respond so effectively to Prolotherapy which rejuvenates the soft connective tissues in our body by stimulating the growth of new collagen tissue which strengthens the joints.

> **Just because you are told you have a rotator cuff tear or injury to the joint itself does not mean you need surgery. Prolotherapy reduces or eliminates the pain and increases range of motion in most cases I have observed.**

Most shoulder problems fall into three major categories:
- **tendonitis or bursitis**
- **injury**
- **arthritis**

Tendonitis

Tendons are tough cords of tissue that connect muscle to bone or to other tissue. Tendinitis is usually a result of the wearing process that takes place over a period of years. Much like the sole of a shoe it can eventually split from overuse. Tendonitis can also occur from one unusual or ballistic movement or fall.

Sometimes, excessive use or injury of the shoulder leads to inflammation and swelling of a **bursa**, a condition known as **bursitis**. Bursas are fluid filled sacs located around the body and joints. They lessen the friction caused by movement of the shoulder. Bursitis often occurs in association with **rotator cuff tendinitis**. Symptoms of shoulder bursitis include mild to severe pain. Sometimes the many tissues in the shoulder become inflamed and painful, limiting the use of the shoulder. In extreme cases the joint stiffens into a condition known as "frozen shoulder"[4] , also referred to by doctors as adhesive capsulitis. Sometimes the bones in the shoulder joint slip out of normal alignment or are forced out by injury, a condition known as **subluxation** if mild in nature and **dislocation** if completely out of joint.

Arthritis

Although it is less common than in the knee or hip, which bear the weight of the body, shoulder pain can also result from arthritis. There are many types of arthritis, but most often in the shoulder it is triggered by an initial trauma. It can also involve "wear and tear" of the tissues of the joint, causing inflammation, swelling and pain. Often people will react by instinctively limiting their shoulder movements in order to lessen the pain, which leads to a tightening or stiffening of the soft tissue parts of the joint, resulting in yet further pain and restriction of motion.

Leading Causes of Shoulder Pain:[5]

■ Repetitive overhead sports motions, such as pitching, swimming, or the tennis serve.

■ Heavy lifting.

■ Excessive force, such as a fall.

■ Degeneration due to aging

■ Narrowing of the space (acromioclavicular arch) between the collarbone (clavicle) and the top portion (acromion) of the shoulder bone (scapula).

■ Abrasion of the rotator cuff surface by the top portion of the shoulder bone (the acromium).

Besides these long-standing problems, doctors are encountering some surprising newer ones, linked to specific causes.

In a year 2000 study, the Consumer Product Safety Commission tracked visits to physician offices, clinics, and hospital emergency rooms related to **backpacks**. Children 0-11 years old had a total of 5,531 visits; 12-17, 6,960 and students ages 18-21, had 773 visits.[6]

Sports injuries among youth are also sky-rocketing, and in one of the most alarming statistics, an estimated 500,000 young athletes, boys and girls, use black-market anabolic steroids to improve their athletic performance.[7] **Steroids**, as we have discussed elsewhere in this book, are extremely destructive to the body's self-repair mechanisms, blocking the normal restorative processes triggered by inflammation. When young people use them, while their bodies are still forming, the results are especially debilitating.

Although there is no "control data" pre-dating our modern era, it is evident that many of the aches and pains associated with shoulder problems represent a new breed of problems for the human race that are directly related to modern devices. Seat belt shoulder harnesses, computer keyboards, telephones cradled on shoulders, and countless other inventions of the Twentieth Century contribute to unnatural constriction and posturing which can lead to cramps, stiff muscles and more serious problems. In some of these examples, entrepreneurs have devised newer products to circumvent such unwanted "side effects"—such as telephone headsets—or medical researchers have come up with tips and guidelines to help people avoid problems.

Shoulder impingement syndrome[8] involves one or a combination of problems, including inflammation of the lubricating sac (bursa) located just over the rotator cuff, a condition called bursitis; inflammation of the rotator cuff tendons, called tendinitis; and calcium deposits in tendons called calcific tendonitis, caused by wear and tear or injury.

The musculature of the shoulder area is fertile ground for trigger points, as is evidenced by the prevalence of "stiff neck"[9] and referred pain radiating anteriorly, laterally or posteriorly from all three of the major scalene muscles into the arms, chest or vertebrae.[10]

Treatment of Shoulder Problems

90 percent of patients with shoulder pain will respond to simple treatment methods such as reduced activities, rest, exercise and medication. Certain types of shoulder problems, such as recurring dislocation and some rotator cuff tears may require more serious treatment. Minor problems, such as mild bursitis, may respond well to non-invasive treatments like ultrasound.

Arthritis sufferers will benefit greatly from exercise, particularly water exercises which can be performed without adding stress to the joints, as well as Tai Chi, yoga or just plain walking. Exercise increases strength and flexibility, increases endorphins (which are similar to narcotics but are natural and healthy) reduces pain, fights fatigue, and helps to maintain a healthy weight — all of which are critical to the treatment of arthritis and its symptoms, regardless of the type or severity. Even people who are confined to a wheel-chair can participate in strength training and sports. The Arthritis Foundation has developed a program called PACE (People with Arthritis Can Exercise) that includes activities that can be performed while seated. Shoulder rolls, arm lifts and leg lifts are some examples.[11] [12]

Rancho Los Amigos Rehabilitation Hospital in Downey California (one of the hospitals I trained at) hosts a multi-tude of competitive sports programs for spinal cord injured or brain trauma patients confined to a wheel chair. Their shoulders are usually the most problematic joint because of its stress from using a wheel chair.

In the case of more serious problems, surgery is often pre-scribed, but as we have pointed out earlier, the invasive and damaging techniques involved in orthopaedic surgery of-ten perpetuates the problems, rather than cures them.

In cases of **trigger point problems** in the muscles and sup-porting tissues, spray and stretch or dry needle injections are highly effective, but must be carefully coordinated and cautiously executed, due to the complex structures which make up the shoulder area, particularly around the neck re-gion.[13]

Most **shoulder sprains** or, more seriously, **dislocations** happen when a person falls on an outstretched hand or sus-tains a blow to the shoulder (especially a downward blow). Approximately 95% of shoulder dislocations are anterior dislocations, in which the anterior static shoulder stabilizers are torn away from the bone.[14]

Until recently it was common in cases of dislocation to immobilize the shoulder, but studies proved that while immobilization helped alleviate the pain of such injuries, it also contributed to a general weakening of the ligaments and predominance of adhesive capsulitis.

In one alarming study[15] of close to 250 patients, about half of those treated with immobilization had recurring dis-locations within the 10 year period of the study. The prob-lem is greater in younger people. This is one of the few areas where older folks have an advantage; because their connective tissues are less elastic, the risk of dislocation is less likely.

Chronic shoulder instability syndrome results from trauma caused by dislocations, or from less detectable micro-trauma caused by repetitive strain on the tissues, or from congenitally loose shoulder joints. Recurrent pain or tenderness in the shoulder joint and weakness in the arm are two of the more common symptoms, but severe examples include patients whose shoulders pop easily in and out of joint. A sequela of shoulder dislocations is stretching the brachial plexus, the nerves that run from the neck down the arm. This process can cause permanent nerve damage and loss of use of the arm.

Orthopaedic surgeons are experimenting with radical new techniques[16], including meniscal transplants from donors and thermal capsular shrinkage, which involves shrinking loose tissue in the shoulder area using heat. While these new techniques are promising, at least in terms of improving on the generally dismal success rates of earlier arthroscopic procedures, they are still highly invasive, and the long term effects are as yet unknown.

Since it's been proven to strengthen the connective tissues, and has the benefit of over fifty years of testing to back it, **Prolotherapy** is arguably one of the best choices of treatment in cases of dislocation, rotator cuff tendinitis, muscle tissue impingement or recurring instability. Before you do anything as radical or irreversible as surgery, and before you accept the grim prognosis of conventional medicine that sentences you to a lifetime of dependence on NSAID's and other pain relief medication, you owe it to yourself to try Prolotherapy. It has proven over and over again to be safe, effective and relatively inexpensive. Read the story of my shoulder surgery in the introduction of this book before you decide.

[1] http://www.ozarkortho.com/patiented/shoulder.htm

[2] http://orthoinfo.aaos.org/fact/thr_report.cfm?thread_id=127&topcategory=shoulder

[3] http://www.ozarkortho.com/patiented/shoulder.htm

[4] http://www.ozarkortho.com/patiented/shoulder.htm

[5] http://orthoinfo.aaos.org/fact/thr_report.cfm?thread_id=127&topcategory=shoulder

[6] Students Should Get in Shape Before Carrying Backpacks, Smith, Angela D., M. D., Swanson, J, Schuetz, T, Schuetz, A.J., American Academy of Orthopaedic Surgeons, Aug. 1, 2001.

[7] http://www.ozarkortho.com/patiented/youth.htm

[8] http://orthoinfo.aaos.org/fact/thr_report.cfm?thread_id=133&topcategory=shoulder

[9] Myofascial Pain and Dysfunction: The Trigger Point Manual, Travell, J.G., Simons, D.G., p. 334, Williams and Wilkins, 1983.

[10] Myofascial Pain and Dysfunction: The Trigger Point Manual, Travell, J.G., Simons, D.G., p. 344, Williams and Wilkins, 1983.

[11] Mayo Clinic Women's HealthSource, Dec. 8, 2000.

[12] www.arthritis.org

[13] Myofascial Pain and Dysfunction: The Trigger Point Manual, Travell, J.G., Simons, D.G., p. 344, Williams and Wilkins, 1983.

[14] Wheaton, M., Prolo Your Sports Shoulder Pain Away! p.252, Prolo Your Sports Injuries Away!, Hauser & Hauser, Beulah Land Press, 2001.

[15] Hovelius, L., Anterior Dislocations of the Shoulder in Teenagers and Young Adults, American Journal of Bone and Joint Surgery, 69: 393-9, 1987.

[16] Advances in Sports Medicine, American Academy of Orthopaedic Surgeons (AAOS), Oct.18, 2000.

"If there is anything better than to be loved it is loving."

—*Anonymous*

7

Knee Pain
Do meniscal tears heal?

*O*nly when we analyze the intricate motions and mechanisms involved in walking, running, swimming, skiing, driving, bending, stretching or climbing stairs do we understand the complexity of the physics involved. Great stresses must be tolerated, even in the course of our daily routines. Even the relatively passive act of sitting in a crowded movie theatre, or contorting into a cramped airline seat, can subject the knee to unnatural tensions. A great deal of power and flexibility is required of the knees in the performance of even the most mundane tasks, and they are beautifully designed to handle it.

> The knee is one of the most important and least appreciated structures in the human body. When healthy, it supports the weight of the torso and allows us to move quickly and agilely. Rarely do we consider what *a marvelous feat of engineering this is.*

Unfortunately, this combination of strength and mobility requires a complex, precisely integrated structure of bone, tissue and cartilage to facilitate such movements.

The phrase **"tensegrity model"** was introduced by orthopedic surgeon Stephen Levin[1] to describe such a structure in the human body. Based on architectural concepts of stability used in the construction of bridges and buildings, the tensegrity system maintains form and function and encloses

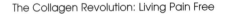

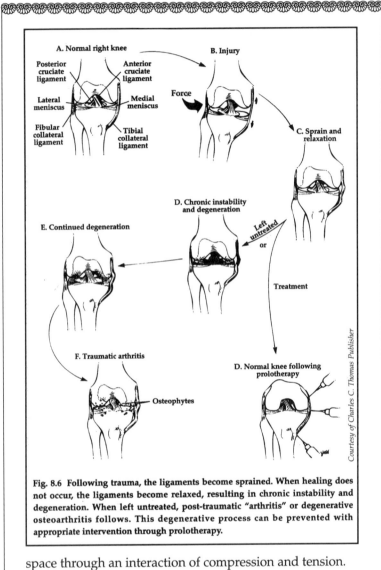

Fig. 8.6 Following trauma, the ligaments become sprained. When healing does not occur, the ligaments become relaxed, resulting in chronic instability and degeneration. When left untreated, post-traumatic "arthritis" or degenerative osteoarthritis follows. This degenerative process can be prevented with appropriate intervention through prolotherapy.

Courtesy of Charles C. Thomas Publisher

space through an interaction of compression and tension.

Biological systems function as tensegrity mechanisms. In contrast to the assumption that the hard parts are piled up on top of each other, living things need to transfer forces, tension and stress in more than one direction. In Dr. Levin's words, "If it functions upside down, it's a tensegrity model."[2]

"Knee Deep" in Cartilage

The knee joint is one of the largest joints in the body. The **patella**, commonly called the kneecap, sits in a groove at the front of the knee. The most common knee problems encountered in clinical practice involve the patella, because its anatomical placement subjects it directly to a variety of bony and soft tissue disorders. A portion of the general population is subject to these disorders, which include:

■ *patellofemoral syndrome (patella mistracks in femoral groove)*

■ *excessive torsional deformity of the tibia*

■ *high or lateral position of the patella*

■ *shallow femoral trochlea,*

■ *atrophy of vastus medialus oblique muscle*

■ *increased quadriceps angle (often in those with wide hips*

■ *overdevelopment of the vastus lateralis muscles*

■ *flat feet*

■ *excessive pronation of the feet (feet turn up to the side*

Behind the patella is a layer of **articular cartilage**—the thickest layer of cartilage found in any of the joints of the body.

Although it is uncertain whether cartilage is directly treated by trigger point injections or Prolotherapy, it does reap benefits from those treatments in adjoining tissue, due to the strengthening of the supporting ligaments and tendons, which keep the joints properly aligned and thereby protect the cartilage from erosion caused by friction.[3]

The upper and lower leg bones are separated at the knee by two discs of cartilage known as the **medial** and **lateral menisci**.

Diagnosing Knee Injuries

Diagnosing and treating knee problems can be as complicated as the knee joint itself. Short of any glaring physical injury like a dislocated patella, it requires a careful examination to determine whether the injury is confined to the elastic tissues, the bony structures, or the cartilage.

X-rays will reveal problems with the bones, and may offer clues to other damage, while MRIs (Magnetic Resonance Imaging) have the ability to reveal soft tissue damage, but problems with cartilage can still be very evasive and hard to pinpoint. Studies have shown that the advanced technologies commonly used to diagnosis injuries are grievously insufficient to do the job.

In one study conducted by Dr. J.A. Lawrance of Oxford, England, MRIs had a success rate of only 11% in diagnosing partial anterior cruciate ligament tears.[4] In yet another study,[5] focusing on the knee, doctors compared the findings of standard x-ray tests and physical examinations on 210 people—all of whom were self-described as pain free at the time of the testing. Although none of the participants exhibited any pain or other symptoms of pathology, and considered themselves completely healthy in regard to their knees, the test results yielded dramatic evidence of physical problems and abnormalities—including an incidence rate of 80% or better for arthritis, patellofemoral crepitus (grinding) in 94% of the women, high percentages of asymmetry and hypermobility, and a dozen other problems to varying degrees.As the authors of the study noted: *"Because patellofemoral crepitus is so common in both symptomatic and asymptomatic volunteers, the importance of this finding must be reevaluated as a surgical indication."*

The conclusion is obvious: by offering "objective" evidence and a technology-based rationale to over-eager surgeons, MRIs, x-rays and other advanced diagnostic techniques contribute greatly to promoting cases of unnecessary or even ill-advised surgery. The end result is more problems for the recipients of these surgeries.

Generally speaking, the most efficient and safe method for diagnosing a knee injury is a simple manual examination, coupled with extensive questioning of the patient to determine exactly what happened and where it hurts.

Some problems caused by surgery:

- increase in pain
- limitations in movement
- ligamental and structural weaknesses
- arthritis or other debilitating conditions
- infection
- more surgery
- knee replacement

Sadly, this damage maybe invariably permanent.

Aside from the non-traumatic problems of the patella discussed earlier, the most common knee injuries are caused by internal or external rotation—often caused by movement alone, without any direct, traumatizing physical contact.[6] Several sports such as basketball and skiing subject the knee to injuries of this sort.

ALTERNATIVES TO KNEE SURGERY

There are certainly instances in life when surgery is called for, but not nearly as often as it is currently performed. Even so-called "minor" surgery takes a drastic toll on the human body, physically traumatizing and permanently altering its structures, often to its detriment.

In a recent randomized, double-blind, placebo-controlled study of Prolotherapy for the treatment of knee osteoarthritis, researchers

While Prolotherapy is not indicated in every case of knee pain or injury, it is one of the safest and most effective treatments in many, if not most, cases.

found that knees treated with Prolotherapy had significantly less pain, swelling and buckling.

Blinded radiographic readings suggested improvement in osteoarthritis severity, and one year after treatment, 8 out of 13 of the knees which had suffered from anterior cruciate ligament laxity were no longer lax.[7]

DON'T MAKE IT WORSE! ARTHROSCOPY, CORTISONE & OTHER BAD CHOICES

The more we learn about many of our traditional medical procedures, the graver the news seems to be. One study showed the rate of success for lumbar spinal fusions to be a mere 16%.[8] Some of the more disturbing failures involved complications like **pseudoarthrosis**— which means the formation of *false joints* in the body where expected bone fusions did not occur—and severe residual pain at the graft donor site.

> Arthroscopy is the standard method of diagnosing joint problems used by orthopedic surgeons today.

The tool used, the **arthroscope**, is a 14 inch long metal tube, as thick as a woman's finger. It is inserted deep into the joint, allowing the physician to peer inside for a close-up look at the problem. As is this wasn't bad enough, the "solution" in arthroscopic surgery is usually to further invade the joint with shavers, burrs, and other medical power tools designed to cut, drill and "strip mine" the body's natural resources.

To understand the theory (and folly) of this seemingly harmless procedure, one needs to understand the physiological composition of the joint. Most of the joints in the body are **synovial joints**, which are flexible and self-lubricating.

The ends of the bones are covered with a protective substance known as **articular cartilage**. These thin coatings are separated by a layer of **synovial fluid**, which further cushions and lubricates them where they meet to form the joint. **Ligaments** add support and hold the joints together. **Tendons** secure the **muscles**, which provide movement to the body. The whole structure is wrapped in a capsule of tissue known as the **synovial membrane**, which also secretes the lubricating and somewhat revitalizing synovial fluid.

The knee and the wrist joints also contain pads of fibrous cartilage, known as **menisci**, which help these overworked joints bear the extra stresses to which they are often subjected.

The articular cartilage which protects the inner surfaces of the joints is a homogenous substance devoid of nerves, lymphatic vessels or blood cells, made up primarily of water, collagen and specialized proteins (**proteoglycans**). Its structure is fairly simple; it contains a small percentage of cells known as **chondrocytes**, which are solely responsible for the maintenance and repair of the articular cartilage, via their ability to synthesis collagen and proteoglycans.[9]

The high water content of the articular cartilage, coupled with the innate compressibility of the proteoglycans, give it the slick, cushioning properties so essential to maintaining healthy, pain free joints, minimizing friction and stress between the bones.[10]

All the available evidence seems to indicate that chondrocytes are fully capable of regenerating articular cartilage throughout the course of a lifetime, which would account for the healthy cell counts even in very old people. However, since they are not fed by blood vessels, they are wholly dependent on nutrient delivery from the synovial fluid; this lack of blood supply puts a damper on their proliferative capabilities.

It is the movement of the joints that loads nutrients into, and waste out of, the cartilage. Despite their limited metabolic resources, chondrocytes can still churn out large quantities of collagen and proteoglycans.[11]

The invasive tools of arthroscopic surgery are used to excise injured ligaments, cartilage and meniscus (which leads to a further depletion of the articular cartilage because the meniscus supplies nutrients to it)—either through shaving or slicing with a high-powered electrical instrument. The immediate result is a temporary respite from whatever pain existed before the procedure— *often followed by more or less permanent weakness and instability in the joint.*

Unfortunately, such "collateral damage" seems more acceptable to the industrialized medical establishment than less invasive *(and less profit-oriented)* therapies like trigger point injections and Prolotherapy. It would be somewhat comforting to know that such intensely destructive procedures are falling from favor, if it weren't for the fact that other, less obvious, but equally damaging techniques are still widespread.

> Although steroids may be useful, repeated injections are deleterious to any part of the body.

The damage steroids do may be permanent and extensive. Effective at reducing pain because of their anti-inflammatory action, cortisone and other corticosteroids assault the body with an avalanche of counter-productive side effects. Even worse, although exercise normally strengthens the body, studies have shown that when cortisone is injected into the knees, and the patient exercises, there is even greater destruction than is wreaked by cortisone shots alone, with cartilage cell counts reduced by over 20%.[12] Steroids inhibit the release of precious Growth Hormone and rob the body of calcium and vitamin D[13]. They also interfere with the development of new tissue growth and disrupt the processes that lead to new cell and blood vessel formation.

Corticosteroids inhibit the synthesis of proteins[14], collagen, and proteoglycans in articular cartilage by inhibiting chondrocyte production, the cells that comprise and produce the articular cartilage.

The net catabolic effect (weakening) of corticosteroids is inhibition of fibroblast production of collagen, ground substance, and angiogenesis (new blood vessel formation). The result is weakened synovial joints, supporting structures, articular cartilage, ligaments, and tendons. This weakness increases the pain, and the increased pain leads to more steroid injections.[15]

A study by Dr. Behrens and colleagues[16] reported a persistent and highly significant reduction in the synthesis of proteins, collagen, and proteoglycans in the articular cartilage of rabbits who received weekly injections of glucocorticoids. They also reported a progressive loss of endoplasmic reticulum, mitochondria, and Golgi apparatus, as the number of injections increased.

Trigger point injections and Prolotherapy offer a radically different approach than either arthroscopic or corticosteroidal therapy. The two latter methods yield temporary relief with their "quick fix" procedures—followed by highly destructive long term side effects including potential irreversible damage.

By contrast, trigger point injections and Prolotherapy deliver permanent improvement, including not only pain relief but strengthening of the treated areas.

For a detailed analysis of knee problems, please read my book, The Knee Sourcebook, published by McGraw Hill. It has more of the traditional approach since it was directed by a publisher other than myself.

---

[1] Dorman, Thomas M.D., Prolotherapy for Knees, Townsend Letter for Doctors & Patients, November, 1997.

[2] Dorman, Thomas M.D., Prolotherapy for Knees, Townsend Letter for Doctors & Patients, November, 1997.

[3] Dorman, Thomas M.D., Prolotherapy for Knees, Townsend Letter for Doctors & Patients, p.73, November, 1997.

[4] MRI Diagnosis of Partial Tears of the Anterior Cruciate Ligament, Dr. J.A. Lawrance, et al, Injury, 27(3):153-155, 1996.

[5] Clinical Assessment of Asymptomatic Knees, Dr. L. Johnson, Arthroscopy: The Journal of Arthroscopic and Related Surgery, 14:347-359, 1998.

[6] Neumann, R.D., Sports Medicine Secrets, Chapter 66, p.291, Traumatic Knee Injuries, Hanley & Belfus Inc, 1994.

[7] Reeves. K.D., Hassanein, K, Randomized Prospective Double-blind, Placebo-controlled Trial of Dextrose Prolotherapy for Knee Osteoarthritis With or Without ACL Laxity, Alter Ther Health Med, 6(2):68-74, 77-80, 2000.

[8] Patient Outcomes After Lumbar Spinal Fusions, Dr. J. Turner, et al, Journal of the American Medical Association, 268:907-911,1992.

[9] The Articular Cartilages: A Review, Dr. H. Mankin, American Academy of Orthopedic Surgeons: Instructional Course Lectures, Volume 19, C.V. Mosby Co., St. Louis, MO, 1970.

[10] Articular Cartilage. Part1: Tissue Design and Chondrocyte-matrix Interactions, Journal of Bone and Joint Surgery, 79A:600-611, 1997.

[11] Nutrition Applied to Injury Rehabilitation and Sports Medicine, Bucci, L., M.D.,CRC Press, p.185, 1995.

[12] Scott, W. Dr. Scott's Knee Book, p.36, Fireside Press NY, 1996.

[13] Rodney Van Pelt, M.D., Prolo Your Sports Injury Away, Ross and Marion Hauser, Chapter 19, p.271, Prolo Your Sports Knee Injuries Away! Beulah Land Press, 2001.

[14] Rodney Van Pelt, M.D., Prolo Your Sports Injury Away, Ross and Marion Hauser, Chapter 19, p.271, Prolo Your Sports Knee Injuries Away! Beulah Land Press, 2001.

[15] Prolo Your Sports Injury Away, Ross and Marion Hauser, Chapter 19, Prolo Your Sports Knee Injuries Away! Rodney Van Pelt, M.D., p.272, Beulah Land Press, 2001.

[16] Alteration of Rabbit Articular Cartilage of Intra-Art
Cartilage Injections of Glucocorticoids, Dr. F. Behrens,
nal of Bone and Joint Surgery, 57A, 70-76, 1975.

icular
our-

"Goals are deceptive-
The unaimed arrow never misses"

8

Carpal Tunnel Syndrome, Headaches and TMJ

*C*ARPAL TUNNEL SYNDROME (CTS)[1] is a compression of the median nerve at the wrist, leading to numbness, tingling, and pain in the hand. The median nerve passes through the carpal tunnel at the wrist and into the palm where it sends branches that control feeling to the thumb, index, middle and half of the ring finger. Symptoms include tingling, pain or numbness in the hand and fingers.

> Research suggests that one person in 10 will develop symptoms of CARPAL TUNNEL SYNDROME (CTS) over the course of their lifetime.

"It's typically worse with reading a newspaper or book, talking on the phone or driving a car, and frequently it wakes people up in the middle of the night with tingling or pain in the hand," says Benn Smith, M.D.[2], co-author of the study and neurologist at Mayo Clinic in Scottsdale, Arizona. "Very often, people obtain temporary relief by shaking the hand or rubbing it, causing the numbness and tingling to go away."

There are a variety of factors that contribute to CTS. "The major risk factors for developing carpal tunnel syndrome are being female and middle-aged," says J. Clarke Stevens, M.D.[3], a neurologist at Mayo Clinic in Rochester, Minnesota. "There are many other causes of carpal tunnel syndrome, such as wrist trauma, diabetes, rheumatoid arthritis and pregnancy."[4]

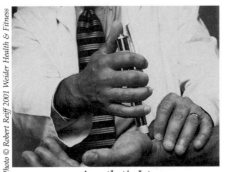

Photo © Robert Reiff 2001 Weider Health & Fitness

Anesthetic Jet

Repetitive motions in industries outside the office also have been linked to CTS, Dr. Stevens says. "There have been a number of studies of factory workers and people in packing plants that suggest that type of repetitive motion does seem to be associated with carpal tunnel syndrome."

The biggest problem with carpal tunnel syndrome is that it is highly over-diagnosed. Doctors unfamiliar with trigger point and referred pain theory often overlook the true causes of problems in the areas associated with carpal tunnel and leap to erroneous conclusions. The most common reasons for misdiagnosis of CTS is weakness in the annular ligament of the elbow, or referred pain from the cervical vertebrae to the thumb, index and middle fingers. A problematic annular ligament when pressed may be a trigger point to the carpal tunnel distribution in the hand. Once the annular ligament is injected with Prolotherapy or trigger point therapy, it is often deactivated and the symptoms of carpal tunnel syndrome disappear.

Traditional methods of treating CTS include wearing a splint at night or injections of cortisone to reduce swelling. If these measures are not successful, carpal tunnel release surgery, which sections the tough transverse carpal ligament and relieves pressure on the median nerve, may be performed.[5] But as we have seen with arthroscopy for the knee, surgery should be the last treatment a patient should ever consider. Countless patients have presented to my office with worse symptoms *after* they had the carpal tunnel surgery.

Prolotherapy to strengthen the annular ligament will in addition often cure chronic elbow pain.[6]

Under no circumstances should a patient consent to surgery for CTS until an evaluation is performed by a physician trained in the referral patterns of pain from ligaments.

CHRONIC HEADACHES

Although the common headache usually responds quite well to aspirin or other "over the counter" medications, those who've experienced the torment of **migraines** or **cluster headaches** are often frustrated by the lack of any effective cure. Drugs like ergotamine developed specifically for such headaches are effective, but the relief they provide is temporary. Until the root of the problem is unearthed and corrected, the headaches will persist, and prolonged drug therapy to relieve them will be necessary, along with the possibility of addiction.

In rare cases, the problem is traced to cysts or brain tumors, but more often it is related to muscular or ligamentary tension. Most people know the phrase **"tension headache"** but not many—doctors included—are aware that neck ligaments refer pain directly to the head. In cases where no cyst or tumor is found but headaches persist, Prolotherapy may be in order. A physician skilled in diagnosing trigger points and recognizing referred pain signals should be consulted in such cases.

In one famous case[7], Prolotherapist Gustav Hemwall, M.D., treated basketball star Kendall Gill of the New Jersey Nets for headache pain that had persisted for 16 years. Pain pills and injections of pain-killers provided transitory relief, but the headaches always returned "with a vengeance" in the words of the long-suffering athlete.

After a single treatment with Prolotherapy, Gill was headache-free for two years!

BARRE-LIEOU SYNDROME

Barre-Lieou Syndrome is characterized by a grab bag of diverse symptoms, all of which are rooted in the sympathetic nervous system, specifically the cluster of nerves located in the posterior cervical area at the back of the neck. It is caused when the sympathetic nerves are pinched by loose, weakly supported vertebrae. These nerves are part of the autonomic nervous system that regulates the body's functions, a myriad of activities ranging from such critical functions as your heartbeat and breathing to countless minor ones.

A list of problems that may be due to Barre-Lieu Syndrome:

- Headache

- Sinusitis

- Chronic Allergies

- Dizziness

- Neck Pain

- Chest Pain

- Face Pain

- Eye Pain

- Blurred Vision

- Ear Pain

- Tinnitus (ringing in ears)

- Hoarseness

- Laryngitis

- Fatigue

- Vertigo

If you have any of those symptoms, combined with neck pain, you may be a candidate for Prolotherapy.

TEMPOROMANDIBULAR JOINT SYNDROME (TMJ)

The temporomandibular joint is where the jaw meets the cranium. The condition known as temporomandibular joint syndrome develops from a combination of inter-related factors, usually starting with poor head posture that contributes to the stretching and weakening of the cervical ligaments and lateral TMJ ligaments. As a result, the lower jaw slips forward, aggravating the situation further by putting additional stress on the ligaments and the joints.

One characteristic of TMJ is the loud popping or clicking of bones rubbing together in the loosened joint, accompanied by pain and stiffness as the muscles tighten, trying to compensate for the instigating laxity.

Conventional treatments include TMJ arthroscopy and various types of surgery, TMJ implants, injections of botulinum toxins[8], and cauterization. All of these are invasive and somewhat risky, and treat the immediate problem while largely ignoring future consequences.

Prolotherapy is a highly effective treatment for TMJ Syndrome, particularly when the related neck ligaments are treated along with the TMJ ligaments. By strengthening these two sets of ligaments, Prolotherapy can eliminate not only the existing TMJ (and any neck-related) problems, but also helps to circumvent recurrences as well.

In summary, if you suffer from chronic pain or any connective tissue trauma or injury, before you resort to treatments such as surgery, cortisone injections or other therapies that you are not in favor of, you owe it to yourself to find a Prolotherapist and discuss your options. After all, as I have said over and over again, it is safe, effective and relatively inexpensive.

If you want to start living your life pain free, check out Prolotherapy, and let the healing begin…

---

[1] Smith, B, Stevens, J. Clarke, Heavy Computer Use Link to Carpal Tunnel Syndrome Debunked, Neurology, June 12, 2001.

[2] http://www.mayo.edu:80/mcs/Medical_Staff/smith-be.html

[3]http://www.mayo.edu:80/cerebro/division/cv_staff.stevens.html

[4] Smith, B, Stevens, J. Clarke, Heavy Computer Use Link to Carpal Tunnel Syndrome Debunked, Neurology, June 12, 2001.

[5] Smith, B, Stevens, J. Clarke, Heavy Computer Use Link to Carpal Tunnel Syndrome Debunked, Neurology, June 12, 2001.

[6] Hauser, R, Prolo Your Pain Away, p.111, Beulah Land Press, 1998.

[7] Hauser, R., Prolo Your Pain Away, p.89, Beulah Land Press,1998.

[8] Cheshire, W., Botulinum Toxin in the Treatment of Myofascial Pain Syndrome, 59:65-69, Pain, 1994.

"The best things in life are not things"

"In the darkest hour the soul is replenished and given strength to continue and endure."

– *Heart Warrior Chosa*

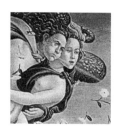

9

Prolotherapy Success Stories

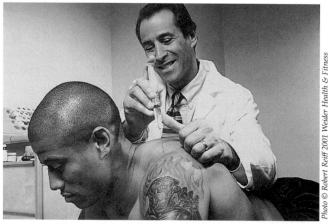

The angel (as Johnnie calls it) dancing on his skin

Photo © Robert Reiff 2001 Weider Health & Fitness

ohnnie Morton Jr., wide receiver for the Detroit Lions was originally pessimistic about trying prolotherapy. He just happened to be in my office escorting a friend who was undergoing treatment. Johnnie figured he had tried every kind of therapy in the book for his chronic pain. He is a top athlete on a professional football team in the NFL, he figured, the teams trainers and doctors had every available resource at their disposal to treat his pain and injuries, right? And nothing had worked. Sure he had some temporary relief, but he figured living with pain was an inevitable price you paid in professional sports. He was understandably skeptical at trying yet another therapy.

Thankfully my power of persuasion must have been on that day. After talking to Johnnie he agreed to try prolotherapy. Johnnie suffered from both a painful sprain where the gluteus muscle attaches to the pelvis and a badly sprained thumb joint from getting clipped during games. After only two Prolotherapy sessions on each trigger point, Johnnie played his first pain-free season in ten years. He was so pleased with the results that he now comes to me first with whatever ails him and is referring other athletes to me for care.

It is important to understand that the actual initial relief Johnnie obtained was from the trigger point effect of the injections not the proliferation of collagen. Prolotherapy implies proliferation of collagen, a process that takes 6-8 weeks to heal. Most of the time when a patient receives, Prolotherapy, he or she is benefiting from the trigger point injection effect.

One of Johnnie's referrals was his teammate David Sloan. David is the starting tight end for the Detroit Lions. In addition to David's skill on the field, he was voted one of Muscle & Fitness NFL's Best Physiques in October of 1999. When David came to me this past Spring of 2001, he suffered from metarsalgia, commonly known as "turf toe". Metarsalgia is a painful condition resulting from training on the turf. While running, the foot gets repeatedly caught on the turf and jams the structures in the big toe. David has received many treatments for this including surgery, and later, Prolotherapy. The surgery didn't seem to do the job. As of this writing, however, David attributes his reduction in his pain to Prolotherapy and the other non-surgical treatments received.

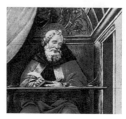

Marc Darrow, M.D.
Joint Rehabilitation and Sports Medical Center
Los Angeles, CA 90025

Dr. Darrow:

I just wanted to let you know how pleased I am with my Prolo therapy. I spent almost the entire month of January in bed taking pain medication for my moderate to severe back pain. That month was very depressing for me. I finally stopped all pain meds except for Ibuprofen and tried to force myself to do things. Sometimes I felt well enough to go out, but often just the idea of driving the car kept me home.

On my first visit with you, you explained the whole process and told me I could begin after stopping the anti-inflammatory drugs for a few days. I went home and told my husband this simply sounded too good to be true.

I am a registered nurse with years of emergency room experience at UCLA Medical Center. I have suffered with back pain for 15 years. The idea that a series of dextrose injections could take away my pain and possibly keep it from reoccurring sounded rediculous to me. To my surprise I was pain-free after the first injection and have remained that way. I hope many patients will hear about the work you are doing and will be able to experience this "miracle." The whole approach of the clinic is great, the coordination with the other doctors, the exercise program, and the emphasis on wellness. Keep up the good work and thanks so much.

Name Omitted

"The greater the difficulty, the greater the glory."

– Cicero

Marc Darrow, M.D.
Joint Rehabilitation and Sports Medical Center
Los Angeles, CA 90025

Dear Dr. Darrow:

Approximately six weeks ago I started Prolotherapy. I have had on and off back pain in the lower lumbar area for approximately 15 years. After a recent car accident the pain became very acute. After only three shots, the pain ceased altogether. But most amazingly, I started developing major shoulder pain that was very debilitating. After two shots with Prolo therapy the pain is totally gone. This pain was a deep ache that would bother me while driving a car. The results have been amazing.

Thank you,

Name Omitted

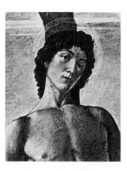

The consciousness of love can cure anything.

– John-Roger

While preparing for a bodybuilding competition still six weeks away, I was in the middle of an intense leg workout. Squats were part of the routine that day, topping out with a descending set from 700 pounds. I was on my second rep with 700 at the bottom of the movement when I felt my hip literally explode. I stayed stuck at the bottom, and now realize that I went into shock almost immediately. I fell, but eventually pulled myself to my feet. My leg went numb, and I knew something serious had happened.

In the days that followed, my leg turned black and blue. I never considered backing out of the show, and did my best

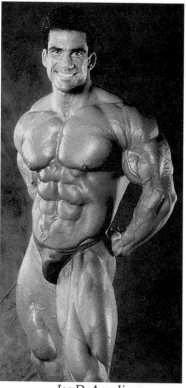

Joe DeAngelis
Mr. Universe and Mr. America

to train around the injury. Sitting and standing were unbearable. In the few days following the injury, my wife had to help me dress. Getting in and out of the car became a dreaded experience.

After the competition, the injury stayed aggravated. Even after the most feeble leg workouts I would be limping for hours. And strangely, I developed a baseball sized rock-hard lump on the side of my thigh. After about six months of this pain, I was introduced to Dr. Darrow at the Joint Rehabilitation and Sports Medical Center, Inc.

Dr. Darrow told me the trigger point effect of his injections might relieve the pain, but there was nothing he could do to reduce the lump on my hip. And the possible Prolo-

"A cheerful heart is good medicine."
– Bible, Proverbs 17:22

therapy effect might even grow some new collagen and assist the healing. I didn't care if it was trigger points or Prolotherapy because the results were miraculous. After six months of pain and the inability to squat 225, I performed repetitions with 500 lbs.! This was after only four treatments. Not only that, but that big rock on my thigh disappeared. Now I'm back to 700 lbs.

While I never admit even to myself how bad the situation may have been, there was always the feeling that those heavy days of squatting and deadlifting were over for good. Prolotherapy literally gave me a new lease on my training life."

Mr. Universe and Mr. America, Joe DeAngelis

Marc Darrow, M.D.
Joint Rehabilitation and Sports Medical Center
Los Angeles, CA 90025

Dear Dr. Darrow:

On January 27, 1999 I got into a car accident that injured my lower back. I tried everything from herbs to acupuncture. Everything seemed to do well, but being a dancer I am prone to re-injuring myself. After three months of misery, I finally decided to try Prolotherapy. It was a bit uncomfortable at first. It completely increased not only the strength, but gave me a sense of recovering that lies ahead. It was the strongest decision I have made for myself in my career and I don't think I could have continued dancing without it.

Sincerely,

Name Omitted

"Resolve to keep happy, and your joy shall form an invincible host against difficulty."

– Helen Keller

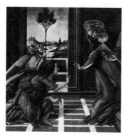

Marc Darrow, M.D.
Joint Rehabilitation and Sports Medical Center
Los Angeles, CA 90025

Dear Dr. Darrow:

I just wanted you to know how quickly my back problem is healing. When I came in to see you in incredible pain, bent over like the hunchback of Notre Dame, I didn't believe I would ever have a strong back after 25 years of intermittent spasms and lower back pain. Although its only couple of weeks since you injected me, 90% of the pain and weakness is gone. I can stand straight and feel more like I want to feel.

Very gratefully,

Name Omitted

Marc Darrow, MD, JD

"God heals, and the physician hath the thanks."
– George Herbert, Outlandish Proverbs.

Joint Rehabilitation & Sports Medical Center
Los Angeles, CA 90025

Dear Dr. Darrow:

"Prolo works! After injuring my shoulder (hyperextension/overuse syndrome) near the tail end of the Long Drive competitive season, I was beginning to wonder if it would ever get back to normal. Progress was inching along at a snail's pace when I was utilizing massage, heat, icing, manipulation, and various rehabilitative exercises.

After only one injection, my shoulder was probably 80 percent recovered after three days. I could do most of the upper body exercises I used to do prior to the injury, and was pain free with my golf swing. I found that very impressive.

After receiving treatment on both my right shoulder, which was the one originally injured, and the left one, which I wanted healed as well, the long drive season started again. Prior to my injury, my best drive was 385 yards. After my injury, but before treatment, I was incapable of hitting over 300 yards. In my first event after treatment, hitting a standard length club to ease into the competition again, I hit a 320 yard drive. I have already qualified for the Southern California District and I feel absolutely no pain in either shoulder. It's pretty amazing."

My gratitude to you,

Name Omitted

Although there may have been an additional proliferative effect, the quick healing seemed to be from the trigger point effect of the injections.

"Happiness lies, first of all, in health."
– George William Curtis

Marc Darrow, M.D.
Joint Rehabilitation and Sports Medical Center
Los Angeles, CA 90025

Dear Dr. Darrow:

I came to your office in October 1999 suffering from bursitis in my hip since April, and lower back pain since August. I finally decided to seek medical attention after suffering countless sleepless nights due to pain. After your diagnosis and explanation of my condition, I began my physical therapy twice a week. The positive atmosphere, dedication, and camaraderie of the staff had made this rehabilitation process a pleasure. Since I began injection therapy, my back pain has diminished dramatically. I can see a definite improvement in my rehabilitation by receiving your injections. I have many pain-free days and nights, and have increased my back strength over 100%.

Thank you for your care and help.

Sincerely,

Name Omitted

Marc Darrow, M.D.
Joint Rehabilitation and Sports Medical Center
Los Angeles, CA 90025

Dr. Darrow:

I am so grateful to you, Dr. Bill, and Dr. Jason for helping me out of the chronic pain I had suffered with for so long. The injections were a godsend. My hip, lower back, ankle, and heel are 90% better. Thank you all for being so brave and innovative with your treatment.

Name Omitted

"The universe is full of magical things,
patiently waiting for our wits to grow sharper."

— Eden Phillpotts

September 18, 2001
Marc Darrow, M.D., J.D.
Joint Rehabilitation and Sports Medical Center
Los Angeles, CA 90025

Dear Dr. Darrow:

   I am so glad to have met you earlier this year. Last year I injured my right shoulder while playing tennis. For months I tried to let it heal by itself, but to no avail. I had pain doing simple tasks such as combing my hair or reaching for my wallet. I finally relented and saw an orthopedist who had it x-rayed. He concluded I had arthritis and there was nothing he could do. I was pretty upset because at age 43 I felt I had many years left to play tennis. That's when I met you. You said you could fix it with a weekly series of Prolotherapy injections. To make a long story short, you were correct. After seven treatments I was back on the court playing pain-free.

   However, as you know, that terrific state of affairs didn't last long. Two weeks later I tore two ligaments in my right ankle stepping on a tennis ball while going for a cross-court backhand shot. It blew up like a balloon. After I got an MRI the orthopedist said I would probably need surgery. I told him about you and that I wanted to see what you thought first. We decided to give Prolotherapy a chance. That, combined with an ankle exercise board and heat treatments, and use surgery as a last resort. Well, once again, you worked your magic and two months later I'm back playing tennis with reckless abandon. I don't even need an ankle support. I couldn't be more pleased. I think your book, *The Collagen Revolution: Living Pain Free* should be mandatory reading for anyone who suffers joint pain, no matter what their age. It sure opened my eyes. I plan on playing tennis for another 50 years or so. Thanks for your help Dr. Darrow.
Sincerely,
Bill Strong
Beverly Hills, California

"When one door of happiness closes, another opens;
but often we look so long at the closed door that we
do not see the one which has opened for us."

– Helen Keller

Marc Darrow, M.D., J.D.
Joint Rehabilitation and Sports Medical Center
Los Angeles, CA 90025

To Dr. Darrow:
   I would like to convey the following results of our Prolo therapy experience. I first saw you in January of this year for a chronic and very painful hip problem. At first I was very leery and scared about doing the injections. In the end the pain and discomfort got to me and I agreed to the injections. We had two sessions. After the first, the pain was significantly diminished. After the second session to date, the pain has not recurred. My daily life has so improved I can now walk for hours with no problems, and have gone back to aerobics three times a week. I would like to thank you and acknowledge your "gift."

Sincerely,
Name Omitted

Marc Darrow, M.D., J.D.
Joint Rehabilitation and Sports Medical Center
Los Angeles, CA 90025

Dr. Darrow:
   Yippee, hooray, right on. Pain is gone. Prolo has me dancing again. My knee is healed.

Name Omitted

*"Early to bed and early to rise,
makes a man healthy, wealthy, and wise."*
–Benjamin Franklin, Poor Richard's Almanac

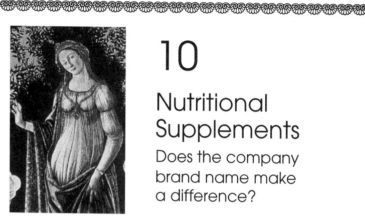

10

Nutritional Supplements

Does the company brand name make a difference?

I practice Holistic Medicine. By that I mean that I consider the mind and body to be one entity. I do not
buy into the Cartesian Dualism that conventional western
medicine is based upon which treats the body and mind separately. To this end, I believe it is vitally important that we
provide the body with the nutritional support necessary to
help heal joints and soft connective tissue.

While we have talked a lot about the importance of pain
and inflammation in the healing process, healing also involves "a complex myriad of biochemical and cellular reactions. Research suggests that modulation of these reactions
can be achieved nutritionally, thereby hastening tissue healing and recovery time."[1]

The past 20 years has seen an explosion in the nutritional
supplements marketplace. In the 8o's you had to seek out
herbal and nutritional supplements at "alternative" health
stores. As the 60's generation aged, the same questioning of
conventional wisdom that was brought to bear on our gov-
ernment and cultural life was directed towards the health
care industry. This occurred as a whole generation of aging
baby boomers looked to alternative health care solutions and
preventative treatments. The markets responded and homeopathic, herbal and all sorts of nutritional supplements have
flooded the market to the point where you can go to almost
any drug store and buy Echinacea, CoQ10 or any other num-

ber of promising supplements that promote health and well being. While this ready availability is a great thing, what is not so great is that there is no regulation of the nutritional supplement industry. In other words, what you see, is not always what you get.

Because the industry is not regulated by the FDA you can not be guaranteed that the product contains the active ingredient it claims to, or the quantity of the supplements is what it purports to be. *There is no quality control.* Until there are some kind of standards and procedures for these industries, I prefer to deal with companies I trust and know to be the cutting edge leaders in the professional nutrition marketplace. They must have exceptional quality control and strong biochemical leadership.

One of my favorite companies (which is Located in San Clemente, California), *Metegenics,* has been in business since 1983, and proven to be a leader in the fields of scientific research and discovery all geared towards enhancing our genetic potential through nutritional support. Their research is sound, and I trust their quality control. If you can not find Metagenics products where you live, you can visit our website at http://www.JointRehab.com and order from us. I was introduced to Metagenics because of their educational materials and knowledgeable and friendly tech hotline. They are the only company that spends enormous amounts of time in doctor's offices teaching us what we did not learn in medical school- basic nutrition. I thank them for supplying me with information for this book.

There are some key nutritional supplements that have proven to be effective in healing chronic pain and injury associated with the musculoskeletal injury and myofascial pain. They will be discussed in general terms as they relate to healing the connective tissue.

Brief Overview of Inflammation and Healing

When injury to a ligament or tendon occurs, a sequence of events begins at the cellular and biochemical level that initiates healing.[2] Inflammation is the body's initial attempt to heal itself. Redness, swelling, pain, heat, and loss of function are classic signs of inflammation. The biochemistry of inflammation that produces these manifestations is induced and regulated by a large number of chemical mediators, including **eicosanoids**, cytokines, kinnins, complement proteins, histamine, and monokines.[1],[3]

> *Eicosands are produced from omega-6 and omega-3 polyunsaturated fatty acids.*

Linolenic acid, which occurs abundantly in vegetable oils, *is the predominant omega-6 fatty acid.* It is classified as an essential fatty acid (EFA) because the human body must have it, but cannot synthesize it. *Dietary linolenic acid is primarily converted to arachidonic acid (AA),* the direct precursor of pro-inflammatory mediators. [1] AA is the major fatty acid released in response to tissue injury and contributes greatly to the inflammatory process.[4] AA can be directly obtained from meat, eggs, and a few plant products including, most notably peanut oil.[1]

Alpha-linolenic acid (omega-3) occurs primarily in green leafy vegetables, soybeans, spirulina, walnut, canola, and flaxseed oils. Various forms of anti-inflammatory therapy involve regulating the production of some of these chemical mediators.

The actions of both omega-6 and omega-3 – derived eicosanoids are necessary to maintain balance and homeostasis during an inflammatory response.[3, 4, 5]

Nutrients for Modulating the Inflammatory Response

With increasing complications and hospitalization due to serious side effects from NSAIDs and anti-inflammatory medications it makes sense to find safe and effective alternatives. Natural substances including fatty acids, various herbs, bioflavanoids, and proteolyctic enzymes have been shown to possess substantial anti-inflammatory and pain relieving properties.[1]

Essential Fatty Acids

Gamma-linolenic acid (GLA) found in hemp, borage, black currant and evening primrose oils belongs to the omega-6 family, but has an almost identical chemical structure to alpha-linolenic acid (omega-3), and is therefore beneficial for many of the same purposes.[6]

Numerous research articles and clinical studies have demonstrated the efficacy of 0mega-3 fatty acids and GLA as anti-inflammatory agents.[6,7,8,9,10] Research also indicates that enhancement of omega-3 status improves pain tolerance.[4,11]

Herbs

A number of chemical compounds (*phytochemicals*) found in common herbs demonstrate pain and inflammation-reducing properties.[12]

> Bioflavonoids- a broad class of phytochemicals found largely in citrus fruits, tea, and wine –may reduce pain and inflammation.

Ginger and Tumeric

Ginger and tumeric, two popular herbs used in the East Indian system of medicine known as Ayurveda, have long been used in folk medicine for a variety of both acute and chronic inflammatory conditions.[13] Several animal and in vitro studies have demonstrated significant anti-inflammatory and anti-oxidant activities for both ginger and tumeric.[12,14]

Cayene Pepper – (*Capsicum annuum*) has been shown to possess powerful anti-oxidant compounds, reduce platelet aggregation and improve blood circulation.[15]

Boswellia – A gum resin from the *Boswellia serrata* tree is a traditional Ayurvedic remedy used for inflammation. Boswellic acids have been shown to inhibit the complement system, a set of enzymes that work with antibodies to attack foreign cells and bacteria.[16]

Bioflavonoids

Bioflavanoids a broad class of phytochemicals found largely in citrus fruits, tea, and wine –may reduce pain and inflam-

mation. Their therapeutic applications are broad, and their roles in mitigating injury, pain and inflammation include antioxidant activity, inhibition of enzymes involved in AA metabolism, inhibition of leukocyte infiltration into the site of inflammation, and protection of collagen and hyaluronan in connective tissue.[4,15]

Proteolytic Enzymes

Supplemental proteolytic enzymes are derived from plant and animal sources. Common proteases include *bromelaine* from pineapple; *papain and chymopapain* from papaya; the fungal protease from the *Aspergillus oryzae* fungi; and trypsin, chymotrypsin, and pancreatin usually of porcine (pig) or bovine (cow) origin.[1] A great deal of the research that describes an anti-inflammatory effect of proteolytic enzymes centers around acute (e.g. sports) injuries, although post-surgery and degenerative joint conditions have been studied as well.[4,17,18,19] In most cases the patients that received the enzymes demonstrated significantreduction in pain and inflammation and faster recovery rates compared to the placebo groups (the duration of healing was reduced by half in some instances).[17,18,19] And unlike traditional anti-inflammatory drugs, essential fatty acids, herbs, bioflavanoids, and proteolytic enzymes appear to exhibit no significant side effects or toxicity.[9-16]

Nutrients Involved in Connective Tissue Repair

Following injury of the connective tissue (ligaments, tendons), it is critical to supply the raw materials and proper nutrients that support tissue recovery and new tissue synthesis.

The collagen fiber, the major component of our connective tissue, consists of long protein chains that are made up of amino acids. Collagen is dependent on the supply of nutrient building blocks such as amino acids, vitamins and minerals that are needed for the many enzymatic reactions involved in tissue rebuilding.[1]

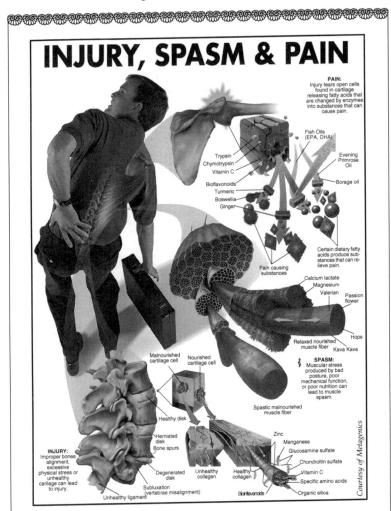

INJURY, SPASM & PAIN

PAIN: Injury tears open cells found in cartilage releasing fatty acids that are changed by enzymes into substances that can cause pain.

Trypsin
Chymotrypsin
Vitamin C

Bioflavonoids
Turmeric
Boswellia
Ginger

Fish Oils (EPA, DHA)

Evening Primrose Oil

Borage oil

Certain dietary fatty acids produce substances that can relieve pain.

Pain causing substances

Calcium lactate
Magnesium
Valerian
Passion flower

Hops

Relaxed nourished muscle fiber
Kava Kava

SPASM: Muscular stress produced by bad posture, poor mechanical function, or poor nutrition can lead to muscle spasm.

Spastic malnourished muscle fiber

Malnourished cartilage cell
Nourished cartilage cell

Healthy disk

Herniated disk
Bone spurs

Zinc
Manganese
Glucosamine sulfate
Chondroitin sulfate
Vitamin C
Specific amino acids
Organic silica

INJURY: Improper bones alignment, excessive physical stress or unhealthy cartilage can lead to injury.

Degenerated disk
Unhealthy collagen
Healthy collagen

Subluxation (vertebrae misalignment)
Unhealthy ligament
Bioflavonoids

Courtesy of Metagenics

Amino Acids

Collagen fibers are made up of long chains of amino acids, of which one third is glycine. It is critical to provide your body with the nutritional support that the amino acids provide as they are utilized by the body and help result in the synthesis of new collagen tissue.

Glucosamine and Chondroitin Sulfates

Glucosamine sulfate is derived from the chitin of crab shells, whereas the source of chondroitin sulfate is usually bovine trachea. The primary therapeutic indication for these two substances is in the treatment of degenerative diseases of the joints. Glucosamine plays a critical role in the formation of tendons, ligaments, skin, nails, heart valves, blood vessels, bones, and articular surfaces of joints. Glucosamine sulfate halts the progression of joint degeneration and promotes the regeneration of cartilage by stimulating the production of proteoglycans. The mechanism of action of chondroitin sulfate is similar in that it provides substrates for proteoglycan production and the formation of healthy joint matrix. Unlike the NSAIDs, glucosamine does not inhibit the enzyme cyclooxygehnase or the synthesis of prostaglandins. It is ineffective in suppressing the enzymes involved in inflammation. In studies comparing glucosamine sulfate to NSAIDs, long-term reduction of pain was more substantial for patients receiving glucosamine sulfate.[20]

Vitamin C

Vitamin C is required for collagen fiber synthesis, a process vital for tissue repair and healing. A deficiency in vitamin C is associated with poor collagen formation, less stable collagen due to insufficient hydroxylation, and delayed wound healing.[21]

Bioflavanoids

Bioflavanoids are thought to benefit connective tissue by binding to elastin, thereby preventing its degradation by elastases released as a result of inflammation.[22] Most bioflavanoids also act as antioxidants that help to prevent damage to tissue.

Antioxidants

A number of conditions such as chronic inflammatory disorders and connective tissue damage are associated with free radical activity. The main rationale for supplementation with antioxidants in injury is to reduce the damaging effects of free radicals and benefit tissue healing and repair.[4] Both Vitamin C and E are major antioxidants that quench free radicals in most tissues.

Nutritional Support for Muscle Relaxation and Rest

When there is injury to a ligament or tendon, patients tend to favor or self-mobilize the injured area to avoid pain and further injury to damaged tissue. This places stress on the associated muscles, often resulting in muscle strain, sprain, spasm, and or cramping, all of which can influence healing negatively. Calcium, magnesium, and various herbs promote relaxation of the muscles and help to reduce the psychological anxiety and stress that can be associated with injury.[1]

Calcium and Magnesium

Muscle cramps may result from altered neuromuscular function due to a lack of calcium and magnesium homeostasis, and supplementation of these minerals has proven effective in reducing muscle cramps.[23, 24]Whenever a patient presents with persistent or severe muscle pain, a magnesium deficiency is usually suspect.

Passion Flower

Passion flower is well known for it's tranquilizing and sleep inducing qualities. Without sleep it has been found that healthy college students have many of the pain symptoms of fibromyalgia. The pain disappears once normal sleep patterns are resumed.

Valerian Root

Valerian is one of the most relaxing herbs available, and is recognized for its efficacy in treating nervous system disorders and calming the entire body.[25] Better still, unlike other sleep aids, valerian does not leave you with a "hang -over " effect the next day.

Kava Root

A popular herb native to the South Pacific islands, kava is widely used for it's anti-anxiety effect. Kava may also be of value in pain control and in inducing muscle relaxation, exerting local anesthetic and analgesic activities likened to aspirin or morphine in potency. [1,3,26]

As you can see, proper nutrition is a key component in helping you heal, rejuvenate and prevent connective tissue injury.

Many of the herbs, amino acids and nutritional supplements described here are available in most large drug stores. But if your looking for quality control, premium potency and nutritional products that are on the cutting edge of scientific research, be sure to choose a product line prescribed by your doctor. You can visit our website http://www.jointrehab.com to purchase these products.

---

[1] Treating Injury and Supporting musculoskeletal Healing; Dr.Mark Percival;p:1;Applied Nutritional Science Reports,2000;Advanced Nutrition Publications, Inc.

[2] Guyton AC.Textbook of Medical Physiology 8th ed. Philadelphia: WBSaunders;1991

[3] Salmon JA, Higgs GA. Prostaglandins and leukokortrienes as inflammatory mediators. *Br Med Bull* 1987; 43(2):285-6

[4] Bucci LR. Nutrition Applied to Injury Rehabilitation and Spirts medicine. Boca Raton,FL;CRC Press; 1995

[5] Simopoulos AP. Omega-3 fatty acids in health and disease and in growth and development. *Am J Clin Nutr 1991;54;438-63*

[6]Erasmus U. Fats That Heal. Fats That Kill 2nd ed. Burnby BC, Canada;Alive Books;1993

[7]James MJ, Gibson RA, Cleland LG. Dietary polyunsaturated fatty acids and inflammatory mediator production. *Am J Clin Nutr* 2000;71 (Suppl);343S-48S

[8]Blok,WL, Katan MB, van der Meer J. Modulation of inflammation and cytokine production by dietary (n-3) fatty acids. *Jnutr 1996;126:1515-33.*

[9]Kunkel SL, Ogawa H., Ward PA, et al. Suppression of chronic inflammation by evening primrose oil. *Prog Lipid Res 1982;* 20:885-88

[10]Meydani SN. Effect of (n-3) polyunsaturated fatty acids on cytokine production and their biologic function. *Nutr 1996;* 12:S8-S-14

[11]Kremer,JM, Lawrence DA, Petrillo GF, et al. Effect of high dose fish oil on rheumatoid arthritis after stopping nonsteroidal antiinflammatory drugs. *Arth Rheum 1995;38(8);1107-14*

[12] Srivastava KC, Mustafa T. Ginger (*Zingiber officinale*) in rheumatism and musculoskeletal disorders. *Med Hypoth* 1992; 39;342-348

[13]Weiner MA, Weiner JA. Herbs that Heal. Mill Valley, CA: Quantum Books;1999

[14]Flynn DL, Rafferty MF. Inhibition of humanneutrophil 5-lioxygenase activity by gingerdione, shogoal, capsaicin and related pungent compounds. *Prostaglandins Leukotr Med 1986;* 24:195-198

[15]Havsteen B. Flavonoids, a class of natural products of high pharmacological potency. *Biochemical Pharmacology* 1983;32(7):1141-48.

[16]Knaus U, Wagner H., Effects of boswellic acid of *Boswewellia serrata* and other triterpenic acids on the complement system. *Phytomed 1996;3;77-81*

[17] Trickett P. Proteolytic enzymes in treatment of athletic injuries. *Appl Ther 1964;Aug:647-51*

[18] Shaw PC.The use of a trypsin-chymotrypsin formulation in fractures of the hand. *Br J Clin Prac* 1969;23(1):25-26

[19] Rathgeber WF. The use of proteolytic enzymes (Chymoral) in sporting injuries. *SA Med J* 1971; Feb 181-83.

[20]Validate Your Pain! Exposing the Chronic Pain Cover-Up; 2000 Chino, Alan F. Ph. D. , Davis, Corrine D. M.D. p. 168-169; InSync Communications LC and Health Access Press http://www.insynchronicity.com

[21]Schwarz RI, Kleinman P, Owens N. Ascorbate can act as inducer of the collagen pathway because most steps are tightly coupled. Third conference of Vitamin C 1987;498:172-84

[22]Tixier JM, Godeau G, Robert AM, et al. Evidence by in vivo and in vitro studies that binding of pycnogenols to elastin affects its rate of degradation by elastases. *Biochem Pharmacol* 1984;33(24)3933-39.

[23]Dahle L., Berg G, Hammar M, et al. The effect of oral magnesium substitution on pregnancy –induced leg cramps. *Am J Obstet Gynecol* 1995; 173(1):175-80

[24]Hammar M, Larsson L, Tegler L. Calcium treatment of leg cramps in pregnancy. the effect on clinical symptoms and total serum and ionized serum calcium concentrations. *Acta Obstet Gynecol Scand* 1981;60(4):345-47

[25]Witchl M. Herbal Drugs and Phytopharmaceuticals. Boca Ratn, FL. CRC Press, 1994

[26]Singh YN. Effects of kava on neuromuscular transmission and muscle contractility. *Jethnopharmacol* 1983: 7:267-76.

"Look at everything as though you were seeing it for the first time or last time. Then your time on earth will be filled with glory."

—A Tree Grows in Brooklyn

11

The Doctor's Role in Healing

*M*y job is to cure people of chronic pain; and I love my job. I love the work that I do because there is no greater satisfaction for me than lifting peoples' spirits. When a person who has suffered from chronic pain heals, he or she is not only healing the tissue trauma, but the totality of the trauma that living in pain has caused the mind, body and soul.

The approach I take to healing is threefold. I call it the Trinity of Healing, and focus equally on all three aspects. (1) Treat the physical body that needs the repair, (2) Treat the mind that lives in that body and deals with the pain, and (3) Treat the external things that are going on in that person's life that either affect or are affected by this pain.

Pain is a function of the interaction of these three things. As a doctor, it is important to remember that each of these three aspects must be considered, and given adequate attention so that the patient receives the most thoughtful care in order for complete healing to be achieved. I cannot emphasize this enough. If you do not treat the totality of the trauma, you are merely treating symptoms, and not truly healing and curing the problem of chronic pain.

I have found it to be extremely rewarding, both for the patient and myself, to enter into this quest for wellness as an agreement; an agreement that we are equal partners on the road to recovery and healing. I see it as a journey, a road we will travel together. I insist that it be a fifty-fifty partnership, and that my patients play an active role in their recovery.

The patient's willingness to enter into this agreement is crucial. This includes approaching treatment with a positive attitude and believing that he or she can and will get better. That is not to diminish the pain they have suffered already. I know all too well how depression and pessimism can settle in when you have been hurting for so long.

In every partnership, there must be trust. The only way trust can be formed is if a friendship is created. I truly care about what happens to my patients; both with their ailments and their life separate from that. Once my patients become aware of this, they are able to place their trust in me and they are motivated to work with me, putting in their one hundred percent of the fifty percent of the work they committed to as we heal and head down the road to recovery.

I view only a small part of my job as the actual physcal modalities. Yes, it is important to be technically correct as a physician. But, to me, that is just the beginning. Although patients are paying only for the procedural modalities, I make it my self-appointed responsibility to work on other levels. To do this I must truly listen and understand them. Not the easiest task in all cases, I must admit, and I certainly don't have it perfected.

You may be thinking, easier said than done. And I agree. One of the first casualties in the battle between doctors and so called "managed care" insurers has been the doctor/patient relationship. The whole paradigm has shifted. Before managed care, the question was: What is best for the patient? After managed care the most pressing question for insurers is what is best for the bottom line? This has lead to an unhealthy state of affairs and leaves both doctors and patients frustrated. Doctors frustrated that they have to get approval for treatment from accountants who have never been to medical school, feeling that in order to survive financially they must squeeze in as many patients as possible, and see them in the most efficient manner, not necessarily the most beneficial. The strains on both doctors and patients have begun to fray nerves and there is a movement underway to demand a "Patients Bill of Rights". In the meantime it is up to you to take responsibility for your own health and well being. If you feel like your doctor isn't hearing you, or that you are unhappy with the relationship, find another doctor! One who will listen. Because it is only when we listen, that we can hear, and then heal.

I agree with Dr. Alan F. Chino, Ph.D. and Dr. Corrine D. Davis M.D. in their book *Validate Your Pain!*, "...paying attention to – and validating – the human experience of chronic pain will bring about a significant healing effect. Outcome from 'proper' physical treatment administered by an unfeeling, uncaring, dispassionate robot will be far inferior to that provided within the context of a caring, compassionate team of human beings. [1]" You hold the key to your healing. I am but a partner on the path.

I work at being an effective healer for people with pain because I myself have lived with chronic pain. I think of it as the price I paid for the many sports injuries I've suffered throughout the years. I know what living with chronic pain can do to you, physically, emotionally and spiritually. There is a miasma of misery that can cloud your view of everything when you tolerate pain and suffering as part of your everyday experience. I had tried everything to rid myself of my pain with no success. Suffering from chronic pain can sure lend nicely to the development of a pessimistic attitude.

My closed minded misery almost cost me the opportunity to be cured. If I had not been in so much pain I doubt I would have agreed to try Prolotherapy. I mean I was a doctor and had never heard of this? But the pain was screaming, I was desperate and I put my skepticism aside. In suspending skepticism, I found relief. Miraculous relief. I found Prolotherapy and it changed my life. I had no choice but to to help others the way I had been helped.

In my practice I have I achieved an 85 to 90% success rate curing my patients with Prolotherapy. I use the term Prolotherapy more than trigger point injections because as you have read, every injection of this type is really a combination of both, no matter what solution is used, or if only a needle is used without a solution.

There is a saying, "Physician heal thyself," and I do. All the chronic injuries that I sustained through my active participation in sports throughout the years have been injected (many by self-injection). This has made a dramatic change in the quality of my life.

One of the most satisfying aspects of my job is being able to prevent unnecessary surgery. I pride myself on saving my patients from the knife. It is rare that a patient undergoes surgery after Prolotherapy. Why would anyone go under the knife and change the natural anatomy of their body by removing a part of it?

I love to take away a patient's diagnosis and educate patients that in most cases, their diagnosis is either wrong or is not even the cause of pain. An example of this is the common disc problem. One-half of all people with no back pain have disc problems and findings on MRI, CT Scan, or x-ray that a surgeon would love to "fix". This is one of many instances where technology in diagnosis can prove harmful.

A big part of my job is opening up the doors of perception so that patients can see that they have the ability to move past the restraint of a physical diagnosis and into a place of healing. I have noticed that people who are positive in their consciousness get better faster than the others. Some people have come to identify themselves with their pain and derive purpose from it. This greatly prohibits them from healing.

I am not saying you have to love your doctor, or vice versa, but if you feel that your doctor is not responsive, not hearing you, or worse, not helping you, you owe it to yourself to find another doctor. But you must also own up to your responsibility and start the healing inside yourself. Be prepared to give up all those things that get in the way of your health. Get involved in you own recovery. Don't expect a doctor to do it for you.

Satisfaction in my work depends on patients getting better. I share my patient's highs and lows. I am as excited as they are when they start to feel better, and am as discouraged as they are if the treatment is taking longer to kick in than they had hoped. I am very involved and get very attached. I put myself in the place of the patient, which is easy to do because, after all, I have been there.

May Peace and Health Be With You.
Marc Darrow
Los Angeles, CA

References:
[1] Chino, Alan F. and Davis, Corinne D. Validate Your Pain!: Exposing the Chronic Pain Cover-Up. Florida: Health Access Press, 2000.

"The Constitution only gives people the right to pursue happiness. You have to catch it yourself."

–Ben Franklin

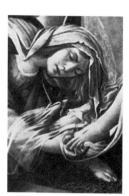

Resources

American Assn. of Orthopaedic Medicine - You can get a list of physicians who utilize Prolotherapy
http://www.aaomed.org/

American Back Institute of New Orleans on Prolotherapy
http://www.backpaininstitute.com/serv03.htm

Atkins Center for Complementary Medicine
http://www.atkinscenter.com/center.html

Back Pain - Article
http://www.powerup.com.au/~dominion/ff/k31.htm

Chronic Pain Solutions: A News Guide - Prolotherapy
http://www.chronicpainsolutions.com/articles/djuricsummer99.htm

Dr. Cohen on Prolotherapy
http://www.sover.net/~samallen/cohen.htm

Dr. Weil on Prolotherapy
http://www.pathfinder.com/drweil/archiveqa/0,2283,1476,00.html

The Doctor's Medical Library
http://www.medical-library.net/specialties/prolotherapy.html

Effects of smoking on collagen production - Article
http://www.steinorthopaedic.com/healthylinks.htm

Evaluating Your Prolotherapist
http://www.caringmedical.com/evaluating_your_
prolotherapist.htm

Fact, Fiction & Fraud in Modern Medicine
http://www.dormanpub.com/home.htm

Health Plus Web: Alternative Health Directory - Definition
http://www.healthplusweb.com/alt_directory/
prolotherapy.html

HealthWorldOnline - Article
http://www.healthy.net/library/newsletters/Update/
prolotherapy.htm

ProloNews.com - Archives of the Prolotherapy e-newsletter
from Ross Hauser, M.D., and Marion Hauser, M.S., R.D.,
(Authors of Prolo Your Pain Away)
http://www.prolonews.com/

Prolotherapy - Article
http://www.esomc.com/prolotherapy.html

Prolotherapy - Alternative Health Directory
http://www.healthplusweb.com/alt_directory/
prolotherapy.html

Prolotherapy - from phys.com
http://www.phys.com/fitness/sports_injury/sportsmed/
prolotherapy.html

Prolotherapy - Dr. C. Everett Koop's Story
http://www.wheatons.com/Prolotherapy_Endorsement_
by_DrKoop.htm

Prolotherapy.com - information, books, articles
http://www.prolotherapy.com/

Prolotherapy Discussion Board
http://www.prolo.net/

Prolotherapy: Everything you need to know
http://www.wheatons.com/Prolotherapy.htm

Prolotherapy helps whiplash victims
http://www.chronicpainsolutions.com/articles/djuricsummer99.htm

Prolotherapy is for Pain
http://www.prolodoc.com/all_about_prolotherapy.htm

Prolotherapy or Ligament Reconstructive Treatment by Injection http://treatingpain.com/prolothe.htm

Prolotherapy On-Line Articles
http://www.prolotherapy.com/documents.htm

Tech Mall - Article
http://www8.techmall.com/techdocs/TS981125-7.html

Trigger Point Injections - Article
http://www.lilesnet.com/rptc/trigger_point_injections.htm

Trigger Point Injections - Policy review
http://www.gamedicare.com/policies/220.htm

Trigger Point Injections - Position paper
http://www.dringber.com/tpoint.html

Thinking Person's Guide to Perfect Health
http://www.sonic.net/~nexus/sclero.html

What is prolotherapy?
http://www.sfpmg.com/pain/page2.html

Other Centers Offering Prolotherapy

Allen Thomashefsky, MD, PC Santa Barbara, CA and Ashland, OR
http://www.drtom.net/

American Back Institute - New Orleans, Louisiana
http://www.backpaininstitute.com/serv03.htm

Caring Medical Rehabilitation Services - Oak Park, Illinois
http://www.caringmedical.com/aboutcmrs.asp

Center for Sports & Osteopathic Medicine - New York
http://www.bonesdoctor.com/prolo.html

Comprehensive Medical Services - East Meadow and New
York City http://www.drcalapai.com/rtap.html

East-West Medical - Atlanta, Georgia
http://www.docbridges.com/index.htm

Eugene Sports & Orthopaedic Medcine Center - Eugene,
Oregon http://www.esomc.com/index.html

Joseph Valdez, M.D., M.S - Pasadena, Texas
http://www.valdezmd.com/index2.htm

Kab S. Hong, M.D.,P.C. - Elkins Park, Pennsylvannia
http://www.prolotherapy-us.com/

Milwaukee Pain Clinic - Dr. William Faber
http://nutriteam.com/doctor.htm

Pain Management & Rehabilitation - Irvine, California
http://www.folandpainmgt-rehabmd.com/indexProlo.htm

Paracelsus Clinic - Federal Way, Washington
http://www.paracelsusclinic.com/

Piedmont Physical Medicine & Rehabilitation - Greenville,
South Carolina http://www.prolotherapy.ws/

Prolotherapy for Pain - Palm Bay, Florida
http://www.prolotherapyforpain.com/prolotherapy.html

San Francisco Center for Pain Management
http://www.sfpmg.com/pain/index.html

About Orthopaedics
http://orthopedics.about.com/?once=true&

Alternative Medicine Center http://www.healthy.net/asp/
templates/center.asp?centerid=1

America's Health Network http://www.ahn.com/

American Family Physician - Cardiovascular Screening of Student Athletes
http://www.findarticles.com/m3225/4_62/65106196/p1/article.jhtml

American Fibromyalgia Syndrome Association
http://www.afsafund.org/

Cell phone radiation is linked to cancer - Click here for a free electromagnetic radiation exposure test
http://www.radar3.com/

Chiropractic America http://www.chirousa.com/

ChiroWeb http://www.chiroweb.com/

Dr. Koop's Health; Wellness Center
http://www.drkoop.com/

Doctor Directory
http://www.doctordirectory.com/

Doctors in LA
http://www.la-doctor.com/main-directory.htm

Fibromyalgia Network
http://www.fmnetnews.com/

Guide to Alternative Medicine - Chiropractic
http://www.knowledgecenters.versaware.com/notoc/getpage.asp?book=alternativemedicine&page=061000009.asp

Health Answers
http://www.healthanswers.com/home/pubHome.asp

Directory of health links
http://www.healthlinks.net/

The Health Pages
http://www.the-health-pages.com/

HealthWave Directory
http://www.healthwave.com/

Introduction to Muscle Physiology
http://ortho84-13.ucsd.edu/MusIntro/Jump.html

Introduction to Muscle Physiology - Chiropractors
http://www.malacti.com/Chiropractors_USA.htm

Less Pain Better Golf - devoted to the concept of playing better golf with less back pain
http://www.lesspainbettergolf.com/

Medical Information http://www.americasdoctor.com/

MedicineNet.com- Doctor-produced healthcare information
http://www.medicinenet.com/Script/Main/hp.asp

MSN Health http://health.msn.com/

MSN – Sports & Fitness
http://content.health.msn.com/living_better/fit

MSPWeb - Sports Medicine links
http://www.mspweb.com/

The Physician and Sports Medicine
http://www.physsportsmed.com/index.html

Spinalinks.com - Chiropractor Directory
http://spinalinks.com/

Sports Medicine - links from About.com
http://sportsmedicine.about.com/health/sportsmedicine/
?once=true&

Sports Medicine http://www.medfacts.com/

Sports Medicine.com http://www.sportsmedicine.com/

Sports Medicine Bulletin Board
http://sportsmedicine.about.com/health/sportsmedicine/
mpboards.htm

Sports Medicine Education Programs
http://sportsmedicine.about.com/health/sportsmedicine/
?once=true&

Sports Medicine Foot Facts
http://sportsmedicine.about.com/health/sportsmedicine/
msubfeet.htm

Sports Medicine News
http://www.ivanhoe.com/sportsmed/

Sports Medicine Newsletter
http://cac.psu.edu/~hgk2/

Sports Nutrition
http://sportsmedicine.about.com/health/sportsmedicine/
msubnutrition.htm

WebMD
http://my.webmd.com/

WebMD – Ask the experts
http://webmd.lycos.com/ask_our_experts_summaries/fit

Weitz Sports Chiropractic and Rehabilitation - Santa Monica
http://www.drweitz.com/

WholeHealth MD
http://www.wholehealthmd.com/

World Wide Chiropractic Directory
http://webmd.lycos.com/ask_our_experts_summaries/fit

Your Health is Your Business
http://www.siu.edu/departments/bushea/

YourSpine - Chiropractic Help OnLine
http://www.yourspine.com/

Glossary

Acupuncture - a therapy initiated in China over 5000 years ago. Much like trigger point therapy, needles are inserted into acupuncture (same points as trigger points) points to promote healing, and reduce pain. Repeated needling with acupuncture needles may proliferate collagen and promote healing much like Prolotherapy.

Acute Pain – New onset. Common kinds of acute pain are low back pain and headache which can last for several days or more. Term does not refer to the intensity of pain but the timing.

Arthritis - Breakdown of the structures in and around a joint. Bones hypertrophy as cartilage is destroyed.

Arthroscopy – A highly invasive surgical therapy which involves the use of metal scopes to diagnose damage, and drills, shavers and other tools to cut and remove tissue and bone from the joints.

Articular cartilage - The glassy cartilage covering the ends of bones. Without it bones grind and cause pain.

Avascular – An area of the body such as cartilage that is not fed well by blood. Vascular refers to vessels.

Bursa - Sacs of fluid that protect tendons, muscles and ligaments from rubbing on bone.

Bursitis: "Itis" refers to inflammation of the term it follows. In this case inflammation of the bursa.

Carpal tunnel syndrome (CTS) – An impingement of the median nerve at the wrist often caused by repetitive motion.

Cartilage - Connective tissue made out of collagen. Found in the joints and covering bone where it acts as a smooth surface for gliding. See also Articular cartilage.

Chiropractic – Hands on therapy that balances the body. Newer forms of chiropractic such as AK relieve pain and promote mobility and healing without forced adjustments.

Chondroitin sulfate – A nutritional supplement that is a building block of cartilage.

Chondromalacia patellae - Breaking down of the cartilage on the back of the knee bone. A type of arthritis.

Chronic Pain – Pain generally lasting more than 3 months. Patients are often disabled by their pain and may suffer severe depression and anxiety, & drug abuse.

Collagen - A major structural protein, the glue that holds our bodies together. Collagen is formed with molecular cables that strengthen the tendons and vast, resilient sheets that support the skin and internal organs.

Connective tissues – The soft-non-bone tissues in the body that hold us together. Examples are ligaments, muscle fascia, joint capsules and tendons.

Corticosteroids – Anti-inflammatory steroids, often injected, which reduce inflammation and pain but in doing so, interfere with the body's natural healing cascade. An example is cortisone.

Etiology - The cause of a disease or pathology.

Fascia — The connective tissue that envelops the muscles and provides support and attachment to the bones.

Fibroblasts – Cells that produce collagen.

Fibromyalgia – A complicated syndrome involving wide spread pain and fatigue, often with insomnia. It is a wastebasket diagnosis for unsolved reasons for pain.

Glucosamine sulfate – A nutritional supplement that acts to reduce joint pain. It is a building block of cartilage.

Inflammation or healing cascade – The body's natural response to injuries. It begins with inflammation (swelling and pain), which triggers an influx of fibroblasts that produce collagen and "rejuvinate" the tissue.

Ligaments – Strong elastic bands of connective tissue that connect bone to bone at the joints of the body.

Meniscus - A cushion in the knee joint made out of collagen.

Muscle – Contractile tissue that flexes and stretches, giving movement to the various parts of the musculosketal structure.

Musculoskeletal – Relating to the framework of the body composed of bones that are connected and supported by muscle and other soft tissue.

Myofascial – Relating to a type of pain in the network of connective soft tissue that covers the muscular system.

NSAIDs – All prescription and non-prescription anti-inflammatory drugs not containing steroids are classified as "non-steroidal anti-inflammatory drugs" or "NSAID's." Examples of NSAIDs are ibuprofen, Motrin, aspirin, Naprosyn, Dapro, Celebrex, Vioxx, and an endless multitude of others. Their side effects include gastrointestinal bleeding with occasional death, and kidney and liver problems.

Patellofemoral syndrome – Painful knee condition occurring from mistracking of the patella in the femur (thigh bone). Common in runners.

Physiatrist – A medical doctor who has a specialty in Physical Medicine and Rehabilitation.

Prolotherapy – Natural simulation of the body to produce or proliferate collagen. The process rejuvenates the musculoskeletal system and reduces or eliminates pain.

Referred Pain- Pain manifested in distant areas away from the active trigger point.

RICE protocol - A treatment in which Rest, Ice, Compression, and Elevation are used after injury to prevent inflammation.

Tendinitis - Inflammation of a tendon.

Tendons – Sheets of collagen that connect muscle to bone.

Trigger points – According to Janet Travel, MD, taut, tender tissue in muscles that refer pain and create dysfunction. They are the same points as acupuncture points. Muscles, tendons, ligaments and joints may have trigger points.

Trigger point injection – Injections that reduce pain in trigger or tender point areas. Trigger point injections may also proliferate collagen secondary to the inflammation caused by needle trauma, and in effect be Prolotherpy. Janet Travel, MD who popularized trigger point therapy, mentions in her book that a patient may be sore for a day or so after injections. It is obvious that this discomfort is a result of needle induced inflammation.

INDEX

A

Accidents
motor vehicle, 92-93
Active trigger points, 74
Acupuncture, 39, 62-63, 184
Acute pain, 51, 184
Alpha-linolenic acid, 161
Amino acids, 164-165
Anesthetic jet therapy, 132
Anesthetics
used in prolotherapy, 68, 80
Anti-inflammatory medications, 26, 45-49, 71
complications from, 46-48
Antioxidants, 165
Applied Kinesiology (AK), 101
Arthritis, 44, 111-112, 184
Arthroscopy, 110, 184
dangers of, 124-126
Articular cartilage, 121, 124, 184
Avascular tissue, 184

B

Back pain, 24, 87-107
lower, 94-103
personality types associated with, 88-89
and pregnancy, 91-92
risk factors for, 88-89
surgeries for, 91
tips for preventing, 94-95
Backpacks
causing shoulder pain in children, 112
Barre-Lieou Syndrome, 133-134
Bioflavinoids, 162-163, 165
Boswellia, 162
Bursae, 111, 184
Bursitis, 111, 184

C

Calcium, 166
Carpal tunnel syndrome (CTS), 131-133, 184
Cartilage, 184
articular, 121
Cayene pepper, 162
Chemical irritants, 69
Chemotactic agents, 69
Chiropractic, 184
Chondrocytes, 125
Chondroitin sulfate, 185
Chondromalacia patellae, 185
Chronic pain, 21-22, 185
dramatic increase in, 43-44

headache, 133
survey on, 49-50
Co-factors, 70
Collagen, 29-41, 32, 67, 185
cosmetic benefits of, 30-32
triple helix, 38-40
Vitamin C and, 38-40
Computerized tomography (CT scans), 110
Connective tissue, 185
nutritional supplements supporting repair of, 163-165
"Corrective" surgery, 100
Corticosteroids, 47, 185
Cortisone injections, 24, 34
Cosmetic surgery, 31-32

D

Degenerative disk disease, 96
Dermatology, 31-32
Discogenic syndrome, 98
Disk disease
degenerative, 96
Disk herniation, 99
Dislocation, 111, 114-115
Doctors
role in healing, 171-175
Dry needling, 79-80

E

Electromyograms (EMGs), 110
Emotional pain, 53
Essential fatty acids, 162
Essential pain zones, 74
Etiology of disease, 185
Exercise, 88

F

Facet syndrome, 99
"Failed back syndrome," 100-101
Fascia, 185
Fatty acids
essential, 162
Fetal stem cells, 70
Fibroblasts, 68, 185
Fibromyalgia, 185
Fibrous tissue
production of, 37-38
Functional proteins, 26

G

Gamma-linolenic acid (GLA), 162
Gate control therapy for pain, 51-52
Ginger, 162
Glucosamine sulfate, 185
Growth factors, 70
Growth hormones, 70

Jonathan Skariton

SÉANCE INFERNALE

Jonathan Skariton was born in Athens, Greece, and attended the University of Edinburgh and the University of Wales, Bangor. He has a Ph.D. in cognitive neuroscience and experimental psychology. Skariton works as a cognitive neuroscientist for the largest fragrance manufacturer in the world. He lives in Kent, England.

www.jonathanskariton.com

SÉANCE INFERNALE

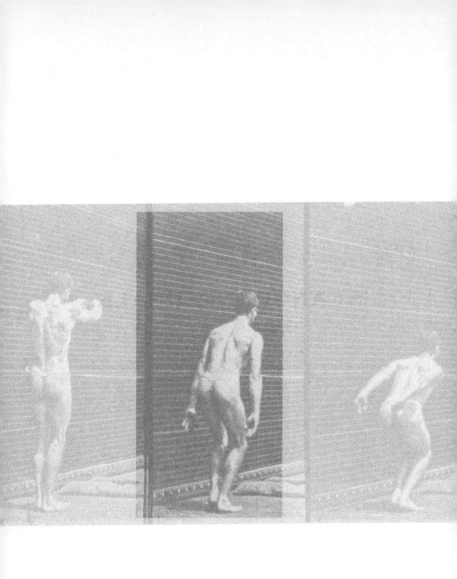

SÉANCE INFERNALE

Jonathan Skariton

VINTAGE BOOKS
A Division of Penguin Random House LLC
New York

For my father

FIRST VINTAGE BOOKS EDITION, JULY 2018

Copyright © 2017 by Jonathan Skariton

All rights reserved. Published in the United States by Vintage Books, a division of
Penguin Random House LLC, New York, and distributed in Canada by Random House
of Canada, a division of Penguin Random House Canada Limited, Toronto.
Originally published in hardcover in the United States by Alfred A. Knopf,
a division of Penguin Random House LLC, New York, in 2017.

Vintage and colophon are registered trademarks of Penguin Random House LLC.

Man in pelvis cloth standing and jumping by Eadweard Muybridge,
courtesy of Laurence Miller Gallery.

"In the Hall of the Mountain King" from *Peer Gynt* Suite No. 1,
courtesy of the Sheet Music Archive.

The Library of Congress has cataloged the Knopf edition as follows:
Names: Skariton, Jonathan, author.
Title: Séance infernale : a novel / Jonathan Skariton.
Description: First edition. | New York : Alfred A. Knopf, 2017.
Identifiers: LCCN 2016048129
Subjects: LCSH: Lost Films—Fiction. | Mystery Fiction. |
BISAC: FICTION / Mystery & Detective / General.
Classification: LCC PR6119.K37 S43 2017 | DDC 823/.92—dc23
LC record available at https://lccn.loc.gov/2016048129

Vintage Books Trade Paperback ISBN: 978-1-101-97050-8
eBook ISBN: 978-1-101-94674-9

Book design by Iris Weinstein

www.vintagebooks.com

Printed in the United States of America
10 9 8 7 6 5 4 3 2 1

Part I

October 2002

1

The receptionist's black leather pumps echoed on the marble floor of the foyer. She escorted Alex Whitman past an ornamental fountain until they reached a bulky oakwood door at the end of a granite-paneled hallway.

Andrew Valdano turned his leather chair to face Whitman.

"Mr. Whitman. Please." He motioned at the chair for guests across the desk. Whitman had already sat himself into it.

Valdano could have been between fifty and sixty-five years of age. His mustache, a lead gray; his ink-black hair retained its color. His dusty complexion peered out beneath custom-made silk.

Valdano's desk was a carved brown mahogany with four seated winged griffins surrounding its base. Behind him, the window looked out on a Los Angeles autumn afternoon. Outside on the building's Gothic façade, granite gargoyles peered out over the city, their claws clasping their grotesque heads.

On the room's walls, framed film posters mounted on duck canvas, reminders of elegant works of the past: *Intolerance: Love's Struggle Throughout the Ages; The Birth of a Nation; M; The Big Parade.* Photographs hung on the walls, of figures who had directed these masterpieces: D. W. Griffith; King Vidor; Josef von Sternberg; F. W. Murnau.

Valdano broke the silence. "Where is it?" He had the tone of someone used to getting what he wanted.

"By all means, skip the opening titles," Whitman said.

Whitman had been hired to track down a copy of *The Cat Creeps*. In this film, an heiress (Helen Twelvetrees) arrives at a remote mansion to claim her fortune and, once there, is terrorized by an escaped maniac ("The Cat") and the predatory would-be heirs, who are also her relatives. Hardly an admirable film; another take on the "old dark house" motif trying to capitalize on the success of Paul Leni's *The Cat and the Canary*, of which *Creeps* was a talkie remake. However, *The Cat Creeps* had been considered lost for decades, and that made it a desirable acquisition, especially for private collectors.

Alex Whitman was part archaeologist, part detective for anything related to film. Whitman had to get himself to the right place at the right time. His almost photographic memory of catalogs, locations, and specifications allowed him to beat out collectors and dealers who wagered thousands of dollars depending on whether a film poster was three-sheet or one-sheet, whether a film reel found in the depths of a dank basement contained a lost scene or undesirable splices. Such pieces, auctioned at Sotheby's or Bonhams, or even privately, were bombarded with bids.

"I left the film cans with your secretary. Eight reels of nitrate film in all," Whitman said. "Let's hope she doesn't blow up."

"Condition?"

"Projectable, given the date. I'm sure your cronies can get rid of the few tears and the unsteadiness of the image in some frames. There are no deep emulsion scratches anyway."

"So you've seen it?"

"I projected it on my living room wall, then decided the wall looked better as it is."

Whitman reached into the pocket of his overcoat and took out a crumpled rolled cigarette.

"You can't smoke in here."

Whitman fished out his lighter and lit the cigarette. He exhaled blue smoke over the desk space between them. A piece of tobacco got caught between his lips and he spat it over the desk, without losing eye contact with Valdano.

Valdano rose from his chair and approached the cabinet to his left, which was flanked by swing-arm lamps. He took out a cut-crystal decanter, turned around, and handed him a glass. Whitman noted the man's pink, ornate nails, manicured to perfection.

"You're good at finding things," Valdano said.

"Only because the film industry has been good at losing things for years."

Valdano ignored him. "Take this piece, for instance. Care to tell me what you know about it, Mr. Whitman?" He motioned to a mounted film poster at the center of the wall to his right. On the poster, towering skyscrapers and magnificent giant structures dominated a sepia-colored landscape. The sharp, jagged lines reinforced its futuristic tones.

"Berlin, 1927," Whitman said. "Originally designed by Heinz Schulz-Neudamm, issued in connection with the release of *Metropolis,* January 10 of that year. The original three-sheet poster was produced by UFA's film studio in Germany. Most of them were destroyed or thrown away after being hung on billboards. Four original copies remain. You own one of the only two existing in private hands."

"An extremely effective and alarming work of art, as is the film, of course," Valdano said.

"Naturally, this is a fake. As is every poster in this room," Whitman replied.

Valdano gave him a mischievous, conspiratorial smile. "How is that so?"

"The size doesn't feel right. Nice framing, by the way. Where did you steal it from, a flea market?"

In fact, the size did seem right. But Whitman reasoned that Valdano was not a fool; he would not leave a film poster valued at more than half a million dollars hanging in his office.

"That's what I like about you, Mr. Whitman. You have an eye for detail. It's a nice facsimile, of course. Faithful, even in size, to the original, which you are correct to assume I keep elsewhere." It was rumored he kept a vaulted storage room inside his house, accessed by fingerprint technology and controlled for temperature and humidity. It contained the rarest of film pieces. Valdano continued to look at the poster. "I suppose you, of all people, should realize it was a copy by mere glance."

Whitman yawned. "Did you bring me here to talk about business or . . ."

The collector pointed to the portrait above the Windsor stone fireplace. The picture was a black-and-white image of a man in his forties, with small ears and kind, wise eyes. The rest of his face was covered in muttonchop side-whiskers and a beard. He was holding a white top hat, a cigarette burning between the fingers of his other hand.

"Do you recognize this man, Mr. Whitman?"

Whitman ran a hand through his beard. "That's Augustin Sekuler, isn't it? The French inventor."

Alex Whitman's father, a film memorabilia dealer at a time when the profession had not yet been defined, had Sekuler's picture in their living room. His father didn't have a picture of his wife or his son, but he did have the Lumière brothers, Thomas Alva Edison, and Eadweard Muybridge.

"Sure," Whitman said. "Sekuler is thought to be the first person to have recorded moving images on film. In fact, his 'Princes Street Gardens Scene' is considered the world's first motion picture film. The images were recorded in 1888 in Edinburgh, Scotland, years before Edison or the Lumière brothers."

"Do you know what happened to him, Mr. Whitman?"

"Nobody does. He was never able to perform a planned public demonstration, because he mysteriously vanished from a train in 1890. His body and luggage were never retrieved. Detectives from three countries were employed to search for him. No trace was ever found. I think at the time of his disappearance he was on a train to Paris."

"That is correct," Valdano said, still lost in Sekuler's eyes. "He was visiting his brother in Dijon. The plan was to meet with friends in Paris before continuing to New York in time for his scheduled exhibition. It would have been the first public demonstration of moving images."

"But Sekuler never arrived in Paris. In fact, he was never seen again. Sounds like a twenties Hitchcock gone bad."

"It's right up your alley," Valdano said. "Have you seen any of his work?"

"I've seen 'Princes Street Gardens Scene.'" He grinned. "All two seconds of it." He adjusted himself in the chair. "The catalogs state his remaining work also includes 'Traffic on South Bridge,' 'The Man Walking Around the Corner,' and 'Accordion Player.'"

Valdano looked at him again with that conspiratorial smile. "That is not entirely correct."

"That's what the catalogs say."

"Of course, your sources are informed, but hardly precise." He pulled out one of the drawers of his desk and revealed two loose pages, which he extended to Whitman.

"I recently acquired these from a New York–based bookseller." As if reading Whitman's mind, he added: "Letters from Carlyle Eistrowe to a friend."

"Carlyle Eistrowe? The occultist?"

"Occultist, writer, mountaineer, philosopher, chess player, painter, and social critic, among other traits."

"Also black magician, drug fiend, sex addict. I remember him on the cover of *Sgt. Pepper's Lonely Hearts Club Band*. He bore a heavy influence on many musicians, like Jimmy Page, who bought his former castle in Scotland."

Valdano smiled. "He's the second one from the left—situated in between Mae West and Sri Yukteswar."

Obsessed with finding the secret to immortality, Carlyle Eistrowe had traveled the world conducting occult rituals and writing "how to" manuals on the esoteric and magic (or "Magick," as he called it) and befriending some of the most significant artists and thinkers of his time, including Augustin Sekuler.

Whitman asked how the letter was related to the French inventor.

"See for yourself."

He steadied his steel-rimmed glasses and gently handled the document. It was a two-page typed letter with two small holes where the pages had once been pinned together. Both pages were discolored by age, and there were light creases from their having been in an envelope. The handwriting was in black ink and seemed slanted, with spikes and troughs. The letter was dated August 16, 1890, and was headed "Blue Claridge's Hotel." The occultist author had crossed out the header and written what appeared to be his own address at the time:

~~Blue Claridge's Hotel~~
xxxxx—illegible address—xxxxx

August 16, 1889

Kathryn Longhorn
12 West Saville Terrace
Edinburgh EH9
U.K.

Dear Kathryn,

I have long foreseen the Alice in Wonderland conclusion of my labours, but I hasten to add this was a signal for the awakenings to the beauty of life.

I do not know of the Diorama you write of. My involvement with the medium came to an end as soon as it had commenced, when an old friend was dear enough to share what are arguably the first moving pictures ever captured. I vividly recall one of these being set in the gardens of Edinburgh's Princes Street. But another, most ingenious one is in preparation; it is called "Séance Infernale," depicting the Fall of Man. I am certain that moving pictures contain the Magickal truth.

The letter went on to discuss Eistrowe's inventory of books and publishing plans, clearly with the intention of enticing the recipient with some involvement. It was signed "Fraternally yours, Carlyle."

Whitman looked up from the manuscript, meeting Valdano's impatient eyes.

"Well? What do you think?"

"You think he's talking about Sekuler. Another film. The 'Séance Infernale.'"

"But of course. What else could it be?"

Whitman remained silent, his calm gaze working along the lines of the letter.

Valdano interrupted his thoughts. "It's safe to say the first of the two specimens Eistrowe writes about is 'Princes Street Gardens Scene.'"

"But it's not clear if he's referring to the same person," Whitman said. "We don't even know if he's talking about a real film. Maybe he's just trying to get it on with this Kathryn woman. Eistrowe was a trickster, wasn't he? Always trying to manipulate people to have his own way."

"I thought you would appreciate that, seeing a little of yourself in his tactics," Valdano said.

Whitman shrugged. "We're all given some sort of skill in life." The blue haze of his cigarette drifted over Valdano's desk. "What do you want from me, then?"

"I want you to find this film for me, Mr. Whitman."

"I'm not interested."

Valdano drummed his fingers on the desk.

"I thought you weren't interested in Victorian cinema anyway. How come you're so keen on this wild-goose chase?"

"Absence makes the heart grow fonder. It will be a remarkable addition to my collection."

"Just give me my money for the Twelvetrees picture and I'll be on my way. I told you *The Cat Creeps* would be my final job for you."

"It was kind of you to let me know. Yet you keep coming back." He sighed. There was impatience even in his sighing. "You've never disappointed me in the past, Mr. Whitman. Except for the *Frankenstein* poster I hired you to find ten years ago. You never did find it for me. However, in light of the circumstances surrounding your life at that time, I am willing to forget about it. Besides, I have no interest in Mr. Whale's works anymore." His eyes hardened for a second. "Even though I can't help thinking you did indeed find a copy, which you kept from me."

Whitman blinked at him, unnerved.

He's bluffing. He doesn't know. He couldn't possibly know.

"I didn't take you for a man bound by family and the unnecessary misfortunes surrounding it, Mr. Whitman."

"And I thought you were a family-oriented guy yourself. I bet you've wrecked four or five this month alone."

In response to this, Valdano pressed a button on the edge of his desk and the gas Windsor fireplace below Sekuler's picture crackled to life. Whitman fidgeted in his chair. He started to sweat. A sense of nausea washed over him as memories of fire fleshed out from the corners of his mind.

"Is everything all right, Mr. Whitman?" the film collector asked, in a grin as wide as that of *The Man Who Laughs*. Whitman swallowed hard, trying to conceal his uneasiness. He avoided looking at the fireplace for fear of going into a state of panic, but he could feel the flames dancing in there, licking their way into the air.

"I'm not sure I'm the man for this job," he managed to say.

The film collector took a checkbook out of the bottom drawer and placed it on the desk. "You didn't cash the check from my *Frankenstein* request. So why do it? Why haggle your way every time we meet to a higher fee when you're not going to cash in on it? You think this is blood money, don't you?" He laughed as if the prospect amused him. "Like you've sold your soul to the devil."

"Maybe I just don't want this job."

"You're lying. The cards are being dealt and your fingers are itching to play." He filled in the check, signed, tore it out, and folded it on the table. "Actions lie louder than words, Mr. Whitman. You see, if you are willing to sit here listening to my rant while perhaps your sole fear in life springs from my fireplace, I bet you'd take this job for free. You would even betray your family for it, if you still had them around."

"Go to hell."

Valdano laughed. "This should pay for your advance, plus all traveling and other expenses." He pushed the slip of paper toward Whitman. "Just another check for you not to cash." He pressed the button on his desk again and the fire retreated to charcoals.

Whitman felt his muscles relax and his breathing return to normal. He swallowed, giving himself a moment to breathe. Then he reached to the desk and slowly unfolded the check, holding it between his index and middle fingers. "You said I keep coming back. This time I won't. Goodbye." He flicked the check back to Valdano's side of the desk and rose from his chair.

"Mr. Whitman," he heard the film collector calling to him from behind. Alex Whitman turned his head and for the first time saw pleading in Valdano's face. Sure, he was trying not to blink, to retain his overbearing smirk of self-importance. But his posture gave him away; it wasn't proud and confident anymore; it was crouching, imploring for help.

Valdano weighed his words carefully. "When you're not drowning in sarcasm and self-pity, you are the best this business has to offer. I may not like you, but I don't have to; you do a damn good job."

Captain Fantastic, Whitman thought. He was intrigued by Valdano's self-proclaimed defeat; surely another of his intricately crafted mind games. Valdano was right: Whitman *was* curious about the lost footage. He ignored the nagging in his gut. In the past, he had come to trust these warning hunches.

"Any family?" Whitman asked, sitting back down on the chair.

"I have not been able to trace any of Sekuler's descendants. This, of course, should not deter you from giving it a try yourself. I have compiled a folder containing all information pertinent to this project. As you will see, most of it has to do with the man himself, as there is nothing known about 'Séance Infernale.' Start from the Science Museum in London and Sekuler's former workshop in Edinburgh."

"What do you think happened to him? Sekuler, I mean."

"Perhaps he meddled in affairs he shouldn't have," Valdano said, staring at Sekuler's picture.

"Do you think Edison got to him?" Thomas Edison had filed his own patent for a working moving-pictures camera just a year after Sekuler disappeared. Conspiracy theories abounded; stealing other inventors' ideas was not new to Edison.

"Would not surprise me. History is not written by the victors; it is written by ruthless patent thieves."

"The title sounds like it's a story, maybe even a linear narrative," Whitman said.

"Almost three decades before Griffith's *Intolerance*? That would be a revelation. But let's not get ahead of ourselves with wishful thinking. We'll be lucky if it's even projectable."

"We'll be lucky if it even exists. I haven't exactly taken on this kind of job before."

"Hence the number of zeros on the check."

The steps from the main hall of Valdano's office building sloped down to a travertine-paved path leading to a marble arch fountain and a bizarre set of statues. The courtyard, unusually for the neighborhood, was partitioned from the outside world by six-foot-high walls and electronic iron gates.

The statues—three ugly winged goddesses with their torsos, arms, and hair intertwined with serpents—were clad in clay. They were clothed in the long robes of mourners and bore brass-studded whips. They were unresting, angry, vengeful. Once convulsed in their anger in the dark world of Tartarus, they were implacable by sacrifice or tears. *Damn hounds of the netherworld,* he thought, *barking like a tortured conscience.* Behind him, gargoyles glared out into the distance. The Gothic building seemed out of place and out of time among the Spanish and Colonial Revival residences of the historic neighborhood.

He thought he heard someone behind him and grasped Valdano's folder tighter. Turning around, he saw only a dog walker. He crossed the silent street, passing the Andalusia and a parking lot, north toward the busy thoroughfare of Sunset. Chateau Marmont loomed over the north side of the Strip. He wondered whether James Dean, trapped in some quirk of time, was hopping through one of its windows to audition with Natalie Wood for *Rebel Without a Cause.*

He went into a friendly looking, low-key bar, hidden behind neon lighting and a lack of door signs. He was in no hurry. He sat at the cigar lounge on the spacious patio and ordered a Grand Marnier. He could just make out the labyrinthine alcoves and staircases, past the stripper's pole, the Mickey Mouse portrait on the wall, and the wall-mounted televisions playing reruns of *The Twilight Zone.*

Whitman took out his Old Holborn and rolled a cigarette. He looked at his lighter and tried to make sense of why matches, but not lighters, caused him to regress to a state of pyrophobic panic. When the waitress brought him his drink, he opened Valdano's folder. He perched his reading glasses on his nose.

The folder contained a typed report on Augustin Sekuler, his life and inventor's career, from his birth in Metz to his mysterious disappearance on the train from Dijon to Paris in 1890. A bibliography and reference list were the main sources of information on the inventor's work. Between the photocopies of citations, there was a photograph of Sekuler, stapled to a piece of paper outlining the main theories for his disappearance. The filmography section was accompanied by photographic stills of each surviving frame of the footage. As a sign of good faith, Valdano had also included Eistrowe's letter.

Whitman took a sip of his drink. The liquor warmed him.

He took money out of his pocket and placed it on the table. Dusting flecks of tobacco from his shirt, he got up and got into the first cab that stopped outside the bar. A dark figure watched him from a distance.

2

From Santa Monica Boulevard at the boundary between Beverly Hills and West Hollywood until Hoover Street in Silver Lake is a high-end fashion lover's mecca; along Melrose's boutiques with tawdry storefronts and fluorescent window displays, salons with funky names in a garish haze of Day-Glo and neon; emporiums of famous designers emblazoning beacons of chic. Among the rows of stores desperately trying to look outlandish, the Crypt was a wolf in black sheep's clothing.

It was cleverly hidden between a new-age bookshop and a parking lot, between pierced noses and Ferraris, on the western stretch of Melrose, inside a mock-Gothic building that used to be a mortuary. No sign on the door indicated it might be a shop.

The Crypt was a movie haunt. Lining the walls, posters of zombies, killer clowns, and alien monsters in exaggerated makeup and far-fetched costumes staggered after scream queens in torn skirts and heels. Pristine film memorabilia was displayed over two stories and a basement, sprawled on Persian rugs and tucked between fine shelves.

Nostalgics mingled with obsessive film buffs, purist poster collectors, and rabid sci-fi nerds. The "reel deal," however, was located below-ground; the basement housed catalogs of select rare titles. For every scrap of Japanese monster flick, German street film, and Italian Giallo, there were people who were willing to put up serious money: pill-popping rock stars, erratic Japanese millionaires, workaholic business sharks, sixteen-millimeter-print collectors, for whom a few cut frames may mean a decrease in value in the region of thousands of dollars. The material—be it nitrate or acetate film, the A4 paper of original typewritten screenplays, or the plastic of a prop—is entirely worthless. People with sound sense would not accept these items even for free. But pity the idiosyncratic mind of the film collector; present him with the original one-sheet poster of *Flying Down to Rio* or "Touchdown Mickey" and he is likely to sell his own mother to attain it. This business was not about buying a piece and selling it at a profit; rather, it was about finding the specific piece that caters to a specific collector's obsession, then holding on to it until he offers everything he owns in exchange.

The studded shop door of the Crypt yielded to Whitman's hand with a jerk. The bell fastened above it tinkled.

The lighting was kept dim. Collector plates and posters embellished the walls. Shelves bowed under the weight of pressbooks and screenplays. Piles of photographic stills and lobby cards were stacked around glass cabinets displaying rare autographed pieces. Some were particularly rare: Chaplin's jacket from *The Great Dictator;* Evel Knievel's helmet; Forrest Gump's box of chocolates; Batman's armor costume; the ventriloquist's dummy from *Dead of Night;* Michael Myers's mask from the first *Halloween;* Robert Englund's original worn blade glove from *A Nightmare on Elm Street;* Jack Nicholson's "Heeere's Johnny" door-wrecking ax.

Weird figures lurked in every corner; life-size props and statues of John Wayne, Katharine Hepburn, and Harry Potter watched the customers through eyes of wax, plastic, or glass. Scattered around the dummies lay antique perfume sprays, evening gloves, cigarillo holders, many of these signed, with their certificates of authenticity. Mannequins and clothes rails held layers of garments worn by famous stars: full-length velvet once sported by Claudette Colbert; chiffon evening gowns pinched at the waist, worn by Lauren Bacall; and day dresses that captured the venerable finesse and charm of Audrey Hepburn's 1950s era. Old club chairs extended an invitation to settle in. Oak chests nearby lay half-open, inviting the visitor to sift through the treasures within.

At the far end of the store, behind a pile of photographic stills, stood Charlie Carmichael, a man of medium height and considerable girth, with the kind of eyes that always seemed to smile.

He had helped Whitman set up and open the Crypt during the eighties, first on the eastern part of Melrose, at a time when thugs and outlaw bikers dominated its graffiti-strewn locality; that was before their move to the Heights, where the crowd gradually got younger and the boutiques and trendsetters started rolling in. Whitman and Charlie had met during a midnight screening of Edwin Porter's *The Great Train Robbery* at the Vogue, on Hollywood and North Las Palmas. That was before the cinema became a strictly night theater during the eighties. The Vogue featured seventy-millimeter projection and would get first run on bookings, even though most A-list films opened at the Chinese. As if spurred by a magic wand, the two strangely found themselves the only people who showed up to see the film; the neon marquee and the beautiful geometric murals on the walls had not attracted any passersby that night. They realized they were laughing with triumph at the same scenes, and an initial conversation on whether the final shot of the bandit firing his gun toward the viewer should be placed in the beginning or the end of the print led to a lifelong friendship.

Together they had mediated the events that had turned their business from hobby-oriented to dealer-driven. And when Whitman moved with his wife to Edinburgh to open a second Crypt there, Charlie had kept the L.A. store running. Charlie never missed the chance to converse with customers, to hear their stories and offer them film information. "What do these people want from me?" Whitman would ask.

Charlie stood talking to a teenager wearing oversize trousers and a scruffy T-shirt. His face was lit up and he was waving his hands ecstatically in the air. When Whitman approached them, he realized why. Clasped in his hands was an eight-by-ten publicity shot of *Freaks,* showing director Tod Browning, a thin man with a wax-tipped mustache and a brooding expression, next to the statuesque blond Olga Baclanova. The photo was signed by both.

Whitman took Charlie aside, next to a replica prop of Johnny 5.

"What did Valdano say?" Charlie asked.

"I'm leaving for London tomorrow. Can you hold the fort?"

Charlie made a whistling sound. "Sure. What's he after this time?"

"A film by Augustin Sekuler."

Charlie frowned, puzzled. "The French dude? I thought he just recorded footage of scenes."

"That's what the history books say. Valdano thinks differently."

"What do *you* think?"

"I don't care, as long as I'm getting paid," he said, although his eyes said otherwise. "His workshop was in Edinburgh, so I'll have to . . . you know."

"You sure you want to go back there? After—" He broke off in sudden embarrassment.

"It was a long time ago."

They were silent, then Charlie said, "Well, what about *The 39 Steps*? We've been sitting on this info for too long; someone might snatch the print."

Whitman took off his glasses and observed them under the ambient light of a solid brass bridge lamp. Hitchcock's 1935 suspense spy thriller was the first in what would become a motif of narrating tales of innocent men on the run. The unforgettable action sequence on the bridge, where Robert Donat jumps from the train to escape, was filmed at Forth Road Bridge in Edinburgh. For the past two months, Charlie had been in contact with a woman based in Edinburgh who claimed her late husband had been in possession of film rolls containing scenes from *The 39 Steps*. Apparently the man had been a stand-in during the shooting and had sneaked into Hitch's tent and taken the film. The woman said her husband had left notes accompanying each roll.

One of the scenes involved a cameo appearance by Hitchcock as one of those killed during the shoot-out in the train sequence. However, his short appearance had already been pinpointed at the beginning of the film, tossing some litter while Robert Donat and Lucie Mannheim run from the theater. If the notes were anything to go by, this would render *The 39 Steps* the only Hitchcock film with two director sightings, one of which had, until then, been lost forever. Neither Charlie nor Whitman could find any mention of this in back interviews or catalogs, but that wasn't what made Whitman skeptical.

"I don't know if it's worth traveling all the way for it. The old woman might be out of her mind. Second cameo, my balls. Ridiculous."

"That's what you thought before we found those extra scenes for *Peeping Tom*. Who'd think Michael Powell had filmed an extra scene involving the girl with the harelip and an extended suicide sequence?"

"We had a good pointer there," Whitman said. "All the inconsistencies across catalogs when it came to duration. Doesn't take a genius to figure out it was either a mistake or a case of missing footage. For the time being, I'd rather have you here keeping an eye on things."

Whitman turned around. "Shop's closing," he told the remaining customers. He looked around him; in the dim light, the outlines of shadows explored the celluloid necropolis.

His glance came to rest on the small shop window. Through the grille he saw a woman and her child just outside. The girl must have been about six years old, and that made it worse. She was pulling and tugging at her mother's hand, urging her to go inside the store. The mother, holding a bag of groceries in her other hand, was shaking her head and resisting, her face saying, *We're not going in there.*

No, Whitman thought. *Don't.*

He moved to the door and locked it so they couldn't get in. "Shop's closing," he shouted, pouring a drink from the Chivas Regal bottle on the table. "Everybody out through the back door. Now."

3

On his way home, Alex Whitman saw his daughter in a stranger's car. But Ellie had been missing for more than ten years. A stone's throw from the arterial road, crossing the parking lot of a gas station bathed in the veraman phosphorescence of mercury vapor, he froze in front of the beige-colored Toyota Celica. The girl sat in the passenger seat, fiddling with the seat belt, waiting for someone in the shop.

She was around five years old, exactly Ellie's age when she had disappeared. She had the same gentle nose and wide hazel eyes as Ellie; her rosy cheeks and curly silk hair were identical to Ellie's. She held a rag doll against her heart; the same as Ellie's raggedy homemade doll. Unaware of being watched, the girl carefully stroked the doll's red yarn pigtails.

The sight opened a doorway in his mind, behind which the incident at the park had never happened. It was as if time had fr—

Now he realized the girl was looking at him. They stared at each other, two strangers amid veraman rays.

He gave one more glance to the girl, who had lost interest in him and was playing with the seat belt, sliding it forward and backwards, side to side and then in circles. He turned south on La Cienega, hoping the traffic would drown his thoughts, which had already been whisked away to the green-laden grass of an Edinburgh park ten years before.

Ellie's disappearance had marked the last in a number of high-profile child kidnappings that had prompted fear throughout the city of Edinburgh, beginning with the kidnapping and death of Danielle McKenzie in February of 1984, followed by a series of further abductions. Police had tried to determine whether Ellie's disappearance could have some connection with the missing girls.

Forty-eight hours after his daughter's disappearance, the Scottish police had yet to come right out and tell Alex Whitman that Ellie didn't have a chance of turning up; but there came a time when he knew without needing to be told. The police had said they were following up on more than a hundred tips, including reports that a man had been in the Meadows and had spoken to children. They had declined to speculate on what might have happened to Ellie, although they said she would have been able to survive outside that night, when it was unseasonably warm.

Darkness was fierce when Alex Whitman got back to his apartment. He went to the bathroom, wrapped gauze around his palm, and ignored the pain.

From time to time, sounds crept into the apartment. A dog howled; an electric guitar rhythmically wept through the opening riff of "Sweet Child o' Mine"; rain steadily tapped against the windowsill. Other than that, his self-constructed dungeon was peaceful, but by no means quiet, for his thoughts raged. He kept replaying in his mind the events before his daughter's disappearance ten years ago in Edinburgh.

Ellie was at an age where the frequency of nightmares had reached a peak. And the night before her disappearance there had been bad dreams. Kate had hurried out of bed and gone to console her, then had stayed in their daughter's bed until sunrise. In the morning, Alex prepared breakfast and dressed Ellie. In spite of the previous night's tribulations, she was cheerful at the prospect of riding her new bicycle in the Meadows. She allowed him to dress her as part of their ludicrous collaboration. "Foot *numero uno*," he said in a badly simulated Italian accent, holding one of her pink socks, and she allowed her limb to be lifted and guided, like a much younger Cinderella. He then switched to an exaggerated version of Pepé Le Pew.

"But, oh, *qu'est-ce que c'est?* What do we have here? Monsieur Belly-buttón is sticking out; we might have to put him back in his place." Attacking her, he buried his face in her tummy, blowing to produce an incredible farting sound. Her fragile body smelled of honeysuckle and cinnamon. Ellie squirmed, tossed and turned in hilarity, yelling for him to stop. When he let her go, she playfully tried to coax him into doing it again.

He helped her into a warm woolen sweater. In what had become their ritual, she brushed her nose against his and, smiling, delicately felt his face with her fingertips like a blind person. Alex closed his eyes and reveled in a sensation that stretched beyond tactile, face-to-identity recognition.

He went to his wife, who had sheepishly let him carry her back to their bedroom as the sun's first rays licked the Edinburgh skyline. Still half-asleep, Kate smiled at him from beneath the bedcovers. She pulled his neck toward her. They kissed and he tasted the smell of sleep from her mouth. He could feel the warmth of the bed on his face. From the hallway, Ellie was humming to herself improvised nursery rhymes and hopping about the wooden floor.

Looking back on the memory, he could pinpoint a specific moment—with the precision of less than a second—when every visual, auditory, tactile external stimulus was perfectly mapped out in his head. These folds and cracks of time were so vivid that time-traveling to that fraction of a second seemed plausible. Whitman remembered himself sitting on the bed, his wife holding his hand, the warm smell of sleep, Ellie hopping around in the hallway. He remembered considering staying in; maybe he could have Ellie occupy herself with the new crayons and the block of aquarelle they'd bought for her. But he dismissed the idea, thinking that Saturdays would never get this sunny later on in the year.

They walked out into the sunny but chilly Edinburgh morning. The Meadows were a short walk down Marchmont Road. It was indeed an exquisite place: a large park crisscrossed by tarmac footpaths, abundant with trees and covered by a well-kept green lawn. Together with the adjacent Bruntsfield Links, it provided acres of greenbelts fastening around the city. In spring, every path was lined with pink petals, while in August, the lower half was overtaken by circus tents, and it was not uncommon to see performers practicing their routines in the surrounding grounds during the day.

In the distance, the jagged silhouette of the Salisbury Crags slanted upward behind Y-shaped trees. Hikers roamed the skyline and summit of Arthur's Seat. Tagging behind self-propelled wheeled vehicles, skateboarders headed northeast, closer to their usual haunt at Bristo Square.

Around them, games of cricket and Ultimate Frisbee. Groups as discrete as tribes: jugglers, readers, lunchers, dog walkers, footballers, rollerbladers. Ellie wanted to go to the Cheese Man's van—that was what she called him. Cheese Man came every Friday and Sunday with cheese directly from France, and ice cream directly from Tesco. Alex told her it was a Saturday. They passed from Jawbone Walk,* opposite the junction with Meadow Place, where the cherry blossom trees faithfully lined the crisscrossing footpaths, and headed toward the tennis courts, since the eastern end of the park never got the early-morning sun and the mist often lingered longer. It was when they reached the west end of Melville Drive, near the tall Masons' Pillars, that the first thoughts of the *Frankenstein* poster flashed through Whitman's mind. Back in California, Valdano was keen on acquiring it.

As Whitman trailed behind Ellie, was someone following them amid the groups of people? Perhaps a faceless figure taking notice of their conversation, the color of Ellie's bike, Whitman's preoccupied eyes. Did that figure stop when they did, in order to pet the fox terrier that was out with its owner?

Whitman entered a phone booth on the side of Melville Drive and told Ellie to ride her bike close to it. She began whining; he assured her it would only take a minute. As he pressed the buttons corresponding to Valdano's phone number, he confirmed that he had visual contact with her. She was having fun, maneuvering her little feet to stay between the pedal belts and willing herself to ride the bike on the pavement. There was no one around her.

As Valdano's secretary put Alex through to the film collector, he

glanced up at Ellie at frequent intervals. Valdano confirmed he was looking for the *Frankenstein* poster; Whitman replied he would look into it.
Of course, he already knew of a source in London, an unwitting owner
who had no idea what he possessed; the one-sheet "style A" poster was
one of only five known copies to survive. He thought about how he
would travel there and acquire the poster for next to nothing, then force
Valdano to bid against other collectors in a secret auction.

Now more people were around Ellie. A jogger went by; a woman
walking her dog; two bearded adolescents in University of Edinburgh
hoodies; another woman, cigarette in mouth, tattoos adorning her arms,
spanking her crying child. On the phone, Valdano said he would pay a
generous six figures for the poster. He gave Whitman a contact number
where he could be reached at any time. Whitman felt in his pocket and
grasped for his pen. He looked through the glass and Ellie was smiling at
him. He smiled back. He flipped the pages of his notepad to find some
white space, and began writing down the number. He turned his head
back up toward the bike. Ellie was gone.

The lone bicycle was on the footpath. He dropped the phone. He
could hear Valdano's voice still asking if he was there. He went out of the
booth; at that point he was more determined than alarmed. He would
scold her, put her back on the bike, and warn her to never (ever, ever)
wander off. She almost never did; but perhaps a shiny object on the
ground or the dog next to the cherry blossoms had gained her attention
and she'd gone to investigate. Maybe she had fallen from the bike and was
resting nearby. He took a few paces and glanced past the only tree she
could have found shelter behind. Nothing.

Stepping back, he looked in all four directions. She couldn't be far. As
long as she stayed away from the traffic, no harm could come to her, and
Ellie had never been fond of the noise and speed of vehicles. He turned
toward Melville Drive again. A few cars drove by; no signs of an accident
having taken place on the asphalt. He tried to relax. She had to be close. A
small child like that was less likely to be seen right away anyhow. Nevertheless, his pace had accelerated, and so had his breathing. He was aware
by now that his restless face and his demeanor were attracting attention.
The terror of what might have happened set in only when he took a deep
breath and shouted his daughter's name with all of his strength.

There may have been a figure casually walking away from him, concealing something in its bulky overcoat, but Alex was on the lookout for a child, not an adult. Now he was leaping, struggling to see in all directions, half-yelling, half-wailing her name. People were turning toward him, maybe mistaking him for one of the red-nosed homeless gentlemen who frequented the park. People were leaving their picnic baskets and guitars and were crowding around him. Within minutes those people knew that Ellie was five; they knew she had last been seen riding her bike next to that tree; that she wore a woolen sweater, that she was carrying a doll. The people surrounding him were no longer tribes; they were no longer joggers and barbecuers and footballers and sunbathers, but prospective parents. Nevertheless, Alex felt alone. He tried to push them aside; they were hindering his sight. He heard the phrase "wee girl" spoken by pedestrian spectators who had been caught up in the upheaval. The atmosphere was stifling, suffocating him.

Everybody was talking, offering information or an opinion, but everything was quiet. He noticed a police car had cruised to a halt on the side of Melville Drive. Two policemen emerged and came over to talk to him. The words "missing" and "girl" coming out of someone else's mouth made him nauseated. He leaned against the tree, Ellie's bike still next to his feet. A voice came through crackling static over the policemen's receiver. Alex told his story and answered their questions, leaving no facts behind. Their reassuring and calm tone had no effect on him short of insult. They repeated Ellie's description over their radio and a distorted reply came back from the station. The law was on his side. Hell, all the men and women in the park were on his side. If she had gone somewhere, they would find her. If she was taken, though . . . he blocked off this thought instantly.

He saw a third policeman, surrounded by spectators, scribbling notes. Yes, they had seen the little girl riding her bike. No, they hadn't seen what happened to her. Her father had been inside the phone booth. Perhaps he should have known better. Children of that age can be strayers, you know.

A young woman was looking at Alex and crying. Among all the people, he saw the French Cheese Man. It hadn't been his day off after all. They divided into groups, men and women united in debilitating cir-

cumstances, and went in separate directions, slowly and effectively combing the area, but to no avail. Someone offered to drive him home, but
Alex declined.

The wind had picked up by now and was slapping his sweat-beaded
forehead. He saw how simple it was: he had come to the Meadows with a
child on a bike, and was returning with the small bike, alone.

4

Whitman unzipped his backpack and set up his laptop on the living room table. He put the notes from Valdano's folder, as well as his own reference materials, beside the computer. He kept the tobacco paraphernalia within hand's reach. He switched on the laptop and began to roll a cigarette as he waited for the word processor to load up.

He sipped on a glass of liquor and rested the cigarette on his glass ashtray. Valdano's research was in accordance with the information from Nathaniel Newby's *History of Victorian Cinema*. Summarizing the findings so far, he typed:

The greatest mystery in the history of cinema involves a train, a disappearance, a grieving family, patent wars.

The history of film has rarely recognized that Edinburgh was the birthplace of the moving picture.

America and France were quick to grant credit for the invention of cinema to either Thomas Edison or the Lumière brothers.

Footage recorded and projected in Edinburgh in 1888 precedes the famous moving images shown in Paris and New York by seven years.

Timeline (from Valdano's folder)

1841—Augustin Louis Sekuler born in Metz, France.

Father—Major of artillery in the French army, an officer of the Légion d'honneur, intimate friend of photography pioneer Louis Jacques Mandé Daguerre.

Education—Attended colleges in Paris and Bourges, undertook postgraduate work in chemistry at Leipzig University. Early signs of artistic nature in Paris taking up oil and pastel painting and art pottery.

1881—Arrived in New York, met group of artists producing circular panoramas— colossal wall paintings facilitating the "you are there" effect when the observer was positioned in the middle of the piece. The die had been cast.

1885—Moved to Edinburgh. Began designing a 16-lens movie camera. Joined the brass foundry of Whitley Partnership as partner of valve department.

1885—Met occultist Carlyle Eistrowe, regarded as Nietzschean super-philosopher by some, a charlatan and devil worshiper by others. Despite Eistrowe's antics in the world, they remained good friends.

November 1885—Filed first American moving-picture patent application, a method and apparatus "for Producing Animated Pictures of Natural Scenery and Life," based on a complex 16-lens camera and projection system. Camera used two strips of light-sensitized gelatin exposed through lenses, sequentially triggered by electromagnetic impulses. At the time, neither Edison nor the Lumières had initiated their work on motion picture research.

December 1885—Married Elizabeth Whitley, the daughter of his partner and friend. They had two children, Adolphe and Zoe.

July 1888—Projected footage from recording of horse-drawn traffic on South Bridge by fixing gelatin positives on glass, which were in turn slotted into a continuous belt that passed in front of an arc light. The first person in history to capture and project moving images. He realized he needed a more heat-resistant medium to project the images.

1888—Carlyle Eistrowe retired from the public eye.

Early 1889—A flexible form of celluloid was made available (since its creation by Alexander Parkes in 1856). Around this time, with help from Eistrowe, Sekuler recorded footage of a moving picture, which he called the "Séance Infernale." Recording to this day remains lost.

1889—Sekuler prepared his equipment for a trip to New York. He convinced Elizabeth and the children to secure a suitable New York venue for the public exhibition of his invention. They finally booked the Jumel Mansion, in Washington Heights. It would have been an extraordinary show of unparalleled innovation. However, the event never took place.

Fall 1889—Sekuler visited Dijon, France, spending a weekend with his brother Albert before returning to New York in time for his public demonstration.

Monday, September 16, 1890—His brother placed Sekuler on a train headed
for Paris, where a banker named Richard Wilson was waiting for him at
the Gare de Lyon. The train arrived in Paris; Sekuler was not on it. He
was never seen again, alive or dead. The police scoured the countryside
between Dijon and Paris; to this day, not a trace of the inventor or his personal effects has been retrieved, nor has his disappearance been explained.
All that survived was two movie cameras and three strips of film, from his
workshop in Edinburgh.

Whitman shifted his gaze from the computer screen to a CD-ROM in
Valdano's folder. Inserting it into the laptop's drive, he discovered that
Valdano had included MPEG files of Sekuler's surviving recordings. He
watched these, one by one, then entered:

Surviving Work

Princes Street Gardens Scene

Adolphe Sekuler, Joseph and Sarah Whitley and Harriet Hartley at Princes Street
Gardens, forming a kind of impromptu conga line, dancing and laughing. Sarah
Whitley walks backwards and Joseph Whitley's coattails are flying.

Notes: Sarah Whitley, Augustin Sekuler's mother-in-law, died aged 72, ten days
after the shooting of the footage.

Shot at 12 frames/second on 14th October, 1888.

Sources:
Royal Edinburgh Museum, 52 frames, runtime 2.11 seconds at 24.64 frames/
second
    National Museum London, 20 frames, runtime 1.66 seconds at 12.00 frames/
second

Traffic on South Bridge

Traffic moving across a road—recognizably Edinburgh's South Bridge. Carriages
pulled by horses. Formally dressed pedestrians wearing top hats strolling on the
street. Bearded man smoking a pipe stopping on the bridge and peering at the
camera.

Shot at 12–20 frames/second.

Sources:
Royal Edinburgh Museum, 65 frames, runtime 2.76 seconds at 23.50 frames/second.
   Note that the original footage comprises 20 frames.

Man Walking Around the Corner

A bearded man in a smock overall walks in front of and passes by a factory-type building.

Uncorroborated evidence concludes this was recorded with the sixteen-lens camera. The same sources claim samples on collodion were sent by Sekuler to his wife. These showed a French workman in his national blouse walking on Avenue Trudaine.

Sources:
Royal Edinburgh Museum, 14 frames.

Left unrestored and unremastered by both museums in Edinburgh and London, due to the poor quality of the images. Sample viewed consists of an amateurish remastering by Valdano's associates.

Accordion Player

Adolphe Sekuler plays the melodeon by the steps of their house, moving his feet to the sound of music.

Sources:
Royal Edinburgh Museum, 20 frames. Unremastered and unrestored as above.

Whitman stopped typing and looked back at "Traffic on South Bridge." He added: "The man seen crossing the bridge may be the occultist Carlyle Eistrowe, a family friend of the Sekulers."

   Whitman looked away from the screen. He took off his glasses and rubbed his eyes. The darkness of the night had crept into the apartment, broken only by the screen's light and the glow of his cigarette. He raised his glass to a toast.

"Here's to you, Muttonchops; I'm looking forward to finding your stash."

Whitman heard a noise from inside the house. He had been feeling tense and uneasy. Sometime during the late hours of the morning he had grabbed the Bowie knife he kept under his bed and inspected every room of the house in search of thieves. All other sounds had ceased.

It was easy to surrender to the painful nostalgia of Ellie's memory. At night in bed, if he closed his eyes, in that gulf of space perception before falling asleep, he could see her, a warm and miraculous fantasy. Wakefulness would take away what he'd glimpsed and he'd experience the loss all over again.

Another sound—as if an object in another room had been dropped. No question about it. Things couldn't be displaced randomly in unoccupied spaces; there had to be a cause; someone—or something—had moved it.

Whitman walked to the kitchen. He moved his hand toward the light switch but stopped halfway. There was a new sound now, a continuous sound, close to him. Whispers. He stood there in the dark, his reconfigured flesh and his hand frozen on the light switch. The whispering permeated the room.

He flicked the switch, the voice in him that wanted to rationalize this repeating over and over, *Forget it—you can't run, you fool. All those things you fear will reach from into the shadows and pull you down there with them.* But it did work, the scatter of light in the kitchen banishing the morbid thoughts, revealing everything as it had always been. No more shadows.

The sound of dripping from the faucet.

He went up to the sink and tightened the water valve. There. But he still wasn't certain.

"Hello?" he called, and that immediately sounded stupid to him. He took a step out toward the kitchen door, nothing but the hollow darkness hovering beyond, and then paused. The apartment was a concave chamber.

Had there been whispering? It would never hurt to check. He picked up a knife from the rack. He held it in attacking position and listened intently. Could there be someone leaning against the opposite wall, similarly listening for him? He quietly moved to the hall.

He searched every room, closet, and storage space in the apartment without finding any burglars. He searched everywhere, except for one room. The spare bedroom would have been Ellie's when they returned as a family from Scotland; it was now an office and projection room. If there was an intruder, he would have to be in there, maybe contemplating whether he could pawn those projectors or that Ernst Lubitsch picture on the wall.

He took a deep breath, preparing to react. By now he was anxious to find out who was hiding in there. Gripping the knife, he tried to ease the office door open with his free hand. For a second the door gave way, but it stopped two inches open.

Someone was behind it.

He instinctively pulled away and threw his back against the wall adjoining the door. He waited another second. Then, his back touching the wall, he slowly put his hand against the door and tried again. It was still obstructed, but the sound, he realized now, was material, as if it was an object.

Stop it. It's not a dead person.

How do you know? You thought you saw your daughter outside a Walmart just an hour ago.

He shoved his body against the door. The door flew open, throwing what was behind it against the room's far wall. When he heard the ring, he realized what it was.

He stood past the door, a quiver on his lips. He stared at his daughter's bicycle, lying on the floor against the wall. The dolly seat had broken from the crash and lay there like unwanted plastic trash. The training wheels were still intact, as was the bell on the handlebars. Ellie had been missing for more than ten years, yet Alex hadn't been able to dispose of most of her belongings; these were still in her room in Edinburgh, exactly as she had left it. The only thing he had taken back to Los Angeles with him was the bike, the token of that day's remembrance. This macabre reminder he always kept in the far corner of the room, next to the desk, where his gaze would sometimes linger. The bike had never been moved. But now it lay at an angle, the seat against the wall, the dolly seat broken and the rest of it slanted.

Still holding the knife, he glanced at the empty room as if it could provide the answers. He couldn't fathom how the bicycle had been positioned behind the door; it made no sense. He examined the window; it was closed shut, as he had left it. He set the knife down and stooped over his missing daughter's broken bike.

As he brushed his fingertips against the bicycle's parts, the possibilities behind this encounter struck him. Had he, in a horrible seizure of grief, come into the room and moved the bike? He didn't want to think what that meant. Madness. Maybe walking in his sleep and moving objects around the house?

He picked up the broken pieces, then what was left of the bike, and moved them to the kitchen, where he placed them inside a plastic bag and began to cry.

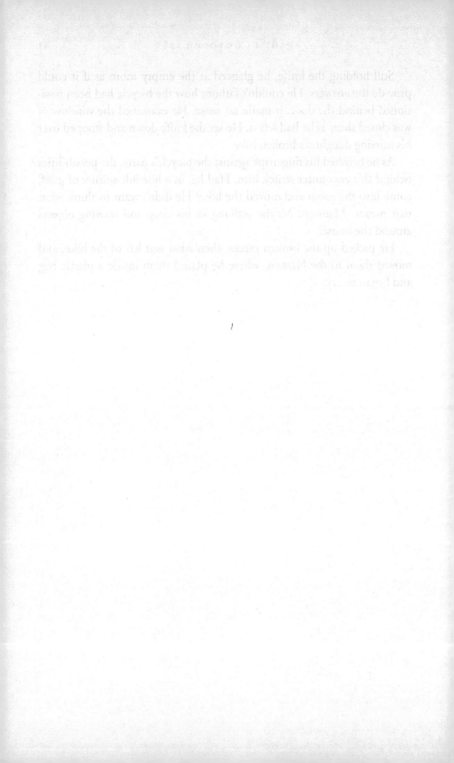

Part II

December 3

Part II

Conclusions

5

When they were home, Elliot used to see them almost every morning, because their apartment was opposite his own. Her mother or the babysitter usually took her out for walks. Elliot did not like the babysitter; he found her reproachful to the daughter.

He used to stand by the window and look up to the road over the steps and sometimes he'd see her, holding her mother's hand with her mitten.

He stood right behind them once in line at the bakery on South Bridge. The girl didn't once look at him, but he watched the back of her head and the braids from her ponytail coming down just below her shoulders in intricate strands.

Another time when they were out, he realized the mother had left the back window unlocked. He slid the window open and crept into the apartment. Their smells reached him. He lay on the girl's bed, and then tried the mother's. He went through her clothes inside the armoire, holding them against his nose and taking it all in. They smelled heavenly. He didn't want to leave.

The first time he saw them, walking out that door, time just seemed to stop. He knew it was a fantasy; he was not crazy. But this was the Grand Plan. His heart, his mind, they were irrevocably caught. He used to think about what would happen if he bumped into them in an adorable "how we met" story, maybe in the process of saving the girl in some heroic act. Then they would discover the things he did; the mother would marvel at them and applaud him, and then she would marry him and the rest would be history. Nothing filthy; that only came later.

There were other times; once he saw the mother go into a young man's house in the afternoon and come out late at night, her hair a mess, and he knew what she had been up to. Elliot followed the man for days after that, always waiting, always on the verge of doing it. One time he sat on the seat behind him on the bus to St. Andrew Square. He watched him for twenty minutes, until he got off. He was this close to doing it. But she never met up with the man again, and he let it go. Until the next young man came along, and the next, and the same thing happened.

Those were the days Elliot tormented himself with the bad dreams. In the dreams, she usually cried before he fucked her and burned her alive. The daughter would watch, silent, expressionless, unlike her dear, bright self.

"See what I have to do?" he would tell the girl, and she would then begin to cry. "See what I have to do so you won't turn out like her?" Then he would let the gasoline wash over the mother. She would apologize profusely. Sometimes he accepted the apology, and the daughter would join him, and he would penetrate them both, soaking in the gasoline, a match nearby ready for action. Most of the times, though, he would watch her being claimed by the flames. She would scream and scream and her daughter would scream and scream and he would wake up soaked in sweat and other nasty things. Those were peculiar times.

6

The body had been pronounced dead, shrouded in questionable happenstance.

It was on one of the narrow passages (called "closes") found on either side of the Royal Mile, running between old buildings. The entrance to the paved close darted from the High Street, flanked by a sandwich shop and an Indian restaurant, and ran through to the stone courtyard of both shops.

Covenant Close. More than three hundred years ago, a copy of the National Covenant was signed in a residence in that claustrophobic lane, preceded by thousands of lives lost. In the early hours of that frosty Edinburgh morning, another life had been lost, turning up dead between the close's stone walls.

Georgina McBride—late twenties, shoulder-length hair, and a detective sergeant's badge tucked in her breast pocket—turned into the close, and that was when she caught the first acrid whiff of combustion. The scene-of-crime van had been parked—illegally—on the road outside the close. The first SOC doctor had already declared death. The SOC officers had taped off the close at top and bottom. A white sheet had been pinned up so that passersby could see nothing but the shadows on the other side. A camera team had just arrived and the mortuary van was standing by. McBride stood for a while on the foot of the close, hesitating, until a deputy waved her in, past the incident tape cordoning off the area where the body lay. In the gathering twilight, the close looked beautiful but desolate.

A lonely place to die.

The deputy escorted her through the close, talking fast as he handed her a clean pair of disposable nitrile gloves.

"M.E. says she's under eighteen," he said.

"I heard she's badly burnt."

He gave a grim smile. "Oh, it's badly burnt all right. But I think you better see for yourself," he said, leading the way farther into the close.

The forensic and photography crews were gathering around a small area, which she guessed contained the body. She recognized a couple of junior CIDs from St. Leonards and some Fettes uniforms, all suited up in the SOCO-trademarked white disposable overalls. They were taking final photographs. She found it bizarre what it all came down to, this bedlam neatly arranged into a fine-grained assortment of puzzle pieces; clean paintbrushes sweeping dirt from the ground into plastic evidence bags, cameras and tripods being repositioned, context photographs being skillfully acquired, everything being bagged, labeled, ordered, and entered into the system. Few things generate more paperwork than murder.

A procurator fiscal was talking to the medical examiner, Dr. Mareth. The M.E. saw McBride coming toward the body and gave her a nod. Dr. Ermis Mareth had a weak chin and a face that looked like it rarely saw the sun. His hair, the color of early-morning summer fog, looked as if it had been used for an experiment with the powers of electricity. Sharp eyes squinted like shards of blue glass behind steel-framed glasses. He always had that hunched, anemic look that hinted at years of hard work. He was the program director for forensic medicine at the University of Edinburgh, and he would frequently serve as forensic medical examiner to the Lothian and Borders Police. It was in this capacity that he had coordinated the pathological aspects of a number of high-profile investigations, like the Lockerbie disaster and the shooting incident at Dunblane Primary School.

On the side of the close, McBride spotted her partner, Detective Inspector Guy Johnson, flicking through the paperwork. She did not acknowledge his presence. She was captivated by the remains that lay between them. As she approached the body, the stink of fire was unmistakable. She looked at the remains and her breath caught in her throat.

The fire had devoured the skin and tissue, turning the body—what was left of it—into a blackened thing of flesh and bone, a charred little doll that resembled a human being only in the most distant of degrees. Internal organs jutted out from the black, shapeless mass that had once been the torso. The larger bones remained, but the smaller ones had calcined, the carbon eradicated from them until they were a crisp gray. Slanted to the top side, a great overseer, the skull lay like a tossed pumpkin. She looked at the hands: small, belonging to—

Oh, God, no, it's a child. It's a child.

Its fingernails were unvarnished and bitten to the quick. The ends of the shafts of the radius and ulna protruded from the exposed tissue of the wrist, the dark amber surrendering to blackness closer to the flesh.

The charred shafts of the tibia and fibula emerged from each of the masses of blackened bone fragments that were the feet. She saw short, burnt stubs protruding from the end of the limbs; she realized these were the child's ribs. There was further damage, lacerations and scabbing; rodents had gnawed at the remaining flesh and bones. She felt a rush of pity and something more: sorrow, or even love, born out of a feeling of intense loss.

The poor, poor child.

She pushed the regrets away; they wouldn't help.

"Thought you would have beat me to it," a husky voice said. D.I. Guy Johnson sneaked next to her from behind. He had called her into the office saying they had a fresh one at Covenant Close.

"Had some things to take care of back at headquarters," she said, her eyes never leaving the remains. She looked up and saw his grim expression, staring at the burnt child.

Johnson was a slim man with a freckled complexion and neat, kempt auburn hair in a cut that hadn't changed in the five years McBride had known him. For all she knew, he had emerged from his mother's womb with that haircut. His mouth was shaped by a short, pointed, gray mustache. He had a long nose, which jutted out between two keen eyes set close together and behind eyelids that often twitched from lack of sleep. His expression was always intent and serious, his demeanor not often so.

Medical Examiner Mareth walked over to them. "Good news is," he said. "We got enough urine to test. Might get some DNA around her."

"He gave the victim a golden shower?"

Mareth nodded. "In all likelihood after the burning."

"Making the humiliation complete."

"How do you know it's a she?"

"Because of the skeleton." Mareth pointed to what was left of the pelvis, obscured by ash but still visible. "The pubic bone of the pelvis is too wide for a male. Then the bone landmarks for muscle attachments—brow ridge, eye sockets, jaw—they are too small; she's female. Judging from the length of the femur and the lack of epiphyseal plate fusion, I'd say she couldn't have been more than six."

"Any evidence of restraint?"

"Her legs and arms had been tied, but that was before the burning."

"How can you tell? I thought the rope would have been burnt with everything else."

"The heat from the fire makes the muscles contract as water evaporates. The stronger muscles bring your arms and legs into a flexed position, resulting in this defensive, bracing posture that we see here, with the hands tightened into fists, similar to those of a boxer in a ring—what we call the pugilistic posture, or boxer's stance. If the limbs had been tied when the fire was set, the arms and legs would have been straight."

"Hard to see how this could happen without fuel oil or something. You'd have to add an accelerant to light her up like that, right?"

Mareth nodded. "We'll run a gas chromo, see what he used."

"Any ID, rings?"

"Everything melted under. No jewelry, as you can see. There is a scar in the abdomen, though. Looks surgical. Can be a point for identification." He made a movement with his head as if making a mental note of it.

"I'll run the details through the missing-persons database," Johnson said. "See if we get a match. Race, size, age—anything that can help the profile."

"Are you sure nothing was taken from the body? Maybe any trace of belongings found about?" McBride said, and Johnson gave her a puzzled sideways look. "Why do you say that?" he asked, but McBride didn't reply.

The stone ground below the body was coated in an unctuous, brownish tan. The same oily substance also lay around the remains.

"What's this brown stuff?" she said.

"Body fat."

"Would make you stay away from sausages in a pan," Johnson said.

"Speak for yourself," Mareth said. "Most important meal of the day."

There was a sound behind them. One of the uniforms was vomiting onto the side of the close. A colleague had propped an arm on his back, trying to comfort him.

McBride turned back to the remains. "Time since death?"

"Normally," Mareth said, "I would need to trace the extent of decomposition in amino and volatile fatty acids from the muscle. These are normally destroyed by fire, but the condition of this body means that the amount of soft tissue may be enough to perform the necessary tests. Based on insect activity on the unburnt tissue, I'd guess we're looking at no more than ten hours. The precise time of death will take longer to establish, for a number of reasons. First, the cold weather will have slowed the rate of decay. Second, because of the nature of the death."

He saw their faces—a perplexed expression he had seen too many times on his students' faces—and explained. "Normally, rigor mortis sets in the muscles because the energy source for muscle contractions has been depleted. This happens around three hours after death, leaving the muscles rigid until the body starts to decompose. But struggling before her death would have hastened the process; energy residues become depleted during the struggle and rigor mortis occurs more quickly."

Johnson pointed at the skull. It lay faceup, flexed to one side among the ashes, its crown marred by a cavernous hole. "Is that a blow to the head?"

Mareth shook his head. "Not necessarily. In fires of high intensity, temperatures will rise enough that the fluids inside the skull will vaporize. The pressure inside the skull will continue to build, since its only outlets are plugged by soft tissue. The surge of gas pressure means there will be a point that the vessel can no longer hold, and then"—he placed his palms facing each other and retracted them at once—"kaboom."

"Christ." McBride considered all the ups and downs of teenage and adult life that the girl wouldn't get to experience: travels, university, driving a car, falling in love. She tried to grasp what must have been going through the girl's mind during the last minutes of her short life.

Put aside the person. Look at the puzzle.

She pointed out of the close, where two bulky trash dumpsters rested on the pavement of the High Street. "Those bins are normally located on the entrance to the close. It's so narrow here that they block the way to pedestrians, right?"

Johnson nodded. "So you're saying . . ."

"He either came through the back of the close or threw the body from the front entrance and over the bin."

"He sure has to be strong to carry her such a long way without her struggling."

She turned, facing Mareth. "Who called it in?"

The M.E. pointed to a short, bald, stocky man sitting on a ledge on the other side of the close. "Albert Mercy, bin man."

McBride walked over to him. "Mr. Mercy, I'm Detective Sergeant McBride. How are you holding up?"

The man was shaking his head in shock. "I've never seen a dead body in my life. I mean, not before they put him in a coffin, you know?"

"We're going to make it as easy and straightforward as possible. I just need you to tell me what you saw."

His eyes were almost in tears, trying not to look behind the D.S., where the body lay. Johnson approached them, taking note of the conversation.

"I went through the close and at first I didn't notice anything wrong," Albert Mercy said. "I tried working the bin and I smelled something burning. I thought someone had thrown one of those bloody cigarettes in there, but there was nothing. Then I saw the child. Who would do that?"

McBride nodded.

"I nearly lost my breakfast," he added, covering his mouth.

"Did you see anybody hanging around here?" Johnson asked.

The bin man shook his head again. "Too cold today," he said, exhaling puffs of frosted smoke. "Even for the homeless."

McBride pointed to his bin cart, which stood unattended at the foot of the close. "We're going to need all the rubbish that you picked up in the area."

He nodded in agreement.

"You find anything like that before?" Johnson asked.

The bin man thought for a second, then pointed east, to the hill overlooking the city. "Dead goats, chickens, near Calton Hill. Some weird people in this city."

"Mr. Mercy, I'm afraid I'm going to need your boots."

The man looked down at his boots, noticing parts of human flesh clinging to them, reduced to ashes from where he'd stood over the body. "Oh, bloody hell . . ."

"It's just so I can eliminate your footprints," McBride said. "You'll just have to sign a form and we'll have them sent back to you."

"Are you mad? Throw 'em away. Burn them. I'll never wear 'em again," he said, at once untying the shoelaces.

Behind them, Mareth was asking the SOCOs whether they were finished with photography. The photographer snapped one more picture of the remains, then nodded assent. The preliminary sketches had already been made, the measurements taken. The evidence technician with responsibility for the close had finished his work around the body and had moved on to the periphery of the crime scene. A pair of medics waited in one corner with a stretcher, ready to move forward. What was left of the body was going to be placed in a white body bag to be taken to the city mortuary for autopsy.

D.S. McBride looked out of the close to the side of the High Street. Tourists would soon be swarming the place, defying the cold and photographing each other next to Mercat Cross, Deacon Brodie's, and the rest of Edinburgh's dark-tourism sites, ascending to the castle in flocks or going down Cockburn Street to buy a Ouija board. In the distance, sirens were headed elsewhere.

"Anything strike you about it?" D.I. Johnson asked her.

"No."

"What was that business about the victim's possessions, then?"

"Huh?"

"You know, when you asked the M.E. whether any possessions had been removed from the body." He placed a hand on the gray hairs of his beard. "You have an idea about this, don't you?"

She nodded. "I think I know who's responsible for this."

7

The airplane was sparsely populated. They were floating high above lush gold and green farmlands. The azure sky spread out over the flat fields, which soon gave way to verdant hills, and then mountains. From his window seat, Alex Whitman turned to the man next to him and watched the soft, cigar-scented puffs of air erupting from his plump lips. He then lapsed into his thoughts.

For the past six weeks he had been following trails that might have led him to inventor Augustin Sekuler and his lost film "Séance Infernale." But the trails had long gone cold. The failure to find a valuable clue spun, *moto perpetuo,* around his brain as he considered the concrete beginnings of his investigation turning into culs-de-sac and locked doors.

Although there were many locations of interest to Whitman's pursuit, he found that clues had long vanished from these places, if they had ever existed. The sixteen-lens camera prototype had been made in Paris, and it was there that the footage for "The Man Walking Around the Corner" had been filmed. Moreover, the building Elizabeth and Adolphe had been staying at in New York had been demolished fifty years earlier, burying beneath solid cement any evidence or secrets.

His next stop had been London: the Science Museum on Exhibition Road, a paradise of steam engines, lunar modules, and robots. He breathed against the glass, staring at Sekuler's cameras. The first was a sixteen-lens camera that took a series of pictures on film with a paper base using sixteen independent shutters fired in sequence. Two viewfinders were above it. In operation, each spool of film moved alternately and was positioned behind one of the two sets of eight lenses, shooting around sixteen images per second.

Whitman was particularly interested in the second camera, which was single-lens. It was believed that this was the camera that had been used to shoot "Princes Street Gardens Scene" and "Traffic on South Bridge" in 1888. Maybe it was the camera Sekuler had used to record whatever came to be known as "Séance Infernale." The technical file next to the exhibition glass said the camera had been made in Edinburgh in 1888 and it was close to the technology used today. The camera body had been constructed by Frederick Mason, a local joiner. The woodwork was unscarred; the light Honduras mahogany of the camera body, its red glow, the dovetail joints, and the applewood of the feet—everything fit like lock and key. The camera used two three-eighths-inch-wide sets of unperforated film wound past the lens via a pair of spools. The film was held fast for exposure by a flat brass plate, the exposure controlled by way of a circular slotted brass shutter that revolved behind the lens in the same way as a modern shutter.

Clickety-clut, open/shut, now you see it, now you can't.

The camera also served as a projector, for which an arc-light source was fitted to the back.

Whitman asked the man in charge whether there were any files in some dusty corner that might have been overlooked. The man was reluctant at first, but once his palm had been pressed with money, there was little of that. The assistant curator accompanied Whitman to the back rooms.

There he found correspondence in the form of a telegram dating back to 1953. It was from Sekuler's grandson, Albrecht Genhagger, who had moved to Switzerland, and asked if his nephew, visiting London at the time, could be shown the cameras by the museum's keeper of photography. It was a residue of information that seemed solid, an imminent hope for making contact. The letter was postmarked Lausanne. It was, at least, something tangible; if the nephew or his family still lived there, maybe they could provide background information on the mysterious father of cinema. The information office in Lausanne did not yield anything to go by; the address was listed under the name Albrecht Genhagger, but there was no telephone number. This was Whitman's last chance; he'd decided to fly to Switzerland and pursue it.

On his way to the airport, he made a stop at the xxx (illegible) xxx, and two streets down, he pressed the buzzer of a terraced flat. He came back out holding the *Frankenstein* poster in a protective black plastic tube. After ten years, he had finally mustered the courage to pick it up from the unwitting collector in London. He wound across the empty lanes of a district he didn't know the name of, holding the poster he and Valdano had been determined to find on the day of Ellie's disappearance.

Finally, Whitman stopped inside a dark, deserted alley lined with garbage bins and filth. Rats scuttled across the wet concrete. He tucked himself behind a stone wall, took the poster out of its tube, and placed it inside an empty metal bin lying abandoned in the alley. He fished out a lighter from his pocket and lit the poster, his face an expressionless blank, even though terror was welling up behind his eyes. That was what a hundred thousand dollars on fire looked like. He just stood there, watching the poster crumble into the flames.

The plane crossed part of Lac Léman and the river Rhône before the captain announced their descent into the city of Geneva. Circularly and with yaws and dips, the plane drew closer to the lakeside city proper.

For Whitman, an interesting point about Sekuler was that the original negatives had been lost. The surviving footage was the result of the printing of the frames on photographic paper and their mounting on numbered card strips. Each card strip was four vertical, sequentially numbered frames. Perhaps the original film had been cut to save the footage, although this was just a guess. Who made the card strips was also unknown.

In a bizarre twist, the larger part of the printed photographic frames was missing. The last recorded frame number of "Traffic on South Bridge" was 129. This would mean that the footage encompassed at least

129 frames. Yet the footage provided by the museum consisted of a mere twenty frames: from 110 to 129. In a similar manner, the footage from the "Princes Street Gardens Scene" comprised twenty frames. The animation sequences released to the public, therefore, constituted less than twenty percent of the originally recorded footage. Valdano was right: there was something odd about this observed discrepancy. The remaining frames could have been destroyed, lost. Or they might still be out there.

It was Edinburgh that Whitman was counting on the most; both the presence of available information on Sekuler's work and the fact that he'd perfected his invention there suggested it was an important location. The exact location of Sekuler's Edinburgh workshop was known; it had been somewhere on Princes Street, the handsome wide thoroughfare that separated the Old and New Towns of the city. Visiting there, Whitman had discovered that the former workshop was under renovation; someone high up in the chain was developing the space as a department store. Whitman had found the construction worker in charge. After bribing the man, Whitman was told he would be notified if "anything interesting came up."

In addition, the first Edinburgh home of the Sekuler and Whitley families on Ramsay Gardens was documented. However, when Elizabeth and Adolphe, Sekuler's wife and son, relocated to the United States, Augustin stayed behind in Edinburgh and moved to another house, presumably for financial reasons; the Sekulers were losing money every day that he delayed the announcement of his invention. It was in the new house that he perfected the cameras. The exact address of this last residence, though, was unknown.

There was a bump, the screech of brakes, and they were on the runway at Geneva airport. The door was opened and the few passengers filed out.

8

A few minutes remained before the departure of the train to Lausanne. Whitman rolled another cigarette. Next to him, a teenage girl struck a match to light one of her Marlboro Lights. He moved away from her. He rested his backpack on top of a garbage bin. As the flames of his lighter caressed the cigarette, he caught something out of the corner of his eye. He turned his head.

Golden yellow eyes slithered in the distance.

"Pluto," he whispered.

The slender figure of the cat stood next to a girl's suitcase, on the other side of the platform. He froze, an amalgam of memories wrapping around his mind's eye. At first he thought the cat belonged to the girl. But then it trotted to a nearby bench, beneath the seats and through the feet of oblivious passengers, and crept out the other side. With its tail lashing from side to side, it darted ahead, up to the yellow line, as if waiting for the train.

The sight was absurd. Stray animals in a Swiss city. In a train station, of all places. Ludicrous. Impossible, even had the animal not seemed identical to . . .

No, it was ridiculous, it couldn't be. They all look alike.

A train worker crossed the platform, spoke into an official-looking phone on the wall, slammed it down, threw a switch, and raced for the door. Time was short. The train idled, doors open.

Whitman finally climbed the steps, boarding the train as the whistle blew. The conductor slid the door behind him. From the window on the other side, he caught a faint glimpse of the cat's silhouette as it scurried into a corridor and lost itself in the shadows. The station's platform flickered past with accumulating momentum and the carriage rattled and bumped in cadence.

Whitman advanced through the aisle seats to his designated carriage. After repeated body motions and efforts to maintain his balance in the narrow corridor, he finally found his seat. He threw his overcoat on the hanger and sat down. Still staring outside, baffled, he fiddled with his backpack and fished out Valdano's folder.

He gazed out the window; he could not concentrate. He opened Valdano's folder and read through the remaining timeline of Augustin Sekuler's disappearance after boarding a train heading to Paris on September 16, 1890:

1891—Edison applied for his first moving-picture patents.

1894—First cinematograph parlors opened in New York.

December 1895—The Lumière brothers staged the first commercially projected film show in Paris. Elizabeth and the Sekuler family immediately suspected foul play, especially as they saw the Lumières and the Edison Company take credit for what the family considered Sekuler's invention.

United States federal law signified a person as dead only seven years after they had gone missing, which prevented Sekuler's family from taking court action against Edison and his contemporaries. It didn't matter if Sekuler had achieved the recording and projection of moving pictures before everybody else; his adversaries would profit considerably more from a missing inventor than from a dead one.

1901—The Sekuler family was eventually forced to ally itself with Mutoscope during that company's patent wars versus Edison. Adolphe Sekuler worked enthusiastically, assembling evidence from his father's workshop, which—in a mysterious twist—had been broken into following Sekuler's disappearance. The predatory lawyers of Mutoscope, however, had a plan of their own, maneuvering Adolphe Sekuler to serve their own purpose. To this effect, Edison's legal representatives tried to undermine Adolphe's findings absolutely, whereas Mutoscope's lawyers handled his testimony only insofar as it attenuated Edison's claims. Adolphe's most important exhibit, his father's cameras, was never produced by Mutoscope, since that would have obliterated both Edison's and their own claims to the invention of the new medium. To Adolphe's dismay, the cameras were left in the car outside the courthouse, even though the attorneys had made him believe that they would eventually be presented.

1902—During the case appeal, when the court ruled that Edison was not the first inventor of the motion picture, Adolphe Sekuler was not there to hear the verdict. In July of the previous year, he had been found dead, with his duck-hunting rifle beside his lifeless body. The official ruling was that it had been an accident, but the Sekuler family—what remained of it—was adamant: it was the product of foul play. They believed competitors—especially Thomas Edison—had forcefully and illegally taken Augustin and Adolphe out of the way.

1999—French police archives revealed a photograph of a drowned man who may have been Sekuler.

2001—Cinema, an industry enjoyed by audiences of all ages, reached the $40 billion mark.

2002—The mystery remained: What happened to the French inventor? What happened to "Séance Infernale"?

Whitman took the black-and-white picture out of the folder and glanced again at the lost inventor. Gentle, considerate eyes, a well-built in-proportion man who stood at six foot three or four. An unparalleled genius who had been seven years ahead of the Lumière brothers, seven years ahead of Thomas Edison.

Seven years.

During his investigation, Whitman had formed a bizarre bond with the muttonchopped inventor. They were trying to communicate through space and time, the clues from the man's life and work, scattered pieces on a film called "Séance Infernale."

There was another reason why Whitman's interest in Sekuler was growing. This was a fact rarely documented in film books, and it had escaped him until he'd found it in Valdano's folder. It had occurred two years before Sekuler's disappearance, when the inventor and his wife and two children were still based in Edinburgh. As with most macabre incidents taking place in Edinburgh, Scottish publishers such as Robert Chambers had documented the event. Accounts disagreed on what exactly happened that night, and documentations included dramatic pieces of description constructed to add flair to the written reports.

Although the sources failed to indicate Sekuler's exact Edinburgh address, they stated that the family lived in a perilous region, full of seedy businesses, dark alleys, and run-down tenements, a place "where wickedness loses its seductive appeal by manifesting in all its depravity." Sekuler was working late in his workshop on Princes Street while the rest of the family was at home, preparing dinner. His wife, Elizabeth, wanted to run some errands at the linen draper's and hosier's shop and tried to convince the children to come with her. Although Adolphe complied, Zoe wanted to nap. Elizabeth let her go back to sleep and told Adolphe to stay and watch over his little sister; she would go run the errands.

As she opened the front door, she saw the figure of a man framed in the light. She thought nothing of it; the man seemed to pay no attention to her, and the entire area was usually busy after hours. She went off on her errand. The shop was closed for the night. She had been away from home for no more than twenty minutes, she later reported. It was just enough time to save her from the fate that befell those inside.

When Elizabeth returned, she found the house windows sunken in darkness. The door was locked. This was atypical, but incidental: she could have mistakenly locked it on her way out. She rapped on the door; there was no answer. She listened to the silence, and could hear footsteps on the stairs. She thought Adolphe was coming down to let her in. But nobody came.

A feeling of terror washed over her and she banged on the door, attracting the attention of passersby. George Macrankin, the night watchman, came to help. He, too, knocked on the door, but to no avail. The commotion had stirred a few neighbors from sleep, and they stumbled out of their houses to figure out its cause. One of the men broke the window of the basement floor and they clambered into the residence. The house was silent. They darted up the stairs, calling to the children.

At the end of the corridor, a cold draft blew through the passageway leading to the children's bedroom. In these narrow premises, they found Adolphe Sekuler lying facedown on the floor. The boy was soaked in blood, which, they realized, was not his own; upon closer inspection, he had sustained no physical injuries. He was in such shock that he was not able to speak for weeks. They combed the house, shouting Zoe's name, but she was nowhere to be seen. By this time, more people from the neighborhood had gathered outside, and some of them entered the home. They held candles high, looking for an intruder, and someone ran to the borough police to fetch help. Zoe Sekuler was never seen again.

Whitman again glanced out the window. After rolling through a whirling valley of golden fields, the train darted out of a tunnel to accost the immeasurable blue expanse of Lac Léman; from down there, the colossal mountainscape cloaked the horizon. A big estate that could have been Les Rives de Prangins loomed over the mountains. Deep-seated vineyards spilled over the contour like wine in water; past the lake, chalets poked their sloping roofs out from the green blanket. The Stendhal syndrome of this display came, in part, from surprise. There had been no sign of the lake or mountainscape about to materialize. Like Alice going down the rabbit hole, the train entered that tunnel and emerged in a magnificent wonderland of mountains and vineyards and castles and the mist of the great lake enshrouding it all.

The conductor, pockets jingling, came around and validated Whitman's ticket. He shut the folder, grabbed his coat and backpack, and got up. The door at the far end of the corridor had been left ajar, and a sudden breeze flew in, ruffling a suited man's newspaper. Whitman held the door open for an elderly woman and she squeezed through with a cold nod of the head.

He traversed into the carriage where the restaurant was located, feeling the cracking barrage blaring from underneath his feet. He ordered a sandwich and sat at a nearby table, jolted by the train's undulations. A signal post flew past, then a dreary, forlorn platform, with a sign obscured by the train's speed and the overcast sky. Whitman had the vague feeling of being followed, watched by familiar faces caught in the glow of their cigarettes, their facial features covered by the strike of their matches; overcoat-wearing characters entering pay phones and pretending to dial nonexistent numbers; faces obscured by sunglasses and newspapers, reappearing in different locations, even in different countries. As he ate his sandwich, he saw nothing suspicious. By the time he moved on to coffee, the train was approaching Lausanne.

· · ·

A few minutes later, his feet touched the concrete platform of Lausanne Bahnhof. He passed through the domestic ticket section and went out the other side, facing the department stores and a McDonald's. The sky seemed unwelcoming, covered by a deep gray haze that shaded the Old Town. The Cathédrale de Notre-Dame, farther up the hills, darkened the city skyline, like a falcon lying in wait.

One word came to mind: order. Everything moved like clockwork in a pathologically tidy manner; even the buildings were constructed with a no-nonsense quality. The people walking hurriedly among the cobbled streets were coral-faced and flush with vigor, as though they scrubbed their faces with tangerines every morning before sitting down to eat a 150-franc breakfast. The men moved their limbs with the confidence of success. It would take the women a mere twinkle of the nose and a whirl of the waist to make any man fall in love.

The sidewalks of Avenue de la Gare were sluggish with tourists. Peak-capped students and happy shoppers fumbled up and down the steep climbs of the pebbly troughs leading up to La Cité. By the underground passageway serving as an entrance to the platforms, behind a mobile canteen, a violinist was playing "Jesu, Joy of Man's Desiring" with the animosity of a true virtuoso. Whitman looked up at the circular clock above the Lausanne Capitale Olympique logo. A quarter to noon.

He went straight for the taxi stand to his right. He gave the driver the address, and a few minutes later the car was humming along the north bank of Lake Geneva, through the quiet semi-suburban settlement of Saint-Sulpice. The taxi rattled along a cobbled section of the main road, then took a left down the hill from a local restaurant. Picturesque parks and delightful beach paths extended along the lakeshore. Terraces, broken by gorges, rose above the lake. He looked over the jungle of sweetbriar flowers, south toward Morges, behind which extended hidden, vine-bordered vistas and valley towns set athwart fast-running streams. The area separated by the beach paths was sprinkled with imposing medieval residences and immaculate mansions. The wealthy hid their spacious garages and magnificent patrician manors behind high stone walls. The dense and soaring trees did the rest. Directly by the lake and the promontory and its pier stood a Romanesque church, its belfry-windowed square tower dominating the rest of the apsed structure. Two centuries ago, on the grounds nearby, Napoleon Bonaparte had reviewed the army that was to distinguish itself in Marengo.

The taxi stopped before a wrought-iron gate. Whitman paid the driver and told him to wait, in the event he was unsuccessful. He was uncertain whether Sekuler's grandson, Albrecht Genhagger, would be there, and even less certain the man would agree to see him. Still, he could have information on Sekuler or "Séance Infernale." Having only an address to work with, Whitman had written a letter a few days earlier. In it he said he would pay the house a visit on that day at that specific time and that he hoped it would be convenient, but he had not allowed time for a reply. He was hopeful, though, for his letter had been written in a manner carefully calculated to gain him admission.

He got out of the car, taking in the freshwater smell of the lake. The sky looked ominous; a storm was approaching. The iron gate was open. Perhaps they were expecting him. He gazed up at the manor, which was surrounded by a strip of land dotted with gloomy trees.

It was a residential Gothic Revival mansion with thick limestone walls and three scalloped arches over the entrance. The multi-gabled louvered cupola, a self-supporting double-shell dome, adorned the steep mansard roof. Below it, curvilinear, gingerbread-type vergeboards accented the steep, carved gables and pointed arches with ornamented pendants. Modillioned with zinc, cornice molding crowned the diamond-paned colored-glass windows in sculptured elegance and Old World charm.

The gate creaked and slid into place with a click. Whitman walked up a path laid with terra-cotta tiles and lined by ivy-covered tree trunks and vegetation. Fountains trinkled with water among small ponds green-laden with hydrophytic plants. The wind pushed him forward. He took up the moss-strewn stone steps leading to the front door. As he rang the bell, he stared at the inscription above the door's corbeled cap: AD PATRES.

With a little luck, he thought. There was no answer, so he rang the bell again. Hands in his pockets, he turned around and gazed at one of the marble statues by the fountains, thinking. The taxi was still waiting outside the gate.

As he was about to ring the bell again, he heard a noise from inside the house. It was a voice—someone shouting—followed by the muffled sound of something crashing to the floor. He thought of ringing again but decided against it. *A little lovers' quarrel between Albrecht and his Swiss wife?* he thought. Whoever was in there did not want to be disturbed.

Unfazed, he traversed the side of the building through the water-soaked bushes, head ducked, prowling for open windows; they were all fastened. He tried the back door, but it was locked. Then he saw what he was looking for: on the west-facing side of the manor, the curtains of a downstairs window were shivering in the breeze. The window, he realized, had not been opened; it had been forced, the glass smashed in.

Perplexed now but curious, he stuck his head into the opening in the curtains and peered inside. The darkness of a dining room stared back at him. All was silent. Taking care to avoid the broken glass, he climbed in and stumbled into the obscurity of the room.

"The Cat creeps," he uttered under his breath. The house smelled peculiar, old. All the curtains were drawn, giving a dingy, deserted feeling. Moving slowly in the dark, he felt his way around the dining table and through the kitchen. His eyes couldn't serve him adequately, but his ears strained in the blackness. He eased through a swinging door and crossed into a living room. As his vision adjusted to the dark, stairs came into focus.

A woman lay on the floor, motionless. Near her, next to the scattered shards of broken glass and traces of blood, lay a handkerchief and duct tape. Whitman approached the woman's body and knelt down beside her. Her eyes were closed. He didn't see the movement behind him; he felt it. He staggered forward, slumping across the carpet. He tried turning around, but by the time he could register the dark figure, everything was going black.

9

Whitman regained consciousness an indefinite amount of time later. A sharp pain pierced through his skull. He moaned, feeling his forehead. He was looking at the blurry outline of a post-and-beam coffered ceiling.

Out of the corner of his eye, a hand extended toward him and he flinched, his head aching even more with the movement. It was a woman's hand. The nails were painted blood red. She was holding a small, Saran-wrapped plastic bag, dripping wet on the inside.

"Ice," a female voice said in French.

He accepted it with something between a "thanks" and a moan. Something was jutting into his thorax. His glasses. Someone—probably the owner of the voice—had placed them there. He realized he was in a different room from the one he had last found himself in. He was lying on a chenille-upholstered sofa, flanked by French chairs with lion tapestry. A finish of subtle gold-leaf details and architectural medallion designs adorned the walls, emanating a rustic charm. It was a living room with antique furnishings, decorated with Victorian drapes and lace curtains. A humpback Victrola stood on the marble top of a Victorian parlor table.

He recognized the Bechstein grand piano that occupied one corner of the room. He had passed through here on the way to the stairs, although at this point he wasn't conscious enough to remember it. He jiggled his glasses in place. Then he stood halfway up from the sofa, his feet touching the Oriental rug underfoot, and faced the woman standing over him.

She was tall and in her mid- to late thirties. Her medium-length black hair had been ruffled from the struggle, and crimson lipstick had smudged on parts of her cheeks. She was dressed in a black skirt and a short-sleeved top. The effects of the struggle had given her the look of an expensive hooker. Her blood-red fingernails were wrapped around the bag of ice over her head. With her other hand she was holding a cell phone. Her green eyes, a hint of icy steel, scrutinized him with quick, nervous intelligence.

"Vous êtes américain," she said.

He looked back at her, his consciousness still lingering, wondering how she knew. He could picture her as a devious vamp princess, clad in fine lingerie and dancing hypnotically.

"You were talking to yourself while you were out," she said.

The iron gate, the locked door, the broken window, the stairs; the unconscious woman, now fleshed out, standing over him.

She threw him his wallet. He made a mental note to later check whether anything was missing.

"You went through my stuff?"

"I had to know whether you were dangerous or it was just a case of unfortunate timing." She put the hand holding the phone on her slim waist. She looked annoyed, tapping her foot on the floor, waiting for Whitman to explain himself.

"I was . . ."

"Attacked, yes."

"Who?"

"Your guess is as good as mine." Her manner was abrupt and hurried, as if she already knew what he was going to say. She looked as if she wanted to call the police and get it over with, then forget all about it, perhaps peel off her clothes and relax in a hot bath. Whitman tried to stop himself from visualizing the last bit.

"I don't like it when people break into my house."

He apologized. "I wasn't . . ."

"I know," she said. "I did the math while you were out. Whoever broke in here knocked us both out. So maybe I should be thanking you?" She didn't wait for him to answer, as though she wasn't expecting a reply to begin with. "Still, it begs the question of why you were here in the first place."

He scrambled to the edge of his seat, the pain still piercing his head, trying to find the words that eluded him.

"So, Mr. Alex Whitman. Before I call the police, you mind telling me what's your business here?"

"I had an appointment with a Mr. Albrecht Genhagger."

She stopped tapping her foot and gave him a surprised look, blinking. "When did you talk to Albrecht Genhagger?"

"I didn't."

She nodded deliberately, as if that explained everything.

"Do you know if he's available?"

"He's been dead for twenty-five years," she said.

Whitman closed his eyes in pain and disappointment. He should have expected this. He pushed his head back so it touched the pillow, and sighed. The final dead end had manifested itself from the darkness.

"What did you want to meet with him about?"

"About a man called Augustin Sekuler."

She cocked her head in recognition and placed the phone back on the table. She had decided to grant him a little more attention.

"Have you heard the name before?" he asked, running his hand across his face.

She laughed. "I've come across it quite a few times."

He nodded, still dizzy.

"My name's Elena. Elena Genhagger."

Whitman furrowed his brow. "Any relation to . . ."

"Albrecht Genhagger was my father."

"Which would make Sekuler . . ."

"My great-grandfather."

Whitman just stood there as the woman told him she was the only surviving offspring of the Sekuler-Genhagger family.

"But . . . how?" he said. "How is that possible?"

"How do you mean?"

"Sekuler's son, Adolphe, died in a hunting accident in 1901. As far as I know, he hadn't married, and he didn't have any children."

She nodded in agreement.

"And Sekuler's daughter, Zoe, disappeared when she was a little girl."

There was again that hint of icy steel in her eyes. "Zoe Sekuler did not disappear for long; she was found soon after."

"My research didn't show anything like that. When was this?"

"It must have been shortly after the patent wars against the Edison Company. Early 1900s, I suppose."

"That's over ten years after her disappearance!"

"More or less," she said. The rough math made sense.

"Nobody thought to ask about this? What happened, I mean."

She shook her head. "Her disappearance was an incident as mysterious as that of her father." She leaned on the arm of the chair, and for a second her silk stockings came into view.

"My great-grandmother was a very eccentric lady. She was a woman of many talents; a Georgian prodigy, you could say. But she didn't really blend in with the crowd, or even with her own family. She never talked about her disappearance. I only got to see her near the end of her life, when she had almost lost it. She'd had two strokes by then. She still had that kind smile. But she wasn't really there anymore."

Whitman nodded. He imagined Zoe's mother wouldn't really have looked into what had happened; by the time Zoe reappeared in her life, she had lost a husband and two children. Then suddenly, out of nowhere, she was being given her daughter back. She would never question the whats and hows.

"I think we could both use a brandy," Elena said. "Then you're going to tell me why my great-grandfather should be of any interest to you, Mr. Whitman."

"Is that what you do for a living? Find movies?" She had sat down slowly, next to him, her skirt gliding up just a bit too far.

"Sometimes." He took a sip of his brandy. It warmed his throat and seemed to relieve the pain in his skull and neck. "Sometimes it's a film prop or an object linked to a particular film. Other times, it's the film itself. People hire me to find the most obscure things."

"You're something of an archaeologist, then. Or a detective," she said with a smile. "Like Indiana Jones, or Philip Marlowe, *non*?"

"I guess you could say that."

"You said people hire you to find things. What is it that you're trying to find, exactly? I assume it's something to do with my great-grandfather."

"I've been hired to find a film which he is believed to have made."

"A film?" she said, furrowing her brow, trying to follow. "Sekuler was not a director; he was an inventor."

"There's some evidence to support it. Inconsistencies in frame numbers of surviving material, as well as a letter from a man named Carlyle Eistrowe, mentioning a film which we believe was Sekuler's work."

She seemed to flinch at this. Sensing her urgency, he handed her the folder with his research.

"In other words," she said, leafing through the notes, "you have hardly any evidence at all." She chuckled. "The name Augustin Sekuler seems to be quite popular nowadays."

"Why do you say that?"

She crossed the room to a stand holding an old mirror. She reached behind it, pulled out a case. Whitman's gaze wandered over her body, lingering on the backs of her thighs. She clicked the case open and fished out a cigarette. *Closet smoker,* Whitman thought.

She placed the cigarette between her lips and bent closer to him. He brought the lighter's flame just close enough to its tip. "A couple of weeks ago, a man phoned here asking questions. What I knew about Augustin Sekuler, whether I would have any material relating to his life, and so on. He seemed quite persistent. I was curious, so the next day I called the contact number he left. The line was dead."

That's crazy, Whitman thought. *Someone is looking for my film?* Or was it just some random film historian, eager to add another trivial fact to another film encyclopedia on Victorian times?

"Do you think there was foul play involved in your great-grandfather's disappearance?"

She smiled, her eyes penetrating his. "You're asking me whether I think Thomas Edison murdered Augustin Sekuler."

Whitman nodded. "As opposed to 'He ran off with the butcher's wife—or the butcher himself.'"

"Few men are virtuous when the reward is only a death away."

"What do you mean?"

She shook her head. "My great-grandfather was dead from the moment he realized his invention. By capturing the moving image, he essentially captured a monster. It is no wonder that the evil men who surrounded him got to profit from his demise. Whether Edison was the culprit . . . I cannot say."

"It would be of great help if you could tell me anything more about Augustin than the few facts I would find in the books or reference materials," he said.

Her icy eyes glared at him as she thought it over for a second. "I could do much better than that, Monsieur Whitman. How would you feel about his wife's memoirs?"

"Elizabeth Sekuler wrote her memoirs?"

"*Unpublished* memoirs," Elena said, smiling. "She tried to offer them to a collection, but her husband's disappearance wasn't considered to be noteworthy. Apparently she felt helpless about the state of things, the disappearance, the incompetence of everybody around her, and the injustice resulting from it. I guess that was all she could do; when nobody understands, or when there is no one around, you can only put it on paper. It's hardly James Boswell, but it could be of importance to your research." She stubbed her cigarette, got up, and opened a cupboard in the vanity. He heard the ruffling of papers and boxes. After a second, she cursed out loud.

"Something wrong?" Whitman called from the couch.

"It's not here," she said. Her face peeked at him from the sideboard. "I keep everything related to Augustin Sekuler in here. Nothing valuable is missing—I checked. None of the jewelry, the paintings, the antiques . . . Given your current situation, I wonder if you know anything about that."

Someone was definitely following his trail. Someone who wanted the film. He could think of no candidate other than his own employer. Whitman stood in silence, the unfamiliar faces in the shadows crawling around his brain. "I have no idea who would be interested in this, apart from my client."

"And who might your client be?"

"That's confidential, I'm afraid."

"I'll have to call the police," she finally said.

"Have you read the memoirs? Can you remember anything that would help my investigation?"

"What do you want to know?"

"An address, a clue, a location, anything. Also, anything suggesting that he was recording footage other than the material we know of."

"I have read and reread those memoirs, monsieur. No film is ever mentioned in there. She does mention Carlyle Eistrowe, though; he was a good friend of the Sekuler family."

"He was a talented man."

"Eistrowe? He was a leading mountaineer, a scandalous poet, and a double agent. He taught the man who would later go on to create the jet propulsion system. He influenced Huxley and Dahl and Fleming, the Beatles and Genesis, Ozzy and Bowie, Somerset Maugham and Hemingway."

"He also tried to raise the devil a few times, from what I hear."

"Dig into any modern occult or neo-pagan system of thought and you'll find his name."

"Was he involved in Augustin's recorded footage?" Whitman asked.

"Not that I know of." She leafed through Whitman's final notes. She made a movement to cross her legs and Whitman glimpsed the luscious shape under her silk stockings.

"It seems your investigation might have reached a dead end." She smiled. "I think we should look more into the Edinburgh connection. If there's any trace left, it's there."

"We?"

"I'm offering you my services. As a partner, an ally."

"I work alone."

"Surely you could use my help."

"Surely not."

"I might remember something from the memoirs."

"Call me if you do."

She laughed. "A man of considerable privacy, Monsieur Whitman. I'm starting to think we are the same, you and I."

He made a movement to get up and his eyes locked on the insides of her stockings. She caught his glance and flashed him a smile that was up to no good. Her green eyes were now sparkling, and Whitman had to do a double take; if there was such a thing as an ancient mystery, it was all in her eyes. By attempting to journey into their wild, he found himself entering uncharted territory.

She shook her head, stood up to face him, unzipped her dress, and stepped out of it. She stood there in front of him in stockings and underwear, as though she was waiting for him to tell her to stop. He could only stare at her. Finally, he placed his hand on her thigh and ran it slowly upward. She moved like a cat, as if her body had learned to defy gravity. She pushed him back on the couch and straddled him.

She attacked his mouth, biting his lower lip and then kissing him on the neck before returning to his mouth, and all the while they were taking each other's clothes off and tossing them to the floor. They grabbed at each other in some sort of emotional desperation. Sweat dripped off their bodies as they went at each other, her hair in his face, her legs wrapped around his torso, her arm clasped around his neck.

A beeping melody broke through their exchange. She didn't want him to stop; she kept telling him to play with her, to touch her. He struggled to place his hand on her mouth, and with the other hand he fished his pants from the floor and reached for his cell phone. She slid off him, a disappointed look on her face.

He apologized and retreated to a corner of the room, a part of him welcoming the phone's interruption. A muffled, distant voice came from the other end of the line.

"Who is this?" Whitman asked.

There was a crackle and the noise of construction.

"It's Tony Dickson, from the stoor at Edinburgh Princes Street. You said I should call if anything came up. There's been a situation here."

"What kind of situation?" he said.

"Well, you knaw how this banger is being restored and renovated, you saw it yoorself."

"Go on."

"Aye, this is the thing. The people doing the renovation wark, they foond something."

Whitman smiled.

"It looks like a trapdoor of soom kind," the man continued.

"Have you looked to see what's in it?"

"It's roosted shut. We've got hold of a maintenance man coming later tonight."

"Have you told anybody about this?"

"I'll have ta. There's a bloody hole on the flare."

"Can you stall it?"

There was a pause, during which Whitman could smell the desire for British sterling emanating through the line.

"You will, of course, be well compensated for your help," Whitman said.

The man complied.

He took a look at his watch. "I'll be there in a few hours," he said, and hung up. In spite of the head rush, his eyes were restless. He turned to Elena.

"Give me a call if you hear anything."

She looked flabbergasted. She could only muster, "I'll call a taxi for you. Where are you going?"

He spotted the ticket desk almost immediately. There was a flight for Edinburgh leaving in two hours, the woman at the counter told him. This left him with ample time for lunch.

He called Valdano, who sounded ecstatic over the latest clue. He was certain the trapdoor contained something Sekuler had hidden, perhaps even the film. He urged Whitman to investigate it further.

Whitman barely had time to gather his thoughts before his cell phone rang again. It was Charlie.

"Believe me," Charlie said, "I'm glad to hear the good news, but what about those *39 Steps*?" Charlie had been calling Whitman from the Crypt regularly for the past two weeks. Their contact in Edinburgh still claimed she possessed a lost director cameo on the Hitchcock film.

"Charlie, how much would the cameo be worth?"

"Less than the ticket across the Atlantic," Charlie replied.

Amid Charlie's reply, Whitman discerned the droning sound of bagpipes in the background. He then understood that Charlie had already planned ahead.

"You're already in Edinburgh, aren't you?"

Charlie laughed. "That obvious?"

Whitman grinned. "Just meet me straight at Sekuler's old workshop on Princes."

10

Elliot had never really thought about women before he started this. He never had anything against them, but they were disgusting, the way some of them would look at him. He had girlfriends now and then; he had to get drunk to do the things they wanted, and even then he had to think about fires during the act. He just didn't think that way—it was something he was born without—and he was pleased with this notion: if more people were like him, he reasoned, the world would be better off.

Elliot was fourteen when his father was killed in an accident. He jumped off the Forth Road Bridge. Elliot was never told the details. Mother—this one time she was drunk—said it may as well have been herself who pushed him off that bridge. She left soon after. She was a promiscuous woman who ran off with a fellow addict.

His uncle Emmett took him in. He was kind. He used to take him bowling. Elliot hated it, but he felt sorry for Emmett; he was alone, like himself. Emmett was around a lot, and that made it difficult for Elliot to do all the things he wanted, all those things he was thinking of. One time Emmett caught him setting fire to a dog. He was dead-on with it; he had a solemn talk with him about how it's not right to do that to animals. After that, Elliot started taking precautions, and it must have worked, because that was the only time he ever came close to getting caught trying to set fires. Uncle Emmett died on Elliot's nineteenth birthday. He didn't care to go bowling again.

When the man from the notary public called, Elliot didn't right away understand. He thought the man was one of those people you must talk to after deaths. Even when the man held up the check for the money Emmett had left him, he didn't right away understand it was his. This was Uncle Emmett's money, not his, he reasoned. The amount was £203,000 and some pence. He got the flat on Blair Street, while Cousin—Emmett's son—was left the house they lived in. Cousin was respectful on the surface, but that was all; he really despised him for having all that money and not knowing what to do with it. He eventually kicked him out of the house.

Elliot hadn't been to the Blair Street basement flat before; it had been in Emmett's family for decades, but nobody had stayed there for as long as he could remember. Once he moved in, he knew he would hate it. So close to the Edinburgh city center; a pub across the street; a nightclub right next to the flat. The first nights he couldn't sleep. But then things started changing. He considered the freedom he had. He was alone, but he was free to do as he wished. Then there was her: living across the hall from him, with her daughter, both of them radiant among the dirty clouds of this macabre city, like moths in a swamp.

He had a job at some company called Boiler and Gas Services. He hated it, but it gave him access to gasoline and a van, which he eventually bought. The van was a great advantage; there was space down the long side in the back for a full-size bed. It could easily fit a little girl.

As time went by, he thought he might forget about the Grand Plan, forget about the mother and her daughter. But forgetting is a process that is always uneven: you may forget a few things one day and forget a few things another day again, but some things never really leave you. Especially people: try to forget someone and you may wake up one night to find that the memory of the person has stayed with you all along, sitting on the foot of your bed, watching you while you sleep, and roaming your room like a ghost.

It started when he was deep-cleaning the flat. It had been empty for so many years, gathering dust. At some point on that day, he'd decided to move the furniture in order to clean the floors. There was a huge chest in the hall, and once he moved that out of the way, he saw something peculiar. There were stone tiles among the bricks of the wall.

The edges of the bricks bordered the outer parts of a mosaic pattern on the wall. Elliot knelt down. He rolled aside the end of the rug, and a hairy spider scuttled out and faded into the shadows. Clouds of dust hovered in the wavering light. He finally decided to roll the rug into a long tube and prop it against the wall. He blew the dust away, revealing the full length of the colored mosaic set into the stone of the wall and the floor. After brushing and blowing, he stepped back to look at it. The pattern was about seven feet long and took up the whole width of the hall. At first he was annoyed; he would have to call someone to come and fix this—or maybe he could put the chest back against the wall so it would cover this weird mosaic.

But then it got him thinking: Was there anything behind this inconsistent, polymorphic pattern? He decided the wall was asymmetric anyway, and a little experimentation had never hurt anyone.

Said experimentation started with gentle tapping, then continued with him trying to push that part of the wall. He ended up getting a hammer and smashing a bit off of it. It was hollow inside. By then curiosity had gotten the better of him, so he tore down the rest. A rush of cold air escaped from beyond.

The moment he shone his flashlight into the hole, he knew that the fading beam would light something irrevocably beautiful. But he had no idea what until he saw it.

11

The fog had gripped Edinburgh. It carried the salt tang of the Firth of Forth, mixed with the sharp, nostalgic scent of ghosts and smoke buried within the city, a force both natural and supernatural. The gaslights along Princes Street flickered amid the fog like tips of ashen fire hovering uncannily in midair. They trembled in the wind, each in the sequence a little dimmer than the last, into the pale obscurity that enveloped it all.

The wind was roaring its way down, snapping Whitman's overcoat about his legs like a hefty flag caught on a fence. He crossed from the vast thoroughfare of Princes Street into the paved street that ran parallel; Rose Street gave a back-way entrance to the store.

Tony Dickson's voice greeted him from inside.

"It's amazing what you find in these auld biggins."

Whitman looked at the aging contractor: safety helmet propped on his head, a shirt and tie underneath his blue overalls. He was the chief, the go-to man; nothing surprised him anymore, not even what he was about to show Whitman.

The air was a mixture of dirt, flooring particles, dust, and grime. It was a large main area with high ceilings. It had once been Sekuler's workshop, then department store after department store; now, demolition debris lay in a rectangle of four big piles near the center of the room. Nails and litter covered the floors, punctuated with gaping holes. Long hairline cracks ran across the walls. Dotted across the room, metal post pins attached to baseplates and crossbeams provided an intermediary between the flooring and ceiling. Four fluted columns textured in faux stone plaster remained untouched in the corners of the room. It was a workman's paradise; trowels, straightedges, framing squares, drills, circular saws, cat's-paws, wood chisels, ratchet wrenches, gauge rakes, hammers, tape measures, all begging to be picked up and have a go at the place.

"You ken wit a mean," Dickson went on. "In my time I've found everything—fram ancient placks to a pocket watch."

"What about this hatch you found?"

"Lad's sawing off the lock reet noo."

They passed through the rusty nails and wire mesh to an empty, grimy back room, until recently a stockroom facility. The floors had been stripped to the underlayer. The floor bulged and dipped. A dead mouse lay in a forgotten corner.

"Mind yer feet, big man," he said. "This way." Dickson explained how, during renovations, surprises often lurked beneath floors, behind walls, and above ceilings.

"I mind we gart a manufacturing plant near Broxburn, aye, and we foond asphalt under the flare that we needed to blooter. Trying the big jessie way in constructing new flats and yer arse is oot the windae." He shook his head. "It didnae work with old biggins. You know, a big pipe mee run through a room, the woolls may be of different heights, aye? And these heid bangers at the council didnae make things easier for us. But this . . . this I never seen before."

At the far end of the room, a man was stooping down a lowered part of the underlayment, using a chain saw on something at full throttle. They joined him.

Dickson motioned at the man and introduced him as "Stan Lee." Struggling with the saw, Stanley muttered something that sounded like a vowel under his breath.

"We're giving it the full warks, you see—gutted, new drainage system, rewiring," Dickson explained. "We were gonna tak out the flare in the

cellar to lay new cundies and also because there seemed to be damp—nae
doot there was a fousty smell to the place, and we needed to find the ruit
of the problem, you see. We thought we would find auld cundies, open
cundies. Maybe even a trickle of a syke, you know these bangers mean
damp. Instead the pneumatic dreels fund this."

It was an iron trapdoor, the size of a Danish casement window, halved
in two cellar flaps with a metal handrail mounted on each of them.

"Must be gey old, eh?"

"How do you make that out?"

"No clue."

Whitman conceded, as if the man had a point. The trapdoor was situated a story or so beneath road level.

It took the strength of both men to pull it up. The trapdoor latched
open with a solid thump, as if it was a living organism taking its first
breath in a century. Darkness lingered within.

"We're gonna need a light."

Whitman instantly pulled a flashlight out of his seemingly endless
Sport Billy coat pockets. At the sight of this, Dickson made a whistling
sound.

"You're gey graithed, aren't ya?" he muttered.

Whitman expected the door to open to a basement or vault space,
but he was wrong. For such a big hatch, it opened to a limited space, no
more than three feet down. There was a grating, and air was coming out
of it. It had been open to all kinds of nasty things, but it was over a shaft,
so it had never flooded within. Whitman couldn't discern anything on
the grating; he shoved his hand into the opening. It was dirty and damp,
numbing him. As his fingers worked through the gap, he felt something.
He grabbed hold of the can and pulled it out, then struggled to turn it
open.

"Whit is that?" The contractor sounded disappointed.

Whitman didn't answer. He ran his fingers through the soft and
mushy material of the film.

"Pictures?" Dickson said. He seemed uninterested, even disgusted, as
if this had been part of a bad joke.

Whitman backed away from the trapdoor and, squatting, placed the
film in front of him. Precisely calculated, the successive wrappings of
the paper rolls had protected it. Each time they were wrapped around,

the picture underneath was protected. He examined the end of one of the rolls. He silently read the words.

"Eastman Paper Film." It might as well have read "jackpot."

Dickson was bending over the hatch, his hands in there up to his arms.

"You a historian or something?"

"Or something."

"A right gunk. Some pictures." He chuckled again. "I thought it been a posie in there; why in God would someone scouk pictures?"

Whitman seemed to remember something, and reached into his overcoat to pull out his wallet. The sight seemed to please and embarrass the contractor at the same time.

"If you tell your employer about this, he's going to take away these things and throw them in the trash. I mean"—he turned the mushy film over—"it's just pictures." He snapped his wallet open and held it close to the man, letting him catch sight of the bills inside.

Dickson nodded.

"I can take them off your hands for . . . say, two hundred?"

The man stood with his mouth agape. With effort, he closed it and swallowed hard.

Even the most ethical man only needs a devil to become a sideshow; there is no man alive who will not give in, as long as it is the right temptation offered at the right time. Whitman was a whiz when it came to the right temptations at the right time.

"No one will know," Whitman continued. "Not with a little floor leveler." He winked at him.

The contractor blinked at the floor. "Three huyner," he said.

Whitman stood for a second, a hint of a grin touching his lips. "Three hundred it is."

He handed a wad of bills over to the man. The man placed the money in his workman's front pocket.

"Nice doing business with you," Whitman said. "If anything else springs up, you know how to reach me." As he turned away, he heard the contractor call out to him.

"These bangers worth anything?" Dickson said.

"Honestly? It's worthless," Whitman answered without turning back.

· · ·

He met up with Charlie at the junction with Castle Street. The fog enveloped them, rising from the wet grass of Princes Street Gardens, hovering amid the faint glow of the streetlights, forming a Gothic gossamer.

"What happens now?" Charlie asked.

Rose Street was busy—workers walking home eased past; groups of students on a pub crawl. Girls out at a hen party blew kisses at Charlie as they stumbled past, then turned their attention to a crowd of young men smoking outside the Black Rose Tavern.

"I called Valdano and told him what I found; my flight leaves tomorrow night. I carry these babies over to him, his minions do their mumbo jumbo, and we see what's in them. If this really belonged to Augustin, then we're on the right track. If it's the film Valdano's looking for, so much the better: I get the rest of my pay, everyone goes home happy."

Charlie bowed his head, staring at the ground as they walked. "Yeah, great, isn't it?"

"You tired or what?" Whitman said. "I thought we were going to check out *The 39 Steps*."

"Yeah, I mean, I want to. I really do . . . but aren't you just a bit curious?"

"What do you mean?"

He stopped walking and Whitman paused, looking into his friend's eyes.

"Well, here we are with maybe the first film ever made—and I don't mean the first footage ever recorded, I mean the very first motion picture. Don't you want to see what's in it?"

Whitman drew from his cigarette. He had been so fervent on tracking down the lost item that he hadn't considered what would happen if he actually found it.

"And I'm not saying that this actually is the 'Séance Infernale,'" Charlie continued, "or whatever its title is supposed to be." His hands were telling the story now, a signature gesture inherited from his Sicilian lineage. "But it's a fact that this place was once the French dude's workshop. That means it's probably his film, and it doesn't matter if it's the one Valdano is looking for. It doesn't change the fact that it's maybe the first of its kind."

"You know that thing you do with your hands? Gets me every time," Whitman said. "I swear, it's like you used to be deaf at some point."

"I knew you would say that. Like I know you will agree to screen the film before Valdano gets his hands on it."

"How do you know that?"

"You said 'Augustin.' You're calling him by his first name. Like you know this dude. Like you share something, some connection."

Whitman coughed on the smoke of his cigarette. He dropped it on the ground and stubbed it with his foot. He cleared his throat. "Even if we wanted to screen the damn thing, we can't. We need equipment. It's paper film, Jabba; put it in any kind of modern projector and we're screwed."

Charlie grinned; he had an ace up his sleeve.

"You've thought this through already, haven't you?" Whitman said.

"Guy I met at USC, he's been working at some film archive right here in Edinburgh for the past three years. He has the right equipment. I haven't told him what we need it for, but I bet he can help."

"Can he be trusted?"

"Does it make a difference? You don't trust anybody."

"I just lower my expectations to the point where they're already met."

"I can make an appointment with him for tomorrow morning."

Whitman looked at Charlie, and weighed their options. "Twenty-four hours," he finally said. "That's how long I can stall Valdano."

12

The fog was receding, but there were puddles all about them as they got out of the Volvo. The parking spaces in front of the city mortuary were taken.

"Something about the morgue, after hours," Johnson said.

It wasn't the morgue, nor the late hour, McBride knew. The Cowgate was part of the lower level of Edinburgh's Old Town, built around the elevated streets of South Bridge and George IV Bridge. As a result, many of its sections were gloomy and dark. The street had once been the loan along which byres of cows were driven out to pasture. Now it was dotted with nightclubs; the only grazing taking place was by the drunks roaming its spaces. But the city was hidden; it still had a lot to give to the attentive viewer. Every now and then an old close in the most visited part of town would reopen. You could have walked past it every day on the way to work and you wouldn't have noticed it, padlocked behind doors or hidden underground. It was right there, for everyone to see, yet it was unknown. But that was Edinburgh, revealing itself only in the constant vigilance of dark, steady eyes.

One of the most famous Edinburgh stories had to do with the construction of the New Town. During the construction, a shopkeeper called George Boyd began to deposit the stone and plank from the building work onto an artificial hill, which would directly link the New Town to the Old. Others soon followed, resulting in the formation of the Mound. Unfortunately for poor old George Boyd, the construction of the Mound entailed the demolition of his own shop.

The façade of the mortuary looked down at them; McBride frowned at the tomatoes being grown on the windowsill. Dr. Ermis Mareth had temporarily set up his forensic medical lab in this building. He met them through a set of double doors, and then guided them into the lab.

The autopsy room was an assault of acrylic, formaldehyde, and moonlight. It was a twenty-by-twenty-foot chamber with a ceramic tile floor. Overhead, the cavernous skylight cast glimpses of the moon on the surgical cart, autopsy saws and scalpels, enameled dishes, organ scales, evidence cabinets. Every inch of the walls was painted with gray acrylic. There were no windows in the room proper; only a gallery walkway and observation glass for the medical students.

The walk-in refrigerator was built into a wall at the far end of the room. Its door lay ajar, inviting. It was flanked by a series of capacious sinks and stainless-steel cabinets. An integrated ventilation system suctioned deleterious odors and pathogens out through a noisy exhaust fan.

The highlight of the room was a transportable postmortem table supported by iron legs and swivel wheels. Shallow channels cut into the tabletop, allowing the discharge of fluids into a wall-mounted dissecting sink. This wouldn't be necessary today; there was nothing left to drain out of the body. On top of the stainless-steel surface, what remained of the girl lay inside a black pouch that looked like an *infernale* cocoon.

Mareth had just walked in, having spent a few minutes in the men's locker room to suit up in the appropriate medical garb. He handed Johnson and McBride two pairs of blue nitrile gloves, asking whether they would need face masks. They both said they wouldn't.

"Two objects can't interact without leaving traces on each other," he said.

"Excuse me?"

The M.E. parked the table near the sink and locked the swivel casters.

He squinted through the frames of the rimmed glasses he wore behind his own mask. His voice was now muffled.

"That's the motto I base my whole working life on, Detectives," he said. "That's why, no matter how smart a criminal thinks he is, I'm smarter."

He gestured toward the autopsy table. His hands were always stained and soiled with chemical compounds, yet he possessed an extraordinary delicacy of touch, as both detectives frequently had occasion to observe.

From the moment she stepped into the morgue, Georgina McBride had been biting her lip. In her law enforcement career, she had seen all kinds of damage done to people, but a child victimized was a different thing altogether.

If you'd caught this bastard, she wouldn't be here.

The medical examiner unzipped the pouch and spread it open, its plastic rustling. A putrid stench of decomposing flesh reached their nostrils. The charred remains of the hand-stitched rag doll now lay across the stainless-steel surface. Each of the bones was marked, the larger pieces with stickers and the smaller ones with string tags, all of them with notations.

"Let's see what we have so far," Ermis said.

There was almost nothing left of her face. Thick sutures lined her forehead; half of her face had been peeled back to examine the skull. McBride wanted to turn away, to jump back and cover her nose and mouth. But there is no cover from that stench, unlike any other, clinging to the roof of the mouth.

Don't do it. Don't fuck yourself.

Mareth switched on a magnifying lamp and positioned it above the body. Both uniforms stepped closer to the table.

"Hairline fractures on right wrist and rib, bruise marks on breast and arms," he said.

"Consistent with restraint?"

"Yes, but like I said, that was before the burning took place."

He pointed to the lower limbs.

"Deeper contusions on the legs."

"Knee marks."

McBride picked up a folder from the countertop and glanced through the girl's autopsy control and initial investigation. She was three foot six and weighed thirty-nine pounds. On a body diagram, the M.E. had drawn the observed contusions.

"But she died from the fumes, right?" Johnson said. "I mean, the perp sets her on fire, she breathes the carbon monoxide, then—bam!—she's down before the flames reach her vital parts."

Mareth shook his head. "Carbon monoxide levels in her blood suggest that the fire wasn't large; it was set with skill and applied so that it progressively burnt first the calves, then the thighs and hands, followed by the torso, forearms, breasts, upper chest, face . . ."

"And then death."

"Heatstroke and loss of blood plasma resulting in death, yes."

McBride watched her partner remove a black ballpoint pen from the holder of a concealed tape recorder. He slipped out a small spiral notebook, ready to scribble. She had seen him fiddle around with pens, papers, key rings, his eyes never on the deceased. She understood why.

He had once told her about the World's End murders. In October of 1977, two seventeen-year-olds who had finished their pub crawl at the World's End Pub, on the High Street, had gone missing. Their bodies were found the following morning, beaten, raped, and strangled. Johnson, and others she knew, had worked the case; they all carried with them the exasperation of a mystery unsolved, and most of them would carry it to the grave. Because a murder investigation is first and foremost a hired investigation; your client may be silent and dead, but he is still screaming out for justice. Sometimes, if McBride listened carefully, she could still hear the victims screaming—not ghosts, nothing supernatural, merely moments in time, trapped in horrible injustice. Screaming.

These cases had sent her back into the vortex of their screams. Sometimes it took all her strength to pull her back to the here and now.

This is what happens when they get away. When I don't catch them.

"Any evidence of penetration?" she asked.

"No scars on her vaginal area or anus. Also, I'm just waiting on the rape kit to be vouchered; looks like she's negative for semen."

"So she wasn't raped."

"No. Whoever you're looking for is sicker than I thought."

"Burning her isn't sick enough?"

"The rape kit's negative, but I found traces of semen in the urine at the scene."

"Meaning?"

"Meaning," Mareth said, "the perpetrator had either just had intercourse before the act or . . ."

"Or he had a little fun of his own during the act," Johnson said.

"So he burns her and urinates on her—he doesn't rape her, but then masturbates over the body?" McBride said.

"Sure sends a message."

"What about the sealing tape?" McBride asked. "The debris in her lungs also contained some kind of cloth, right?"

"Yes, it was cotton cloth. But the amount of it found in her lungs was insignificant, and none of it was found at the scene per se," Mareth said. "It was probably removed before the burning took place."

"He wanted to hear her scream."

"But in such a crowded place? He would risk being seen. Are we wrong here or is this guy careless?"

"Sounds like he's in his comfort zone. He places her in plain sight; he's taunting us. It's like saying, 'This is what I'm doing, and there's nothing you can do to stop me.'"

"Maybe he lives nearby. It would be easier for him to dispose of a dead body." McBride breathed in deeply, producing a sharp pain in her ribs; her body was craving nicotine, but it was more than that. She knew this emotion from the moment she had looked down at the remains in that narrow close; it was dread. Another story of horror had emerged, but not in a living person's home or workplace; this time it had emerged from the dark depths of the city.

"Do we know at least how long ago she died?"

"Based on insect activity, I'd say between fifteen and eighteen hours ago. Looking at the mummification on the parts of the skin that hadn't burned, he must have kept her in a cool place."

"You mentioned something about identifying the victim."

"Well, in such a situation, the identification of the victim is better investigated using dental anatomical findings. Because of muscular stiffness, I had to remove mandible and maxilla in order to examine the teeth."

McBride looked at the electric saw, the spare face mask and the eyeglasses lying on a table adjacent to the body. She shook her head. "So you cut open her face and mouth."

"There was extensive stiffness of the soft tissues that hadn't been burnt, so I had to cut lateral anatomical structures of the face. It's a lateral labial commissurotomy extended to the mandibular rami; it was imperative if we wanted to identify her."

"And?"

"I spoke to our forensic odontologist, who then compared the antemortem and postmortem data. We have a positive identification."

He went to a nearby desk and retrieved a photograph. He held it out for them to see. It was a girl around five years old, straight black hair, refreshing blue eyes, smiling for the camera next to a lit Christmas tree.

"Meet Emma Wallace. Parents reported her missing six weeks ago."

"Are we sure this is her?"

"Ninety-nine-point-five percent sure."

He noted a scraped, stitched area between her thorax and pelvis.

"And the scar agrees with the findings. It's surgical. Appendix removal."

"How old was she?"

"Five. The estimate we gave based on the sutures of the skull and the condition of the heart and blood vessels was accurate."

"Has the family been notified?" McBride asked.

"Parents took a Valium."

"Six weeks ago," she said, mostly to herself. "He likes spending time with them."

"At the time of disappearance, she was wearing black jeans, a white silk shirt, white panties. Her body didn't have any fiber from those clothes, just that from the cotton."

"She was naked when he burnt her."

"Also her watch, necklace, bracelets: none of these have been found. It's logical to assume the killer has taken them."

"Souvenirs?"

"Perhaps."

Dr. Mareth took off his gloves and rinsed his hands in the vigorous stream of water thundering into the metal sink. He dried them with a towel.

McBride looked at what remained of little Emma Wallace. Her organs were gone. Her skin was mirrored back from her body and spread out in folds that revealed grooves of dark purple hemorrhages of different shades. Her remaining eye was a void, and behind it lay the interior of the skull.

"Using an accelerant could mean biology student."

"Or biology teacher," Johnson said.

"You need confidence to talk in a class full of kids. Pyrophiles are socially incompetent. This guy doesn't go out. He doesn't have friends. He doesn't feel comfortable in front of crowds."

"I'd say neither teacher nor student," the M.E. said. "The results from the gas chromo are back: the accelerant used wasn't benzene."

"What was it?"

"Nitrocellulose. Gas chromo and the sample was a dead-on match with the traces found on the scene."

McBride frowned. "Nitrocellulose? Like gunpowder?"

"Similar gun chemical propellant; it's used as a low-order explosive. But the trace we found is single base; it was not mixed with nitroglycerine. This is not surprising: nitrocellulose has numerous other uses. For example, in my lab demos at the medical school, we use it in the sticky membranes in Southern blots—that's a molecular biology test for checking for the presence of a DNA sequence in a DNA sample."

"So we're looking for a biologist-slash-medic?"

Mareth shook his head. "Nitrocellulose has so many other uses. You can find it in the lacquer varnish of guitars, in some types of film, or even in the flash papers magicians use."

"Musician, filmmaker, illusionist. Sure looks like a big list of possible perps, Erm."

McBride stared again at the girl. An emaciated little person sliced in neat straight lines from chin to genitals, from shoulders to hands, from hips to toes, her chest open like a hollowed-out watermelon. The M.E. rolled the zipper back, closing the pouch as he started preparing the body for its return to the freezer. "Last thing," he said, "and this is where it gets truly bizarre."

"It's not been bizarre enough for you so far?" Johnson said.

"We got the carbon analysis back from the soil lab."

"From the debris on her skin?"

"Yes. The different combinations of rock, decaying plant and animal material, and the DNA fingerprint of the living things found in soil mean that every soil sample is unique to where it came from. As such, we can sometimes pinpoint the mud on a suspect's shoe to a particular garden or even a single flower bed. Topography, climate, course of years, botanical and microbiological functions, conditions of watering, and even human activities—all these result in the diversity of soil. Also, there are millions of fossils, external matter, like pollen and spores, and even artificial materials."

"So we got something?"

He nodded. "Preliminary results show the debris from her skin is indigenous to Edinburgh soil."

"Nothing weird about that," Johnson said.

"Edinburgh soil dating back to the 1700s."

They both stared at him, mouths agape.

"What are you trying to tell us, Erm? That we're looking for a time traveler?"

He laughed, rolling away the steel cart bearing the small black body bag. "Not at all. The perpetrator lives and breathes in our own time, Detectives." The metal wheels clattered on the tile. "The truth is we can't specify where the site of murder was; this is precisely because we live in a city where every nook and cranny could hark back to the eighteenth century: graveyards, streams, sewers; a whole setup of forgotten locations of the past."

As he swung the freezer door open, it made a sucking noise. "Trust me, your perp's no time traveler," he said, unmoved by the stench of ice-cold death. A toe tag hung from the bag's zipper pull, and this would need to be updated; all it said now was "Unidentified," in black ink, and the date and Mareth's signature.

After McBride and Johnson had thanked him and left, Ermis Mareth shut the freezer's steel door and walked out into the room proper, his disposable shoe covers making brief whishing sounds on the tile floor. He untied his blue surgical gown and closed his eyes.

He had preserved parts of her organs in canopic jars; he had arranged for specimens of her brain and eye to undergo post hoc analyses. Mareth would not be able to do anything more for the child. Until they came to take her, she would stay with him, lying in her galvanized steel chamber, where time stood still. If necessary, she could stay there forever.

Screaming.

Part III

December 4

13

It was a beautiful, two-storied Scottish baronial mansion on the edge of Holyrood Park, southeast of central Edinburgh. And it was designed to dazzle.

To anyone who claimed the Scottish film industry was a jerry-built business of shabby character and negligible influence, the edifice was a calculated argument to the contrary. It was designed to resemble a sixteenth-century stately home, even though it had been built three hundred years later. It was embellished with pepper-pot turrets and a tower with eyelets and corbeled bartizans, as well as a cap-house with small arch-pointed windows, reminiscent of a Highland croft house. Tall bushes and vegetation fenced the paved courtyard from the street.

The building had served briefly as a school for girls called St. Trinnean's, and its use had been the inspiration for Ronald Searle's books of the same name; notably, the author's niece had attended it.

Housed within the greater area of the University of Edinburgh halls of residence, the imposing St. Leonard's now accommodated conferences, dinners, and film-related events. Restored to its former glory, it was the headquarters of the Archive, or the Arch, a prestigious Edinburgh film society. Joining the ranks of the Archive could be achieved by member invitation only, and this was notoriously difficult to obtain. This state of things had endowed it with an air not so much of mystique but of privilege and awe.

"I found myself at the Arch yesterday," one person would say.

"Well?"

"Lobbied around with the members and enjoyed a special screening of *The Last Laugh.*"

Whitman and Charlie breezed through the glass doors facing the reception desk. The effect of the sixteenth-century façade was carried inside, where dark-wood-paneled walls, painted ceilings, and great sweeping spaces gave the effect of a grand hunting lodge. Chandeliers hung from the ornate Neo-Jacobean ceilings. There were lovely Arts and Crafts painted panels, emblazoned with medallions depicting the likenesses of the Duke of Argyll and John Knox. The hallway was lined with a notice board full of advertisements, followed by the photographs of every individual society member, strung up along the walls of the grand, ornate wooden staircase leading to the first floor. Whitman eyed the message boards: film seminars, screenings, events.

They spoke to the old lady at reception and, after a phone call, were granted temporary clearance. They registered in a thick volume filled with pen scribbles of names, and then were instructed to sit on one of the couches in a waiting area called the "Sea of Tranquillity."

At the far end of the corridor, the door had been left open, as if to entice prospective passersby with visual access to the St. Trinnean's Room. There was sound coming from a PA system; a seminar was taking place. Whitman sneaked a peek through the opening. The room was set up in a theater configuration with seating for approximately sixty people. A beautifully fitted projection screen loomed at the far end. A large loudspeaker graced each side of a big perforated canvas screen. A mustached man in a tuxedo stood on the podium, rambling about *The Joyless Street* and the New Objectivity movement. He was crouching in an effort to hide his height, as if its very sight would impede the spectators' attention. Whitman had hardly managed to take in any other details when the receptionist appeared from behind him and whispered that they would be admitted upstairs.

They passed the winged Pan (or perhaps it was Mephistopheles—Whitman couldn't make up his mind) on the base of the steps, along with gargoyles, demons, hawks, and other evil creatures, and depictions of family arms and emblems, culminating in a shield showing a lion with the words VIRTUTE ET VORTIS inscribed over it. Charlie gave him a look and said, "Puritans, those original owners, huh?" They followed the erratic twists of the staircase.

Once they reached the upper floor, they found what they were looking for past a portrait of Sir David Brewster and a small library. The door before them was shut, and bore a sign with TO PRESERVE AND PROTECT written across it in bold letters. Whitman made a blowing sound and scowled at its sight. Charlie had hardly knocked on the door before Whitman pushed it open. They found themselves in a well-appointed room, which they had overheard the receptionist refer to as the "Pollock."

It wasn't its spaciousness so much as the manner in which the space had been used. The floor was divided so that hardly an inch was wasted. The room was at once a factory, a studio, and an office. The office part occupied one corner with two desks, on top of which rested two computers and four monitors. There was another desk on the other side, but it was obscured by a record player, a bunch of splicers and a rewind, a DVD player, and a Hi8 video player. The rest of the room was in studio anarchy. Everywhere one looked there were projectors: slide projectors, filmstrip projectors, overhead projectors, opaque projectors. A single projector screen took up half of the west-facing wall, flanked by loudspeakers. Cables abounded upon the floor, snaking around C-stands, Super 8 equipment, and sandbags.

"I'll be right with you," a voice called from between four man-size cardboard boxes stacked in the middle of the room. The boxes were filled with carefully sorted tidbits: lithium batteries, RF connectors, wires, cables. The man wading through them had his back turned to Whitman and Charlie. He was bent on finding whatever it was he was searching for, and he had spilled some of the contents on the floor.

"There you are, you little . . ." he said, emerging from the chaos with a VGA cable in hand. Then he saw Charlie and he became conscious that there were other people in the room. The Catalan was short and slight, with a long, acne-ridden face and a snub nose. Although his long, stringy brown hair—graying at the temples and sticking out at odd angles around his ears—was tied, it still hung down almost to the waist. Enquiring cobalt eyes peered behind glasses with a thick black frame. He was dressed in a scruffy shirt and flannel attire.

"Hi, Nestor," Charlie said.

"Charlie Carmichael!" the man said almost simultaneously, and opened his arms in greeting. But halfway there, he saw Whitman and dropped his hands to his sides. His eyes suddenly hardened.

"What the fuck is *he* doing here?"

"You two know each other?" Charlie said. But he knew the answer, and he could imagine how.

Nestor pointed an accusing finger at Whitman. "Fifteen years ago, this prick broke into the vaults at USC and stole the only copy of *Alice in Wonderland* we had."

"Allegedly," Whitman said to Charlie, grinning triumphantly. "It was never proved."

"Yeah, because someone messed with the security cameras."

Charlie turned to Whitman, who was still grinning. "I should have known," Charlie said, shaking his head.

Nestor paced the room in a fit, red with anger.

Charlie whispered to Whitman, "Is there a single person who you haven't screwed over in this business?"

Whitman didn't answer.

"It's not a rhetorical question, Alex. I mean, really, is there?"

"I know you meant it seriously. I'm still thinking. Do you count?"

"Nestor," Charlie said, reaching for the man with the VGA cable, "calm down."

"I am calm, man! If I knew you'd be bringing this snake to my workplace, I would have brought a knife with me today."

Charlie turned to Whitman. "Give us a second."

Once outside, Whitman dug into his coat pocket and fished out a rolled, crumpled cigarette. He plopped it between his lips and gazed at the busy, active freshmen strolling the university area. The minutes passed, and he had another cigarette. When he climbed the stairs back up, he could still hear Nestor shouting from behind the door. Charlie's voice was tranquil, trying to reassure the man with the VGA cable and the memory of an elephant. Whitman didn't knock, just went in anyway.

". . . as a favor to me. Please," he heard Charlie saying.

Nestor nodded, avoiding eye contact with Whitman. "I'll listen to what you have to say. *Only* as a favor to you." Then he pointed at Whitman. "And he better keep his mouth shut or I'll have security remove you both, you hear?"

"Loud and clear, Nestor."

Nestor turned his back to them—presumably so he wouldn't have to look at Whitman. Whitman realized the Catalan wasn't wearing any shoes and his socks didn't match. At first he thought Nestor was staring at the wall; even after he saw him raising his hand, caressing something, it still didn't make sense. Nestor was looking at a whiteboard.

Half the board was taken up by a screenshot of "Arrival of a Train at La Ciotat," a fifty-second silent documentary shot by the Lumière brothers in 1895. In the classical footage, a railway train appeared on the screen, darting like an arrow straight toward the audience, seemingly ready to rush into wherever they were sitting and reduce them to a mangled sack of shattered bones. The effect was, of course, accidental, but what a magnificent effect it was; using the train as a subject, it would grant a glimpse of that platform to the world even more than a century after it was filmed.

The other half of the board was occupied by a film poster. A Scotland Yard inspector with a talent for hypnosis and disguise stared through wire-looped eyes. He was dressed in a heavy black coat and immense top hat, sallow makeup and eerily symmetrical pointed teeth set in a fixed grin, perhaps hoping to hypnotize and frighten his prey into revealing the secrets of the crime with his terrifying smile. LONDON AFTER MIDNIGHT, the letters on the top said in deep black.

Nestor kept running his fingers up and down the poster, eyelids half-closed.

"What is he doing?" Whitman whispered to Charlie.

"No clue."

"This is like a Gary Oldman scene from *The Professional*," he whispered, and made a movement of tearing up imaginary paper.

Nestor sighed. "Shut up, Whitman." He took a sharp intake of breath between his teeth. "Whenever I get stressed, I need to feel something pure, just so I know that some things are worth living for. That's what this wall is: the polarity of the train that was there and the Chaney film that is lost."

"The man of a thousand faces," Charlie said. It was more of a statement than an observation, a carefully placed whisper of conversation among lovers of the same art form, stimulated by the eerie, lugubrious vibe of staring at a long-lost love. Revered as one of the silent screen's most versatile and gifted actors, and the patron saint of art and movie makeup, Lon Chaney specialized in roles that required him to disguise his features and contort his appearance.

"What a pity."

"You know, he wore a set of false animal teeth, which caused him quite a bit of pain, for that role. They were made of gutta-percha, a hard rubber-like material," Nestor said.

The three of them looked at the man with the top hat; they were transfixed by his vampire getup, with the cape, the razor teeth, and the bulging eyes.

"The man in the beaver hat," Charlie whispered to himself.

"I've been trying to find it for the last twenty-odd years," Nestor said. "All trails vanish after 1967; inventory records from MGM's vault number 7 indicate they had it until a fire broke out. A couple of times I came close. There were rumors that a print had survived somehow: a sixteen-millimeter copy was going around, word was, or some collector was sitting on it, afraid to say anything for fear of losing it to MGM, who holds the rights until 2022. Someone told me once that MGM have the surviving material themselves and for some reason they've chosen to keep it secret; another guy said that they were unaware they had it, that it was lying somewhere, forgotten."

Nestor turned and faced them. He seemed to come around. Whitman and Charlie were still staring at Chaney's eyes.

"You remember what I said on the phone?" Charlie said.

Nestor felt his forehead. He looked like he was having a migraine. "Right. The Eastman paper film?"

"Yes. We need to transfer it to a projectable format: sixteen millimeter, thirty-five millimeter, or even digital. Can you help us?"

"I need to see it first," Nestor said, eyes dimming with fatigue behind his glasses.

"First you tell us what you're going to do with it," Whitman said.

Nestor pretended he hadn't heard him. Charlie gave Whitman a look. That was his call to shut up, take the film out of the bag, and hand it to Nestor.

Nestor handled the film with the same care he would show a newborn. He gently placed it on his desk, like a laboratory specimen of immense cultural value. He switched on a halogen lamp and adjusted its spring-balanced steel arm over the film, shining the light over the glossy unglazed surface, whispering to himself. "Positive opaque copy of a negative . . . the bromide photographic paper, the conventional double-weight fiber base, the neutral-tone bromide emulsion . . . It's paper film, all right."

He looked up into Whitman's inquiring eyes.

"I did an internship at the Library of Congress. Worked with the Paper Print Collection there."

"That's impressive," Charlie said. "It's the only collection of its kind in the world."

"So can it be transferred?"

Nestor crossed the room, stepping over cables, to another desk. On top of it was some kind of machine, covered by a shower curtain. He blew the dust off the cover and unveiled it.

"Is that what I think it is?" Charlie said.

"Process optical printer," Nestor answered. He tapped his nails on the sprockets. "Special projection head with interchangeable sprockets to accommodate paper without mutilating it. I can exchange heads and pins that are necessary to advance the film but won't tear it to pieces. You see the aperture plate over here?

"It's adjustable, so I can frame off-standard lines. Paper prints are produced continuously, without taking into account the different densities of the original negative, so I can use the reflected light to illuminate the parts to be worked on and can calibrate the lighting depending on the scene."

"I've seen this before, at the Motion Picture Conservation Center in Ohio," Charlie said.

"This is a modified version of the one they used. Theirs was equipped with a video tap and frame buffer—but the operator still had to align every frame by hand, leading to a whole lotta jitter."

He caressed the gate of the scanner like it was a beautiful woman. "The film path is short and simple; the film wraps around six three-inch particle transfer rollers and over the film gate."

Whitman glared at Nestor and tapped on his watch. Nestor ignored him.

"This paper film has been through a lot over the last century," Charlie said. "Do you think your printer's going to do the job?"

"Check this out," Nestor said. He spoke quickly when he was excited. "The gate is curved, so that even a warped print like yours will lie flat, with minimal tension on the film. The motor control system uses a patented dancer-arm controller, and the position of the dancer arms is read by a Hall-effect sensor that tracks the position of a magnet mounted at the pivot point of the arm."

"Do I look like I understand Martian?" Whitman said.

"This printer could, in principle, make a negative and then recopy to thirty-five millimeter. And they would look like exact copies of the original paper prints. From there you could create backups on mediaplayer or QuickTime files for a computer, if you'd like something handy to see and easily copy. I could do all this, and I could do it well. But I won't." The last few words he spewed with disgust, all the time staring into Whitman's eyes.

"We need your help," Charlie said. He sensed Whitman next to him. "I mean, *I* need your help."

Nestor shook his head. "This is too much, Charlie. I value our friendship, but"—he pointed at Whitman again—"I don't do favors for lower life-forms."

Charlie pleaded with him again, but the Catalan was having none of it. "How could you think that I would ever do this?"

Whitman spoke then. He pointed to the poster of the man with the beaver hat, the armless knife thrower, the deranged doctor, Lon Chaney in *London After Midnight*. "How badly do you want this film?"

"What?"

"Didn't you hear what I said?"

"What do you mean?"

"What would you be willing to do to get your hands on *London After Midnight*?" Whitman asked.

Nestor took a while to answer. Whitman was confident now, carrying on. "Would you, say, help out an old acquaintance with some paper-film transfer?"

Nestor gaped at him, dumbfounded. "Bullshit," he whispered.

Whitman shrugged, grinning; it was a winner's grin.

"Where did you find it?" Nestor asked.

"Some film storage facility on the border of Culver City and Inglewood—mid-1980s we're talking now—at Turner, after their MGM buyout of films."

Nestor banged a fist on his right knee. "I'll be damned. They had it all along, those idiots!"

"It was labeled as *The Hypnotist,* one of the U.K. titles. Remarkably good condition. Nobody ever checks the alternative titles."

"And they just happened to let you in, I suppose, to take whatever you wanted."

Whitman grinned. "Something like that."

Nestor whispered an obscenity. "There's a name for that sort of thing: it's called a felony."

"Sometimes things just fall out of the backs of trucks. It happens. Check the statistics."

"And you sold it?"

"For a hefty sum."

"You motherfucker."

"First I made some copies for myself and Chubs over here, of course. You can have my sixteen-millimeter copy, if you want. But you'll have to do something for me in exchange."

"You're disgusting."

"Finders keepers. You know those dumbfucks at MGM actually thought there was a reel missing. So not only were they unaware of what they had; its restoration was low-priority. They had it marked as UNKNOWN, on one of those long lists in a kind of film purgatory, where it's hoped the titles will one day be restored. The print was complete, of course. If I had left it there, by the time someone found it, it would have been toast. At least my way someone gets to see the damn thing. It's rescued."

"So you're saying the film is better off in the hands of some private collector, who just happens to have no credentials other than being the highest bidder?"

"I'm saying the film would have been destroyed beyond recognition if I hadn't gotten to it first."

"You don't know that. Either way, it doesn't give you the right . . ."

"Look, Slick. Those archivists that you hold so much respect for are nothing more than glorified pencil pushers. They have no interest in film unless its preservation benefits the curator or the institution holding it. They're not looking for film preservation, only self-preservation."

Charlie burst between them. "Now's not the time for this discussion, guys."

Nestor exhaled, still taking in the news of the rediscovery of his missing piece of treasure. He said nothing, but he relaxed a little and some color returned to his face.

"So will you help us?" Whitman asked.

"It's going to take some time."

"We only have twenty-four hours," Charlie said.

"You're kidding, right?"

They both shook their heads at the same time.

Nestor sighed, eyeballing the poster. Chaney's face stared back at him with wide eyes. "I'll start now. Pull an all-nighter. I'm not promising anything."

Charlie smiled. Nestor pointed at Chaney again. "And I want the *London* cans delivered to my house," he continued. "You're going to get me fired over here."

"I thought you would like to share it with your co-workers," Whitman said with a wicked grin. "Maybe send a copy to MGM while you're at it. Make that a VHS copy—just for the fun of it."

"Fuck off, Whitman."

"So what happens now?" Charlie asked.

"What happens now is youse get the fuck out of here and let me work my magic for the night. Have your phone handy. I'll give you a call early tomorrow and we can look over what I've done till then."

Whitman nodded, glancing at the collage of pictures on the wall. At the Grand Café in Paris on the 28th of December, 1895, the arrival of a train was observed by a handful of individuals. The first train on film, approaching La Ciotat, steaming toward the audience and into history. The magic at the time was that a train and a group of people were moving on a screen; the magic ever since has been the extraordinary location of where that camera was placed; all the more in capturing the ordinary glimpses of ordinary people's lives in a long shot, a medium, a close-up.

As long as the film survives, those people on the station platform survive, too, and perhaps remain trapped in time forever.

"The Lumières were wrong. 'Invention without a future,' my ass," Nestor said. "We're still here."

"Yes," Whitman said, "but for how long?"

14

When Elliot saw what was lurking behind the hole, he knew it was an act of God, and that if God was out there, He was with him.

Tunnels snaking around sharp bends, darkness and passages to the left and to the right, like a labyrinth beneath the building, beneath the city, shielded by thousands of tons of solid rock.

A unique hiding place.

He didn't know who had made this or whether anyone knew about it. It was only later that he found out about the vaults of South Bridge, that there were hundreds of vaults like his underneath the Old Town of Edinburgh. That hardly mattered; he had his own hidey-hole.

The whole idea came unexpectedly, a kind of tour de force out of nowhere.

The biggest problem was noise. There was a fine old wooden frame in the doorway through to the passage, but he needed to fit a door on there. It took a couple of attempts, but he struck gold. It was four-inch plywood embedded with a metal pane in the middle, and that would help with the noises, too. (He later tested this by blasting a battery-powered radio at full volume from inside the vault with the door shut. It was a success, but he still soundproofed the walls—one could never be too cautious.) It was a massive undertaking, but he did it. Then he came up with an ingenious addition to the plan. He made what looked like a set of library shelves and nailed it to the doorway, so that to the casual passerby it seemed it was just a piece of furniture on a wall. He even fitted a mantelpiece to cover the remaining part of the wall pattern. He could push it up, and there it was: his own secret passage. He also fitted a set of bolts on the inner side of the door to ensure his privacy.

Two things he found in one of the vault rooms puzzled him. The first discovery was the skeleton. He knelt next to those crumbling remains. It looked like a grown man. Later he stumbled on a gold watch the man must have been wearing: the initials c.e. were still visible, engraved on the back. Some time after this, someone would break into Elliot's flat and find the crypt—but that would come later, when a mysterious figure would see the skeletons of the children with its own eyes. They were hardly of interest; in the darkness, the figure could not find what it was looking for. There was no sign of the film. However, there was the skeleton of a grown man, sitting in the farthest corner, crumbling away into obscurity. Of course, Carlyle Eistrowe had been dead long before Sekuler laid a hand on that skull.

Next to the remains lay Elliot's second discovery: an ancient projector and a box containing what looked like a reel of ancient film. It was pretty grubby, and some of the frames were stuck together. Elliot soaked the film in water and a wetting agent. Adding the moisture and softening the gelatin worked wonders. After that, a soft cloth took care of the surface matter. Incredibly, the projector still worked, and Elliot had a look through the pictures on the frames. It was all very poetic. It was some story about a man and a skeleton coming to life, and the whole thing looked the way old movies usually looked. But then the story was interrupted by other pictures, pictures of a young girl (this was what got Elliot's attention) standing in a weird stance on a chair. She was staring at an opening of some sort, in a chamber-filled room. A subsequent image gave him clues to what she was looking at. Elliot found it so beautiful— the harmony, the balance, the rhythm—he wished to re-create it. He lacked the language skills to be able to say why it was so beautiful, but what he did was he studied it time and again, trying to understand what someone had constructed in this movie. It took him months, but Elliot reconstructed the small room; he applied a reflective coating in a thin, sparse layer on the half-silvered glass side of a mirror and fastened it on the wall of the small chamber; light in there, dark outside; a one-way mirror facing into another mirror on the far end of the wall of the small room. He peeked through the glass into the chamber—a tunnel of his own reflections stretching into infinity. Eventually he tried this with a girl he snatched at Morrison Street and with the one he dropped at Covenant Close, but he found the whole setup incomprehensible. With the girl from Morrison Street he had made an exquisite video, which he had mailed to the authorities. What a stroke of genius that was, an elaborate prank at once teasing the police and warning the city that a great man was on the loose. Yet even with his recording, he couldn't get the light ratio between the inside and the outside of the room to work properly. There was something about that mirror in the film, too, but he couldn't pinpoint what.

Elliot had eventually quit his job; he didn't need access to gasoline anymore. All he needed was nitrate film; it burned beautifully. He decided to find a new job, something enjoyable, something he could combine with pleasure.

When the sun was out, he would park the van at the Meadows. Some children called him Ice Cream Man, others Cheese Man.

15

Night had fallen when they returned to Whitman's flat sometime around ten. The trees that lined Marchmont Road looked uninviting as the wind rustled their leaves. Whitman and Charlie pulled themselves up the two flights of stairs. There was ample mail waiting, stuffed in the corner of the entrance hall; envelopes had been brushed to the side, unopened. Whitman switched on the lights in the living room. He told Charlie that he should take Ellie's bed and they called it a night.

In the bedroom, Whitman dropped his coat on the chair and checked his cell phone. There was a missed call from a U.S. number; Valdano, no doubt. He would be alarmed when he realized Whitman wasn't on board the plane arriving at LAX in the morning.

But Whitman still had time. Afterwards, he would make up an excuse as to the discrepancy. Valdano wouldn't care as long as he eventually had the film in his hands.

Whitman brushed his teeth in front of the mirror.

He looked into the mirror and downward; Ellie was standing next

to him. She was wearing her pink pajamas, the image of a teddy bear
stamped across her upper jammy. She was brushing her teeth, too. Her
movements were strong, methodical.

Whitman stopped brushing, smiled into the mirror.

"What is it, Daddy?" she said, a glowing, smiling mouth behind the
toothbrush.

Whitman turned around, facing the room outside the mirror. No one
was there.

He took off his shoes and sat down on the bed. Its springs made a metal-
lic rustling as they took his weight. God, he was tired. The events leading
to the finding of "Séance Infernale"—Valdano, the incident at the parking lot, the pink bicycle, Pluto—had cut straight through the defenses
he had built after the loss of his daughter and subsequently his wife. He
took off his glasses and rubbed his eyes, fatigue catching up with him. It
had been a long day.

And you're not finished yet.

Something glowed next to the bed. After almost ten years, Kate's wedding ring still lay on the nightstand. He picked up the ring and perched
his glasses back on his nose, as if he didn't remember every fine-grained
detail.

He was going to marry her. He went to one of the best jewelry design
places in the city and asked them to make a ring shaped like a sparrow; she was his little sparrow. In the end, doubt won him over and he
brought Kate in to help with the design. Together they picked out a
stone. She loved wearing it. When they got divorced, she gave it back to
him. He'd spent money on it, sure, but the materials themselves weren't
worth a great deal. The blue emerald and the topaz from a ring of his
grandmother's didn't amount to much. The real value was the time that
they and the craftsmen put into carving it, the time when they were
happy together. He thought about giving it back to her as a present for
what would have been their fifteenth anniversary, but later dismissed the
idea as silly and misleading. They hadn't talked in a while. She tried to
call him on his birthday; he never answered the phone.

In the months that followed their daughter's disappearance, a grieving
Kate had followed Whitman's aberration as it had grown from austere
grief to an idée fixe. He would spend his days and nights hunting down

rare pieces; travels became more frequent, usually in different countries, away from the woman who reminded him of his missing flesh and blood, away from the woman who shouted at him that he had put Ellie behind him. Yet it was this same woman who began arrangements for the divorce papers a few years later, marrying a real estate broker and starting a new family and a new life. Last he had heard, she had two kids, both in kindergarten. Surely their father would never lose sight of his children.

The times Whitman wasn't traveling in some faraway place, he rarely stayed at home. He found himself returning to the Meadows, placidly sitting on a bench and smoking away, hoping to catch a glimpse, amid the fog, of a little girl with freckles and a doll.

Equipped with a couple of photographs and a piece of paper with a list of names and addresses, he had set out every morning before the break of day. He showed the photographs—two stills of Ellie, a close-up and a full-body—to anyone he could divert from their daily routine. He started in that fateful part of the Meadows.

During the desperate times, when no one would stop to listen, he would wave the photos in the face of anyone he could catch, like a lunatic holding a sign warning about the apocalypse. Their faces often made it worse; they couldn't bring themselves to look him in the eyes. They stared at the pavement or nervously around themselves, feeling the crisp sensation of the morning paper and savoring the rich taste of their takeaway coffee. People passed by him with a warning signal in their eyes. *Whatever happened to you had better stay with you, and away from me,* it said.

The list of names had been particularly unsuccessful. He had assembled it from Edinburgh newspapers over the past fifteen years; they consisted of the names of parents whose children had been kidnapped or murdered or had gone missing. He visited their houses and saw how most people's lives had plunged into a dark pit. The parents were sometimes baffled, other times confrontational. One mother called him "a sick man." He lingered by the phone booth he had called Valdano from that day. He hovered around the photography shop across the street and browsed its shelves. He dawdled farther, taking in the Links and Tollcross on one side and Sciennes and most of Newington on the other, expanding the circular area of his investigation in the scale of miles. This analgesic kept him going, almost as effectively as the film pursuits. It also caused a small stir in the papers—the man still looking for his missing daughter—but it was hardly encouraging. The same story was repeated every time, like a broken record, leading yet again to his dazed escapades in the Meadows.

Kate, on the other hand, remained at the house, on a leave of absence from her work. Alex caught sight of her every morning as she sat by the kitchen table, smoking—she had started a year after Ellie had disappeared—and facing the wall. On the nights when Alex came back, she was either in bed asleep or still on that chair, with the same mechanical rote responses and wooden, soporific demeanor. She didn't put the light on in the kitchen, even when it was pitch-dark. She had aged ten years in a matter of a few weeks. Instead of bringing husband and wife closer together, grief for their missing daughter had torn them apart, leaving them with muted conversations and an inability and unwillingness to communicate.

The police had dropped the case of the missing child. No more children had been reported missing, giving no further clues to a trail that had since gone cold.

One day he heard noises coming from Ellie's bedroom. Kate had stuffed everything that evoked their daughter—the dolls, the toys, the horsies and the ponies, the clothes, the bedsheets, the pictures Ellie had drawn that they had placed on the refrigerator door—into black plastic bags. That was what was left of their daughter now: two bulky, impersonal, disposable garbage bags outside of an empty room. He abhorred and felt ashamed of his wife for giving up like that. He confronted her outside their daughter's room. There were accusations thrown, and there was shouting—things that had remained unspoken until that point, perhaps things that needed to be said. After that day their suffering continued separately.

The bench in the Meadows became his favorite spot; it was what he wanted to see when he closed his eyes. He sat there looking out upon the green-laden strips of land, his right hand drumming the splintered slats, the other tightly clasping the notebooks of research. He watched the Meadows as afternoons washed over the city like blood in water.

One day he came back home and saw that Kate had placed her clothes in a suitcase. He went into the bedroom and sat on the bed as she finished packing her things. He stared at the blouses, the skirts, the underwear, the socks. "I'm leaving you," she said. She left all the photos, because they were a reminder of the child. She opened the door and carried her stuff out. Alex remained there for a while, looking at the closed flat door. He listened to the main door of the building downstairs open and close with a thud. He continued staring at it, long after the sounds below had waned.

Film became a sedative. He found things he expected a home to offer him: answers, and the immediate, insistent sense of belonging that went with family. He continued his visits to the Meadows, only he needed to work faster, search further, include more places of interest, spend less time smoking and drinking, and cover more ground. But there came a point at which he didn't know if he was searching for a missing daughter or for a missing film. He was too brutalized by the loss to care about the fine shadings of injustice or unfairness or, especially, rage; rather, the loss set him on a course for his next find, whatever that might be, wherever it may take him.

Through half-closed eyelids, Whitman stared at his ex-wife's wedding ring, his vision blurry from the slow onset of sleep. His last thoughts before surrendering to Morpheus were of hindsight. All the nights his wife had been sitting in the darkness of the kitchen, the muted conversations, the grief; things had worked out for the better. She had a life now, a family, a purpose.

He couldn't recall why he awoke, but it was to the darkness of the room. There was a glimmer from the window as the streetlamps outside lit the curtains with a streak of shimmering light. There was an unusual stillness and quiet, as if the universe had paused to inhale in preparation for the squalls of wind that would roar through the black clouds. The rain seemed to have stopped; not a whisper escaped from its wake.

From somewhere in the house came the creaking of floorboards. The dragging sound of feet scraping across the floor. Whitman rose from his pillow into an almost sitting position and looked around the room, taking in his surroundings. He listened for a sound. There was none except his breathing.

Someone was with him in the room . . .

16

He didn't know when he had realized he was not alone; it was a gradual realization, as if something had gently brushed by him and eased into his field of vision. In the dim light of the window, he looked at the foot of his bed. Someone was there.

As his eyes adjusted to its presence, he saw it had the shape of a little girl, staring at him. Not a sound escaped from her.

"Ellie?"

He flinched as a sharp gust of wind rattled the windowpanes and the curtains swayed. He scanned around the room. Even before turning his gaze, he knew the shadowy figure would not still be sitting at the foot of the bed. The room was empty.

It has been like this for a long time.

The wind howled once, shaking the windowpanes, planting droplets of rain against the glass. He heard the shuffling of feet again. It could be the noises of the old house.

He got out of bed and stood against the window. The wind was shaking the streetlamp below in a violent dance, as if it were going to break it off its hinges. He tucked himself back in between the covers.

He rolled over to his other side on the bed, and he saw her. She was lying next to him, facing him. The image gave him a sheer jolt, sending him flying back until he almost fell from the bed. He looked again and she had somehow changed position to the opposite side, standing up, facing him. She stood unmoving, a shadow obscuring most of her face. Her eyes were full of blood.

She raised her hand and pointed a finger at him.

My little girl. What are you trying to tell me?

With her finger still locked on him, she opened her mouth. But instead of words, smoke began to course from her lips.

He wanted to turn away, but he could only stare at her. Smoke was gushing out of her now, from her nose, her eyes, her mouth, cascades of thick smoke enveloping everything, until he could see her no more. He could smell her; she was burning alive. There were no flames; only smoke. He knew he had to help her, because she was just a little girl, burning alive.

He shut his eyes, forcing himself to wake up, but it did no good; he could smell smoke blanketing everything in the room—the childlike whispers, they were real, and the cold floor, everything was real, and the smoke . . .

Daddy.

How many times had he heard that voice whispering to him? He could hear her amid the smoke, but he could no longer see her.

He moved forward to get to her, and he heard movement behind him. A hand grabbed his shoulder. The back of his neck froze. He began to turn, but the grip on his shoulder became firmer and he stopped. He knew he did not want to turn, that if he did he would regret seeing who or what was behind him.

His cell phone woke him up sometime before 4 a.m. He wiped the sleep from his eyes, his nose wrinkling from the smell of the cigarettes.

"The film's been tampered with," Nestor's voice said from the other end of the line. He breathed the words in a sore voice, roughened by coffee and lack of sleep. "Sorry, getting way ahead of myself there," Nestor continued. He coughed into the receiver and began speaking with no full stops. He must have been speaking for two whole minutes, without any pause, but not really speaking, just blurting out words about the basic tools used in the film conversion.

"Nestor," Whitman said.

"Oh, right. Sorry. Right, then. The film transfer is going fairly smoothly. Most of it is already on thirty-five millimeter, and it's transferring to digital as we speak."

"Just what I wanted to hear."

"I'm keeping backups at the same time on my memory stick. But there's something weird about this footage."

"You mean it's not original?" Whitman asked.

"It's original, all right . . . There's something about it you'll want to see."

"What do you mean? What's happened to the film?" He heard a noise on the other end.

"Security guard. Comes once during the night. Have to go now. I can't say anything more. Come over in twenty minutes. I'm setting up the projector for us now. I'll leave the main door unlocked."

"How do you—"

The line went dead.

"Hello?" Whitman breathed into the receiver. There was no response.

Part IV

December 5

17

A baronial nightmare, the Archive stood in the thick of the lingering fog. Charlie huddled in his coat as the wind lashed at them from all sides. Whitman threw away his cigarette; it kept going out in the fierce wind. His coat was wrapped around him like tissue paper around an open wound.

They climbed the stone steps. As Nestor had promised, the door was unlocked. They entered, welcoming the warmth that came from inside.

A dim light burned in the corner of the hall. They headed for the staircase, barely making out the outline of the handrail. Whitman could feel the winged Pan staring at them in recognition.

In the dreary light, they climbed the winding staircase. They were one flight away from the top when Whitman felt a sudden alarm. The chill that ran through him was unrelated to the wind outside. He stopped short so abruptly that Charlie almost fell into him. He turned around, thinking he'd never seen Charlie flustered before. This was the man who had swallowed sixteen chicken wings in four minutes; that was four wings a minute, Charlie had reminded him.

On the steps was a pool of dark coagulating blood, the edges spreading in rivulets that dropped from one step to the next.

Whitman quickly read the scene. Someone had stumbled here, struggling to get up, smearing blood as he tried to escape. They gave each other a look. They didn't speak as they carefully stepped over the puddle. Whitman kept his hand on the rail, his eyes and ears on alert.

At the top of the stairs, the door to Nestor's workroom was ajar.

Whitman felt the surface of the floor change texture and he looked down at his feet. He saw a thick line of liquid leading inside the room, as if someone had been dragged in or out of the room, bleeding.

Careful not to tread in it, Whitman peeked through the opening, from which a faint light glowed.

They listened. The only sound was the even whir of a clacking projector and the muffled sound of a car engine somewhere outside.

Whitman eased the door open and tiptoed in.

He realized the light was not coming from the projector after all: the room was on fire. The sight of the flames around the desk and projector sent Whitman into panic. He couldn't hear the projector anymore; he couldn't hear Charlie calling his name.

He was jolted back to reality by his friend shaking him.

"Alex!"

"The memory stick," he managed to say.

"What?"

Whitman tried to speak, but his mouth could form no words.

"It's okay," Charlie said. "I understand. Nestor backed up his work, didn't he?"

Charlie helped him out of the room and then ran back inside.

Whitman knelt down and tried to control his breathing. He couldn't. He could feel the flames drawing closer. The fire was a monster, a living being that needed oxygen to survive. Whitman sat there, helpless, his knees pushing against his thorax.

It was in there. On the edge of consciousness, he could hear the fire puffing as Charlie threw stuff around the room to get to the computer.

As consciousness faded and the fire edged closer, Whitman felt a forgotten fear overtaking him. He tried to imagine verdant fields and ocean waters. But it was of no help.

In the darkness, he saw a silhouette taking form, moving along the hallway.

The horror that had plagued him since he was a kid came back into his brain.

From the shadows, the silhouette emerged on all fours.

"Pluto," he managed to whisper, and in the last glimpse of consciousness, in the second before the lights went out, he saw the cat looking at him with eyes of incongruent color, its left ear cocked toward the commotion inside the room.

Alex's mom had bought him Pluto, the cat, when his father left them. The first time he petted the cat's head, tracing the stripes between its ears with his fingers, was the first time he made a friend.

He was twelve years old. He heard voices and running footfalls outside his house. He peered through his bedroom curtains and watched as Eric Sterger and his two buddies, Tommy and Kenny, sprinted by, laughing, hurrying down the deserted lane.

Eric's family lived a few streets away, in a private, high-walled compound lined with trees. If you were a kid living in East L.A. in the mid-1970s, you would have heard about Eric Sterger and his famous Mississippi Bowie, a deadly steel knife with an etched hamon on the cutting edge of its blade. If he took it out of his pocket, the only thing you could do was run. His reputation for cruelty preceded him on the streets. Flanked by his eager-to-please entourage, he strolled through the neighborhood with a swagger. He was accustomed to being a king in his small realm, and in that realm his word was law.

When he saw them on that day, Alex knew there would be trouble. But he couldn't imagine how bad. He waited for a minute, then followed the three kids as they raced to a rutted track that ran along a bush-filled ravine with a stream running through it.

He stooped behind a tree trunk. They were laughing, running around something; it was a small animal. They had formed a circle around it, taunting it, cursing at it, laughing.

He squinted in the light, and that was when he saw it.

It was Pluto.

They had tied a noose around the cat's neck and were taking turns at

kicking it and bringing it back to their feet. Pluto cried as he was propelled and back again, shutting his eyes, preparing for the next blow.

Tommy was standing on one side, Kenny on the other, and in the
middle was Eric. Alex felt his body clench, and something cold rippled
up his spine. Eric seemed relaxed, confident. He was playing with the
Bowie, twisting it around in his hands, his fingers almost caressing the
blade. There was an empty hutch to their side and a steel container next
to it. Kenny and Tommy shifted nervously on their feet, looking from
Eric to the cat, anticipating what their leader was going to tell them.

Alex knew he had to do something.

He knelt and picked up a rock. He shouted at them to stop it, to
leave the cat alone. Eric looked at him, then yanked the rope, tightening
it around the cat's throat, and brought it upward. Pluto was choking, on
his hind legs, mouth open, hissing like a teakettle.

Eric lifted the cat in the air, then suspended it over the single-story
hutch. He dropped it inside and shut the top. He then motioned with his
hand and the other boys separated, forming a half circle, trapping Alex
in the ravine.

He told them again to leave his cat alone. They asked him what he was
going to do about it. Alex didn't reply; he just clenched his fist around
the rock.

They were staring at him, inching closer all the time. This was no
stalemate; it was three and a knife against one and a rock.

Alex did the only thing he could do: he aimed, and then he hurled
the rock at them. It shot forward with a whoosh, grazing Tommy in the
arm. Tommy yelped. The other two flung themselves at Alex, knocking
him to the ground.

"What do we do?" Kenny kept asking Eric. There was a tremor in his
voice. Then Alex understood: Kenny was afraid because he had no idea
what sick plan Eric had in mind.

"What should we do?" Eric repeated, a wicked smile on his face. Then
he told them.

Kenny and Tommy held Alex next to the hutch so that he was facing
the cat.

From the other side, Eric reached for a stick. He ran it along the bars
of the cage in sadistic foreplay. The cat followed the edge of the stick, in
a circular motion around itself.

Eric grasped the steel container with both hands. He steadied it against his chest and unscrewed the top. The smell of gasoline drifted around them. Alex shivered. His head shook.

Eric said something soothing and quiet to the cat.

Oh, my God, Alex thought. *Oh, no. Please, no.*

Eric flipped the container, dousing the cat with the gasoline. "You're going to shine for me now, aren't you, my love?"

Alex's heart and stomach collided as Eric struck a match. He dangled it over the cage, at the same time looking into Alex's eyes. Alex stared into the head of the match, into the center of the flame; it was dancing wildly, a rabid animal ready to be unleashed from its cage.

Then Eric dropped the match into the hutch and stepped back. The blaze swept quickly over the cage. The whoosh mixed with the cat's screams.

With a furious hiss, the cat flung itself against the bars, mouth wide, teeth bared. He banged against them, flew back, and attacked again—and again—relentlessly, without pause, hissing, snarling.

Alex caught a glimpse of Pluto's face just before the flames engulfed him. He saw the resignation in it. It was the look of the lamb.

He tried to shut his eyes, but Eric kept pummeling him on the head with the butt of the knife until he had opened them again.

Eric was laughing, satisfied. "Look, the cat's running around on fire."

The cat banged again and again; its face was starting to bleed with the repeated impacts. The heat was so intense that even the metal-wired hutch broke apart.

Alex stared in horror.

When it was all over, Pluto lay in the stream. He was barely alive, clinging to his last moments, oblivious to any surroundings. His fur coat was gone, the skin underneath livid and seeping. He kept quivering, and that made Alex shiver, too. But for the quiver, the cat did not move, did not stretch an inch. Only the eye moved—that half-burnt eye as Pluto ghost-raised his head. Some blood flowed from the hole where the other eye had been. Around the cat floated bits of clotted, half-burnt fur. A hint of the smell of burnt meat hovered in the air, and Alex felt a weight settle in his neck, just below his Adam's apple.

He felt relief when the cat took his last breath and closed his eye. He stayed there staring at the charred remains for the rest of the night.

• • •

The fire puffed again from inside the workroom, and the feline intruder jolted.

Whitman raised his head and saw Charlie come running out and shut the door.

"It's out of control."

With relief, Whitman saw that he was holding a memory stick.

Charlie stopped to take a breath, coughing from the smoke. "Give me your cell phone," he said, his hands on his knees.

"What for?"

"Aren't we calling the police?"

Whitman put his index finger next to his temple and made a circular motion. "You nuts? With all the blood in here? Our fingerprints are all over the place."

"We don't have anything to be afraid of."

"That was before it turned out to be *Towering Inferno* day in there, Jabba. I'll be damned if I'm going to get busted for taking back what's mine."

Charlie helped him up. "I don't know about this, dude. Nestor might be in danger. Besides, we don't know if the building really is empty. You wouldn't wish burning on anyone, would you?"

Whitman nodded and handed him the phone. "Make the call. Anonymously."

18

The unthinkable happened. It was shortly after Elliot constructed his hiding place—1990, it must have been. He came back one day and found that the lock to his door had been forced open. After he established that no one was still inside the flat, he began noticing subtle hints of another person having been there. It wasn't that anything was missing (he couldn't care less about the valuable objects in the house), but small deviations from normality surfaced here and there: a vase had been moved; a wardrobe door had not been fully closed; a hair on his bed. But the observation that solidified his suspicions was the rug: one tip had been slightly moved and was curled at an angle to the floor. That meant, in all likelihood, that someone had entered his carefully devised hiding place. In the vault, the ancient projectors and film were still there, in their own hidey-holes. Evidently the burglar had failed to find them.

Hundreds of scenarios of dread filled his head that night. A burglar had broken in, found the vault, found the burnt remains of the girls (how many of them had there been? Fourteen? Fifteen?), and was in the process of calling the police. All it would take would be an anonymous tip and the flat would be crawling with policemen and crime-scene scientists. He became so paranoid then and there that he didn't even wait until the morning. He left the flat, rented a place in Carstairs, and then kept changing addresses for a substantial amount of time. But he couldn't stay away forever—not after he realized no harm had been done: no police, no anonymous tips. The only problem was that there was no more room in the flat's vault; he would have to find places to dump every new victim from now on. Yet he hardly cared about the risk; the important thing was that he was free again, free to return to the vaults, free to continue. The person who had broken in—for some obscure reason—had not given him up. And that made him a friend.

19

It was still dark when they got back to Thirlestane Road. They perched their coats on the hanger in the hall, still thinking of the events at the Archive. The flat smelled musty and cloying, like pear drops. Darts of moonlight filtered through the window grilles of Whitman's flat, turning the walls to an assortment of shadows, like a macabre Gothic projection.

"Your house really smells," Charlie said.

"Huh?"

"Has smoking completely killed off your nose?" Charlie said. "It's that sweet and sickly smell, you know, like the sweat of a diabetic."

"I forgot something in the fridge. Just crack open the living room window," Whitman said. He took off his glasses and rubbed the bridge of his nose. It had been a strange night. The Catalan archivist had disappeared. Whitman thought about the blood on the staircase, and the nagging sensation in his gut turned into a terrible sense of foreboding. It reminded him of the familiar faces following him throughout his travels, and also of the mysterious breaking and entering at Elena Genhagger's house in Switzerland, where the perpetrator had taken Elizabeth Sekuler's memoirs. Until that time, unlawfulness had been the only danger Whitman had known. Every time he deceived another player in the game, he had remained unmoved, because he was the third man—granted, not as well dressed or as mysterious as Harry Lime, but an impervious, safe third man.

The events of that night had revealed an unknown, impending danger; a fire had broken out, destroying the Archive. Nestor was missing because of his involvement with the film; that much was clear. Now the paper film was nowhere to be found, its only trace left in Nestor's memory stick.

Whitman twisted open a bottle of Grand Marnier and searched for aspirin in his slingbag. Instead, his fingers found a bottle of codeine pills left over from a time he'd had a broken tooth. He stared at the bottle for a second, then opened the cap and placed one in his mouth.

He checked his phone: three missed calls—U.S. number. By now, Valdano would have realized what was going on. The plane would be at arrivals at LAX, but Whitman wouldn't be on it. Oh, there would be anger. Failing to track down the film in the first place would have been one thing, but finding it and then letting it be taken from his hands—that meant trouble. Valdano would not be happy with the digital copy. Whitman could picture him tossing the memory stick in his face.

"Shall we?" Charlie's voice interrupted his thoughts. Whitman looked up and saw that he had already switched on the laptop and slipped the memory stick into its USB port.

They moved their seats close to the small screen, sharing conspiratorial glances with each other, two kids fascinated with the magic of moving images, eager to relive the redemption that comes only from becoming one with these curious frames. Within seconds they were watching a film made long before either of them had been born, a film that had been entombed for more than a century and was now waking up from a deep sleep, ready to take its first breath after an eternity.

Like the rest of Sekuler's work, the film footage had no title sequence or any other hint of provenance or ownership. The image was jittery, even though everything had been filmed from a stationary camera, positioned as if it were the audience in a play. It wasn't until D. W. Griffith came along that audiences started seeing close-ups and panoramic long views. But none of this mattered; the image in front of them was marvelous. The quality and care rivaled that of works by Segundo de Chomón, Émile Cohl, and Georges Méliès, who would step in almost a decade later to claim the title of pioneer of early fantasy film.

It was a one-scene shot, using Edinburgh Castle and the Princes Street Gardens as backdrop. It was nighttime, and the moon was shining from far away. Two people in olden costumes entered the shot. The first was dressed in a robe of white linen, with a girdle embroidered in gold and silver. He was carrying a coffin while the other man looked on from the side. The robed man dropped the coffin on the ground and began to speak to the second man. While they were engaged in conversation, a skeleton rose out of the coffin. Turning around and seeing this, the first man sauntered back and pushed the skeleton back down; he dressed the skeleton in white sheets while continuing to engage in their conversation.

Whitman's breath caught in his throat as he realized the man carrying the coffin was Augustin Sekuler. There he was: the inventor, the at-once auteur and actor, pulling the skeleton out of the coffin, performing some kind of magic in theatrical fashion.

In response to its dress-up, the skeleton began to dance in a playful manner. With a twist and turn of his hands, Sekuler made the skeleton turn into a woman—played by his wife, Elizabeth—then back into a skeleton again. Following this, the skeleton melted, until only its head remained. It then began growing and growing, until it had reached twice the height of the inventor. Finally, a neck sprouted from its head like a flower from the earth and the skeleton returned to normal size.

Whitman and Charlie stared as the main character tried to grant his wife one final kiss. To the average observer today it would look fake, but the camera tricks were well executed for the time. That last bit was argu-ably the best: Sekuler attempted to give his skeletal wife a kiss, but some-thing went wrong; as if jolted by the surge of an electrical current, the skeleton danced around wantonly. In collaboration, Sekuler performed an assortment of tricks with the skeleton while the other man watched in awe. It wasn't clear who the other man was. In all likelihood it was Joseph Whitley, Sekuler's father-in-law, or Frederick Mason, the wood joiner who had helped the inventor construct the cameras. Whitman couldn't place the face from the grainy image, but he was certain he had seen the man before.

The main body of the film looked like an early take on the Frankenstein tale, made at least twenty years before Edison's official version. The story seemed to be that an Edinburgh man had recently lost his wife, so he hired an alchemist to retrieve her coffin in order to try to bring her back from the dead. But the film was actually about Sekuler, the cinematic magician, making an impossible trick of disappearance on camera.

Whitman and Charlie watched it again, then a third and fourth time.

"Well? What do you think? Stop-trick extravaganza?" Whitman said.

The film was entirely based on the stop trick, which at that time was a complicated thing to do at high speeds. Sekuler, however, had evidently achieved a fluid way of editing that allowed him to use it even when his characters were running and jumping, without the footage looking absurd. The effects of the many disappearances, done in a pure stage-magician style, were still amazing; even more so on that Thursday morning in Edinburgh, inside a flat that smelled of absence, in 2002, more than a hundred years after the footage had been shot. Both as an experiment and as charming entertainment, "Séance Infernale" surely was a successful film, and it offered a glimpse of what the cinemagician had in his bag.

"There's something about it."

Charlie couldn't put his finger on it, but there was an element of the footage that he found perplexing. He put it down to its age; innovation at such an early stage in filmmaking, long before proper filming techniques and standardized linear narration, could seem unorthodox. But there was something else. "I think I saw something," he said, squinting his eyes.

"What do you mean, 'saw something'?"

"Rewind it and play it back."

When they reached the point where Sekuler brought out the coffin, Charlie pressed Pause.

"There it is," he said.

"I don't see anything. Where? What is it?"

Charlie positioned his index finger on the screen, pointing to the coffin being hauled by the main character. Now Whitman saw it. The inscription on the side of the coffin.

"Can you make it out?"

"I think so. It looks Latin."

"*Cerca Trova,*" Charlie whispered, still squinting. "What does that mean?"

"Seek and you shall find."

"What does that have to do with the coffin?" Charlie asked, pushing Play again. The cinemagician continued carrying the coffin.

"Maybe it doesn't have to do with the coffin."

Onscreen, Sekuler was assembling his equipment, his back turned to the coffin. The skeleton gradually rose from it.

"What do you mean?"

The skeleton began to dance and frolic around like a marionette.

"Nestor mentioned something on the phone ab—"

On the screen, something had happened. Both of them noticed it simultaneously; something had jumped out at them, a momentary flicker. They gave each other a look.

"Rewind it."

Charlie pressed the Rewind button and paused the footage about ten seconds before the flash came on. He used the arrow keys to play the film frame by frame. Their eyes locked on the screen.

The inventor was carrying the coffin on every frame, with turtle steps, while the other actor looked at him in awe. Then the screen went black for three frames. The frame after looked like static, from which bizarre shapes seemed to be displayed to the viewer: a wooden board with slightly raised metal bits, as if different pieces from a game of dominoes had been stuck together, then more static. Charlie pressed the right arrow to proceed to the following frame.

It was a girl. She had curly hair in pigtails and wide, piercing eyes. She was inside a darkish room, in a seated position, seen *en profil* from the camera's view. In front of her lay some kind of chamber.

"What the hell is this?"

The girl was staring blankly before her, into a rectangular structure that could have been a window or a painting on the chamber's wall.

"What is she looking at?"

In the frozen frame, the girl kept her vigil, staring, entranced. More black frames, followed by another image. The same girl. Eyes staring into the structure. The camera had moved slightly to the side, bringing into view what she was seeing.

What the rectangular structure on the chamber wall was remained unclear, but it became evident that one could see through it, as if it was a window. Through it, the girl was looking at a peculiar alcove or staircase, stretching deep inside the chamber.

"Are those stairs?"

Whitman shook his head. "No." It became clear. Embedded on the staircase were multiple, consecutive images—reflections—of the girl in a seated position, stretching into infinity.

"It's a mirror." Whitman pressed the left arrow a few times, culminating with the initial hidden frame. "Okay, she's located inside a basement. We see her *en profil* for now, staring into something—we don't know what it is, but we know it's some kind of steel structure, a room within the basement."

He pressed the arrow forward, until the camera view had changed. The camera angle was such that the observer assumed the point of view of the girl. "There is a rectangular feature fastened to the room. We're looking straight into it—through it, in fact. At first glance, the rectangular feature seems like it's a window."

"But it's not?"

Whitman shook his head. "What do you see through the window?"

"The girl. And behind her, there's a staircase going up?"

"That's not the girl. That's her reflection. When we look through the rectangle, what we see is the far end of its inside."

"And at the far end there is a mirror."

Whitman ran his fingers through his beard. "Exactly. But here's the clincher: the rectangle through which we see the mirror is another mirror—a one-way mirror."

"So the image of the girl is reflected in the second mirror—the one inside the chamber . . . and then that reflection is reflected once again, on the other side of the one-way mirror?"

Whitman nodded. "Back and forth. Continuously. And this is what we get: a tunnel." He couldn't understand exactly how it worked, but the visual outcome was identical to the effect produced when you place an object between two facing mirrors: if the mirrors are parallel, the observer can see a weird tunnel created by a progression of smaller reflected images of the object, sinking endlessly into infinity. Children have been trying this for years inside elevators with mirrors on either side.

It was completely out of place; the image had nothing to do with the rest of the film. They were frames inserted among the others, undetectable to a casual observer. Sekuler had weaved hidden images through the frames of his movie.

They rewound the footage and watched it again.

"What—" Charlie began, but midsentence he realized Whitman had not spoken in minutes. He turned to his friend. Saw his face, his eyes locked on the girl. He saw the yearning and finally understood. "Alex."

Whitman wasn't listening. His eyes had turned misty.

"It's not her, Alex," Charlie said.

"She . . . she looks . . ."

"I know. I'm sorry. She looks like her. But she's not."

"Who is she?"

20

D.S. Georgina McBride eyed her desk. It had become a murder scene. Photos of loci, pictures of victims in life and death, crime scenes and locations. Around her, the soft *clack-clack* of computer keyboards; officers were using the SCRO computer or the Home Office Large Major Enquiry System, HOLMES. The steadfast detectives typed in data and checked, cross-referenced and examined. Names, witnesses, locations—anything that could help ongoing investigations. Another girl had been reported missing: Amanda Pearson, fourteen years old, last seen at the Ocean Terminal shopping complex in Leith.

McBride was standing over D.I. Johnson's desk. There were empty coffee cups everywhere. Johnson had popped to the watercooler, and two uniforms were perched on his chairs: Police Constables Elwood and Dowd, breathing proof of yin and yang. Elwood was slim and lean as a knife; Dowd flirted with 250 pounds of fat beneath his belt buckle. Johnson had joked that Dowd's wasn't a beer belly anymore: it was a beer factory. Elwood was shy and reserved; Dowd couldn't control his mouth, blurting whatever remark popped into his head. Although they were both in their early twenties, almost fresh out of the academy, this was evident only in Dowd; Elwood looked older, with a constant fatigue evident in the crow's-feet at the corners of his eyes.

"How does someone not see or hear a little girl being abducted?" McBride said.

"Sometimes the bad guy gets the advantage," Dowd said.

"Amanda's friend Cassie Milos was the last person to see her alive. Said she was alone for a minute, maybe less."

He works fast, McBride thought. *He's perfected his M.O.*

D.I. Guy Johnson sneaked up to them from behind, a glass of cold water in one hand and another cup of coffee in the other. He offered it to McBride, but she turned it down.

"Hey," Elwood said, tapping her once on the shoulder. "Don't look so disheartened. We win some, we lose some."

For a moment they were silent. McBride pointed back to the screen. "What if we've got a perv who uses the girls as sex slaves in a sadistic manner, then, when he gets tired of them, he burns their bodies; that way he makes it look like a sacrifice or the work of a deranged mind, but also gets rid of every trace of sexual assault."

"You still think these cases are linked?"

"Which cases?" Dowd cut in.

"You're too young to remember," Johnson said. "They took place between 1984 and 1990. Fifteen girls, four to fourteen years old, burnt to death, mostly in public dump sites. Perp even sent the police a video of one of the victims."

The videotape had been sent to the police station in the late 1980s. It showed a girl, tied up in a basement, screaming, before an unidentifiable person burned her alive.

"The case is still open," McBride said.

"Wait, do you think it's the same killer? That's a hell of a cooling-off period."

"It has happened before: for example, in America, the BTK Strangler reappeared after a sixteen-year hiatus," Dowd said.

"True, but he didn't kill anybody during that time, he just taunted the police."

"Still, the burning, the victim's possessions removed . . ." McBride said. "I mean, that's a very specific signature, isn't it?"

Johnson shook his head. "If this is the same perp, what has he been doing for the past ten years?"

McBride had her own theories: that he'd been overseas, perhaps as a merchant or sailor, or on some army or RAF posting; that he'd been in jail for an unrelated crime. Theories, that's all they were. "Can you check the M.O. against girls missing in different counties? It might explain the long absence."

"You really think that's likely?"

"If it is the same guy, then he spends time with them. There's a good chance the girl that disappeared from Ocean Terminal is still alive."

"If it's the same guy," Dowd said, "we're going to find her burnt up somewhere."

"How can there be people as sick as this?"

P.C. Dowd shook his head. "Sometimes things are just weird. Remember the time we found the video of the woman pissing on a sheep?" He rolled over to his desk in the swivel chair and woke up his computer screen from the screen-saver mode. "This is kind of similar. Some of these art-house freak films make my skin crawl." Using the computer mouse, he clicked Play.

"Where did you get this? It doesn't look like part of the pervert's video collection," Johnson said.

"No, no. From the fire at the film society in Newington early this morning."

"The Archive? We weren't there."

"We were. It's in the same place as the halls of residence for the university. Some psycho set fire to the building. One person missing. He was working there late. This is a video we got from one of the computers there."

He clicked Play and a string of black-and-white images came onto the screen. The uniforms and detectives were unaware that they were among the first people to see the footage in more than a century. On the screen, a man was carrying a coffin while another stood watching. They were in Princes Street Gardens, Edinburgh Castle looming in the background.

"Looks old. And just plain weird," Elwood said.

"This is even weirder. Check it out. It looks like there are actually two movies, one embedded in the other."

"How do you mean?"

He pointed to the screen. "See, this is one. The guy carrying a coffin."

"Yes."

"But there are random frames inserted between the frames of this film."

"Like images?"

"Looks like it. Some pretty weird gunk." He paused the film and ran it frame by frame so they could examine the hidden images.

"What's that?" McBride asked, pointing at a series of frames that looked like dominoes stuck together.

"Your guess is as good as mine. Probably frames destroyed by bad weather? You know, I would never have found this. The pictures flash on the screen at such a frequency that you wouldn't normally see them. But my computer's media player returned to the old settings by accident; I think it has to do with the number of picture frames the player shows every second."

He moved the frames forward with a push of the arrow key. The image on the screen was in black and white. It showed a little girl, sitting on a chair. She was around five years old, dressed in a light dress, her tangled blond hair falling on top of it. Her eyes were what startled McBride: the girl was staring straight in front of her, as if she were in a semiconscious trance.

McBride stopped.

I've seen this before somewhere.

Dowd kept moving the images forward. The girl was in a dark room or a basement, looking into a rectangular shape placed on the outside wall of a small metal room; it was not clear what she was looking at, but in the next frame McBride caught a glimpse of the inside; through the rectangle she could see what looked like a stairway or corridor stretching into the wall. Countless consecutive reflections of the girl lost in infinity.

Is that a mirror?

Then the picture went black.

"What happened?" they said, almost in unison.

"It stops after that," Dowd said. "It looks like someone was working on it, maybe digitizing it. I'm guessing that's how far they got."

"The guy who works there? The one who disappeared?"

"It would explain why it's been left unfinished."

"Not a chance in hell," McBride suddenly said, more to herself than anybody else. It didn't make sense, though; it couldn't.

She went over to her desk and turned her computer on. She clicked on the folder containing the video evidence converted from the VHS exhibit of the 1980s case. She had to scroll through an endless array of video files. She eventually found it. A girl, around the same age, restrained on a chair, looking into a rectangular window—and inside, countless of her reflections stretching into nothingness. She had seen the girl's face a thousand times, pored over it and others as part of case evidence. Her name was Katie Mitchell, last seen on Morrison Street sometime late afternoon on September 15, 1986. The video evidence from the old case—involving a victim of her perp—was almost identical to the bizarre secret frames in the film from the Archive. It was as if the person who made it had watched the old one and decided to remake it. The cases had seemed entirely unconnected until now.

She turned to Johnson, who was talking with the others. The door flung open and a mass of fat hesitated at the threshold. A police constable stood with his eyes cast down—a sign that shouting had taken place before he came into the room. It didn't take long for McBride to understand who had been doing the shouting.

"Superintendent Breitner wants to see you," he told no one in particular, but McBride knew it was her who was wanted.

She got up and went to the door, from where she could hear the superintendent boiling.

"McBride! My office—now!"

"I already told you what happened," she said.

"Then tell it to me again."

"I'm just looking to see if I find a nibble from this guy."

"Let it go."

The superintendent's office was squeaky clean, except for his "frustration corner"; there, he seemed to adhere to the turmoil of the rest of the precinct: cabinets half-open, revealing piles upon piles of paperwork that would need to be neatly filed, ordered, and sent to some high-rank place. Superintendent Martin Breitner was a sizable man who walked with a swagger that rivaled a bullfighter's. He had a full head of thick black hair—no gray, no sign of dyeing. His facial features conformed to a geometry that made him seem like he was smiling, even now as he simmered in anger.

D.S. Georgina McBride, arms crossed, was sitting in one of the two chairs across from his desk. Phone messages were stuck to the lower part of his monitor, probably the last hour's worth. The office walls were adorned with framed newspaper articles of Breitner's achievements: Tony Blair shaking his hand; some Dundee chief inspector he had saved during a hostage negotiation gone wrong; establishing the newest training center at the Scottish Police College for junior station inspectors. There were various plaques and badges for dedicated law enforcement, as well as a ribbon; McBride had never asked about the latter.

His computer was up and running, and it had taken over his desk. The photo of his family had been moved to the far side of the desk and turned the other way, facing McBride.

Problems at home, Martin?

"I can't."

"There is no connection between the two cases," he said. "Every time you get like this . . ."

"Which time?" She was waiting for him to mention the Sterger case, one of many in which the perpetrator had walked because of insufficient evidence. McBride had worked the case, and she had gone in too early.

She bit her thumbnail, looking nervously behind her. "I have to get back out there. Perp's still out there."

"I can hold you for as long as I want, Detective."

"You think I don't use these tactics myself, boss?"

He slammed his fist on the desk, rattling the keyboard and knocking the family picture onto the floor. "I know your tactics bloody well, Detective!" He straightened his tie and composed himself. "Did you tell the suspect that you would take his children away from him?" He made no effort to retrieve the picture.

McBride sat there, blinking at him. "We're turning every one of our cases into a witch hunt," she finally said. "Now if you don't mind, Superintendent, I'm busy."

"Not if I can help it." He drummed his fingers impatiently on the desk, as if daring her to reply.

"There's another girl that's disappeared," she said.

He nodded. "Amanda Pearson. She was last seen near Ocean Terminal in Leith."

"So much for change, huh?" McBride chuckled. Leith was brushing the dust off its shoulders. It was more than a scrub and a sweep; the corporate world had decided that a cultural and commercial embourgeoisement was in order: converted waterside flats, fashionable bistros, a concentration of Michelin stars, bars, and street culture. Yet the old seaman's town was still there; sometimes you could hear its soft whisper from the water. "Things left behind are never things forgotten," it whispered. Nowhere was this more evident than at the port's old watering holes: floors tinted with drips of Guinness, swarthy figures with heavy fists crouched on barstools, palms wrapped around a pint. Their empty stares would linger on the front door, as if checking on the weather outside their sanctuary, while nearby, perhaps a dark figure was targeting little girls.

"It might be connected to the girl we found at Covenant Close."

He threw his hands up. "There you go again with the conjecture."

"Let me talk to the girl's parents."

The superintendent's thickish brows rose outward from twin creases above his nose. "Have you been listening to what I've been saying for the past five minutes?"

She sighed.

"Stick to your case. We've got our hands full. There's been some shady business at a film society in Newington."

"The Archive?"

He nodded. "Half the building was in flames and one person's missing. Suspect's still out there. We're still working on IDing him from the building's security cameras."

"Let me help out, then. I'll pay them a visit. You can talk to the girl's parents."

"Someone else is on the case."

She hissed a breath through her teeth.

"It's the Sterger case all over again," he said.

"What the bloody hell is that supposed to mean?" She made a motion to get up but sat back on her chair. "That case, I stood by it and worked it to the book. Played by the rules. And the guy walked."

"Look, McBride, I know your preference for these cases, and I know you genuinely want to help these victims. But you have to work within the channels. This means that sometimes the bad guy gets away."

"I'm not going to leave anybody behind."

"All I'm saying is, just take a leave for today, take it easy for a while. Go home, get some rest. Nobody is going to blame you for taking time off to clear your head."

"I don't need this," she said, on the verge of exploding, but Breitner silenced her with a wave of his hand and a shake of his head.

"I'm not giving you a choice."

She snorted and rose out of her chair. She opened the door and paused. "You know what? Sometimes heads just have to roll." She walked out of the office, slamming the door on her way out.

21

It had been an awful night.

The mother went out to have some drinks; at first this only slightly alarmed Elliot. But then she returned, drunk, tripping on the steps to the door. To make matters worse, she wasn't alone. There was someone with her, a young man he had never seen before. He was drunk, too, or appeared to be; these boys, you don't know what the hell they're up to—he might have been pretending just so he could get her into bed.

Her speech was slurred and the things she was saying made no sense. Elliot was angry at her, for being a prospective whore, for not being able to restrain herself. How could she have betrayed him like this? He kept staring through the peephole for so long that his eye began to hurt. But he kept on; pain was not something he worried about.

The door of her flat closed behind them, but he could still hear voices. Evidently, they were in her living room, joined by another voice. The door opened after a few minutes and the babysitter made her exit. The melody that excited him so much kept playing in his head.

Alla marcia e molto marcato (♩=138)

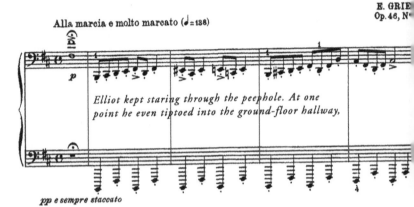

p

*Elliot kept staring through the peephole. At one
point he even tiptoed into the ground-floor hallway,*

pp e sempre staccato

*inches from her door, just so he could eavesdrop
on them. There were moans of pain; he knew what she was*

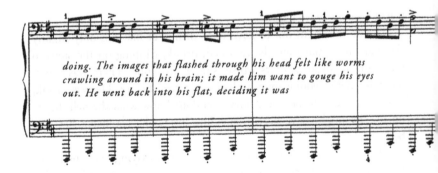

*doing. The images that flashed through his head felt like worms
crawling around in his brain; it made him want to gouge his eyes
out. He went back into his flat, deciding it was*

*wiser to let her have her whorish fun. Just wait. Nothing was
going according to his Grand Plan. Nothing. The mother was a
fucking whore. And that Pearson girl. She wasn't like he had*

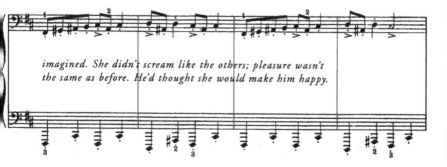

imagined. She didn't scream like the others; pleasure wasn't the same as before. He'd thought she would make him happy.

Nothing. He clenched his hands and placed them on his temples. He couldn't deal with the state of things, with those feelings,

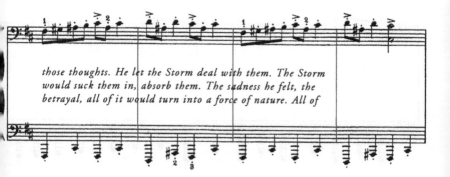

those thoughts. He let the Storm deal with them. The Storm would suck them in, absorb them. The sadness he felt, the betrayal, all of it would turn into a force of nature. All of

the things he could not control, he could consume. With each step he took toward the bedroom, it grew. Need. Need the fire. Make me free. Finally, a clever idea entered his head.

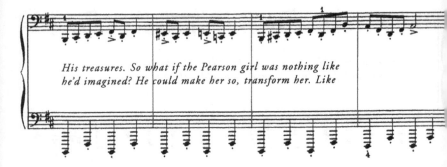

His treasures. So what if the Pearson girl was nothing like
he'd imagined? He could make her so, transform her. Like

playing dress-up. He went into the bedroom and knelt beside
his bed. He fished out the cardboard box. He crossed his legs,
and his trembling hands took turns holding each of the

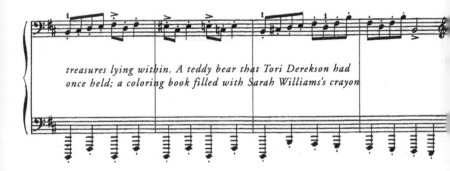

treasures lying within. A teddy bear that Tori Derekson had
once held; a coloring book filled with Sarah Williams's crayon

drawings; Kathryn Larallie's belt buckle, shaped like a
princess; a small snow globe (containing an Alice in
Wonderland figure) from Katie Mitchell's coat pocket;

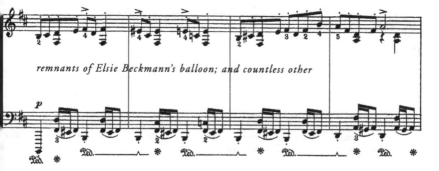

remnants of Elsie Beckmann's balloon; and countless other

souvenirs. Two of these inflamed his interest the most:
the hair clip—still with a string of hairs that had come off her

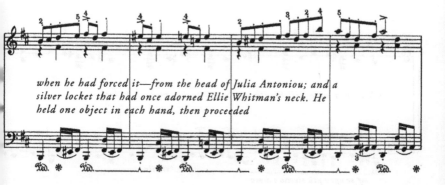

when he had forced it—from the head of Julia Antoniou; and a
silver locket that had once adorned Ellie Whitman's neck. He
held one object in each hand, then proceeded

to the hallway leading to the vault. The door wouldn't budge
at first; it was one of those days when it felt like the
whole world was against him and nothing worked. The Storm.
Let the Storm deal with it. He breathed and he shook and

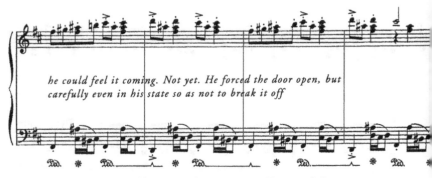

he could feel it coming. Not yet. He forced the door open, but carefully even in his state so as not to break it off

its hinges. He wouldn't want that. Be smart. He crossed the passage into the vault, the girls he once knew lining either side, taunting him like the little bitches they were

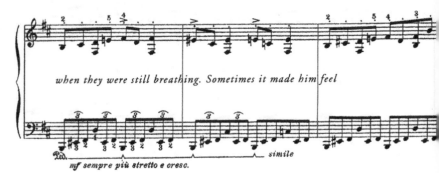

when they were still breathing. Sometimes it made him feel

better just having them around. But they weren't really around anymore. He stormed into the vault, where the Pearson girl

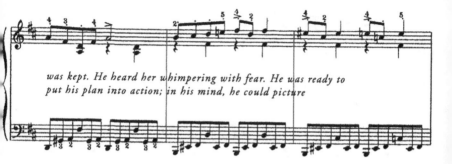

was kept. He heard her whimpering with fear. He was ready to
put his plan into action; in his mind, he could picture

her wearing the locket and the hair clip. Just as it seemed that
everything would fall into place, it all went wrong.

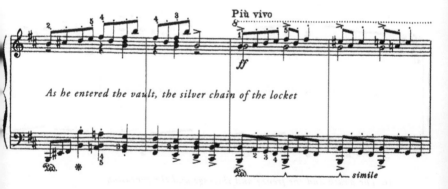

As he entered the vault, the silver chain of the locket

somehow became tangled with one of the girls' hands (they were

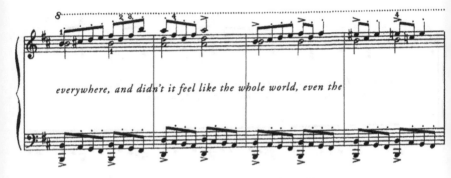

everywhere, and didn't it feel like the whole world, even the

girls, was conspiring against him?) and it put him off-
balance. The chain was caught on one of their skeletal

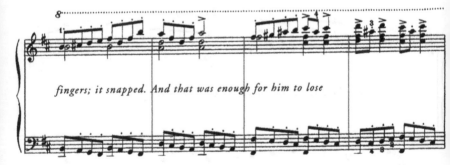

fingers; it snapped. And that was enough for him to lose

it. The wrath and the frenzy and the rage and the confusion

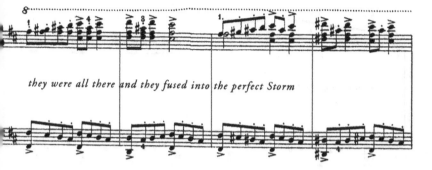

they were all there and they fused into the perfect Storm

a vast and beautiful and horrifying and perfect perfect Storm

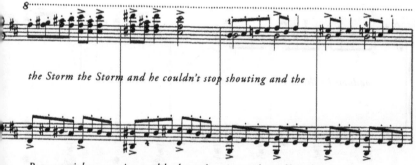

the Storm the Storm and he couldn't stop shouting and the

Pearson girl was crying and he kept shouting at her telling her he
was going to burn her alive that she's going to scream into the

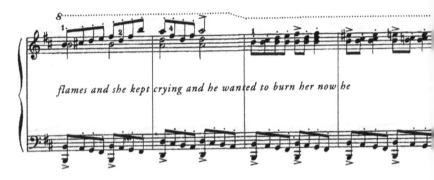

flames and she kept crying and he wanted to burn her now he

wanted to burn her so much but he knew he must wait and in his

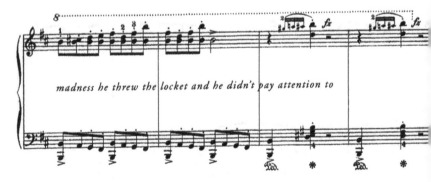

madness he threw the locket and he didn't pay attention to

where it landed even though just in his subconscious he saw

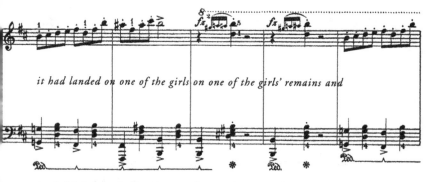

it had landed on one of the girls on one of the girls' remains and

he didn't know which girl it was but he decided to leave it there

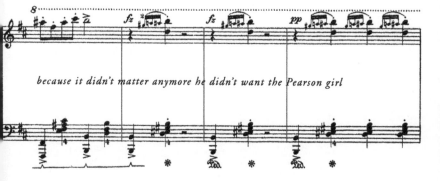

because it didn't matter anymore he didn't want the Pearson girl

anymore because the Storm had come the Storm was there the Storm

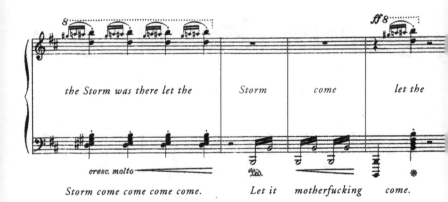

22

On her living room television, a scene from a movie was on mute. Georgina McBride knew the story. This was the part where Shelley Duvall is forced to accept that her writer-husband has lost his marbles.

McBride's boiler system switched on, producing the sound of hell's hammers from the pipes. The radiator next to her quivered as the valves trickled to life. It wasn't half as cool-looking as the Overlook's, but, damn it, it was safer.

Onscreen, Duvall was expecting to see the beginnings of a novel as she flicked through pages her husband had been typing feverishly. Instead she read a single sentence, repeated over and over: "All work and no play makes Jack a dull boy." *The Shining* had been McBride's favorite novel as a teenager; the film adaptation, not so much.

She flicked the remote control and the television turned to standby. Was that the kind of person they were looking for? Did he use axes to crash through wooden doors? Did he talk to imaginary barmen?

She got up from the couch, crossed to the other side of the living room, and placed her hand on the radiator. Too soon. Same ol' Georgina

McBride. Watching the pot that never boils; busting the crook who later walks.

Her doorbell rang. She looked at the mess on the floor, then crossed into the hall. She tiptoed to the door as the bell rang again.

There was a murmur. Fingers pushed the door's mail slot open. Instinctively, she kept to the side of the door, back pressed to the wall, but then she realized how silly this was.

"You sleeping it off?" a familiar voice said.

She turned the bolt silently and yanked the door open. Guy Johnson, who had been peering through the mail slot, stood up.

"You checking up on me?" she said.

He smiled at her from behind tired eyes. She knew he had five cases going to court next week and at least as many that needed to be filed and sent in some semblance of order by yesterday. Five cases of burglary, she recalled; one body at Covenant Close; one missing person at the Arch fire. He shuffled his feet and followed her indoors.

"What's the word, Guy? Is it going to be a busy day?"

"It's been pandemonium so far, and it's not even noon."

She nodded consent. The CID was undermanned as it was, and the latest abduction was bound to make things even tougher.

She offered him a beer, but he turned it down. She moved the magazines from an armchair and motioned for him to sit. She took the sofa for herself, tucking one leg underneath the other.

"What's happening with the Archive case?"

"Breitner's put me in charge," Johnson said.

"Meaning it's your arse on a sling should there be a fuckup."

"Perish the thought, D.S. McBride. Which reminds me . . ." He opened his briefcase and pulled out two black folders. "Fresh off the press," he laughed, handing them to her. He scratched the side of his chin, uneasy. "Let's hope no one's looking for them back at headquarters anytime soon."

The folders could prove to be a breakthrough. The print was her ally. With this, she could reconstruct things—movements, motives, thoughts. But even knowing what she was looking for, it would take time and effort. Her eyes were stinging, and she kept rubbing them, which only blurred her vision. She opened the first folder and skimmed through the documents. It was the typed incident report on the Archive investigation.

"I don't understand what makes you tick with this thing. Twenty-four hours ago you were hell-bent on the Covenant Close incident. Don't tell me you're trying to tie this in with your serial killer story. It hasn't even been six hours since the fire at the Archive."

She didn't acknowledge the question, just kept looking at the paperwork. "CCTV in the building yield anything?"

"For some reason, there is an unaccounted-for gap in the CCTV recording. We suspect it might have been due to a power shortage."

"Is there any useful footage around that time?"

He grinned. "Turn back a few pages and see for yourself."

She flipped the pages until she came across a black-and-white picture of two men entering the main door of the building. One of them was plump and stocky, and his face was hidden underneath a hood. But the other one was clearly visible. She made a mental note of the man's characteristics: late thirties to early forties, gangly, thin, with a wretched build like that of a marionette, big eyes that looked even bigger through steel-rimmed glasses, beard. The scruffy clothes and the inquisitive look made him seem like a journalist on the dole.

"Do we have an ID?"

"Guard at the Archive recognized him," he said, looking at the picture. "His name is Alex Whitman. Of Los Angeles, California. But. Former Edinburgh resident."

"Does he have a record?"

Johnson hesitated, then said, "I wouldn't want to spoil the fun for you. I know how much you enjoy glowing over my neatly typed pages." He winked, but she didn't see it.

She skimmed through the man's file. "So, he moved away from Edinburgh in . . . 1990. What a surprise."

"Clutching at straws. So did about a hundred other people."

"So did our serial killer."

Johnson chuckled. "All right, I'll play along. Similarities?"

"The report from Amanda Pearson's friend says she went to the south side of Ocean Terminal and saw Amanda's handbag on the pavement."

"Okay . . ." Johnson prompted, waiting for the connection.

"Sensing there was something wrong, she ran to the information point to report it. But when security accompanied her back to the scene, the handbag was missing."

"It's obvious the perp came back to pick up the bag," Johnson said. "Or the girl was hallucinating. Or lying."

"Just look at all these cases," she said, holding the folder in front of him. "The victims are missing personal items. A balloon. A locket. A handbag. Our perp's been keeping souvenirs."

He nodded, flipping through the file, not bothering to read the details. He got to the victim's photograph, took it out of the folder, and held it in his hands: revealing top, heavy eye shadow, too much lipstick for a girl that age. He finally shook his head. "The girl's too old. Coincidence." He put the photo down and slid it back to McBride. She took it and sat there looking at the picture of the last victim. It could tell her everything she needed to know.

"Child predators have a specific age group they target," Johnson said. "A perp who targets six-year-olds might think a fourteen-year-old girl is too old. The same goes for a man attracted to teenagers—he'd probably be as disgusted as we are by the thought of molesting a girl that young."

McBride felt her stomach clench. She tried to ignore it.

"So how do you explain the recent increase in missing girls in the past months?"

Johnson shrugged. "Copycat. The movies. MTV. Marilyn Manson."

"Has anyone checked out the parents?" she asked. It was not a stereotype, merely statistics.

"Clean as a whistle. Solid alibis from work at the time of her disappearance. For both of them. We've also looked into close relatives: nothing suspicious."

"Then it must be our guy," she muttered.

"Don't be daft," he said. "Those girls went to different schools, had different friends, came from different backgrounds." He counted each finger like a bullet point. "The girl at Covenant Close is one thing: that's the only M.O. you have reminiscent of past incidents. Amanda Pearson, on the other hand, is a missing person, not a dead one. Let's not forget that. Most importantly, the burnings from your serial killer stopped in 1990. I don't know why, and I'm not interested in finding out. Maybe the guy died, or he skipped town."

She tapped on the papers lying on the table. "For all we know he has found a hiding place to store the bodies. Just look at the records from the neighboring counties. Bizarre disappearances start exactly three months after the last girl disappeared."

She looked at the papers, making the calculations in her mind. A series of disappearances and burnt bodies popping up in Edinburgh until April 1990. Then, nothing. Like the perp had vanished off the face of the earth. A close look in other jurisdictions, though, gave a different picture. August 1990: six-year-old girl goes missing in the Livingston area. November 1990: ten-year-old boy disappears in Dunbar. The list went on.

McBride looked into Johnson's eyes; they were the honest, hard eyes of a real cop.

"A goin' foot's aye gettin', McBride. The problem is girls will always disappear. They have done since the beginning of time, and they will do until long after we're dead and buried. What if, say, we were to try the exact same comparison you just did with a geographically unrelated county—in the south of Wales, London, or, hell, I don't know, Paris? It would show the same thing; kind of like staring at clouds in the sky expecting to find one shaped like an animal."

McBride was silent.

She'd seen something.

A series of disappearances and burnt bodies from 1984 to 1990; then a series of disappearances, no bodies found. She saw the list of disappeared girls and one of the names . . .

That name. She'd seen it before.

Ellie Whitman.

She looked up. Johnson hadn't noticed it; he had taken her silent concentration for protest over his argument.

"I think I'll have that beer," he said, reaching for the can of Tennent's resting on the table.

He reached into his coat. "I want to show you something," he said. He handed her a medallion lock.

"I carry this wherever I go."

She frowned. "Your daughter's?"

"Fife. Christmas Eve, 1976. One of my first cases on the job. A kid sees his father get beaten to death by a drug dealer on the High Street. The guy used a hammer, smashed in the father's head because of a row with his girlfriend minutes before. A few months after, the case had been shelved. Perp had disappeared off the face of the earth. Every year, I call that kid—now an adult—to tell him I haven't forgotten, that I'm still looking. He stopped answering my calls two years ago."

He took another sip of the lager. "Some people just want to let sleeping dogs lie, McBride. Remember what Mareth always says: the brain is the most fragile of organs."

McBride nodded. She disagreed, but she didn't say anything, out of respect for Johnson's willingness to share something so personal.

She looked up from the files, studying him for a few seconds. In her mind's eye she could see him slamming back one whisky after another in a feeble attempt to get the taste of death out of his mouth.

"You want to grab a bite before you head back out?" she asked, squinting at the clock.

He said he really should be getting back. Then he hesitated, as if he was debating with himself whether to let her in on something.

"What is it?"

"You didn't hear it from me. In a few hours there's going to be a raid at Whitman's house." He smiled. "Pending the warrant, of course."

She almost laughed. "Rub it in, Detective. You're responsible for the fuckups now."

"I'll be back in the afternoon to get the files," he said.

She nodded. "I won't get you in trouble."

He took another bottle from the table—some American beer—and popped it open using his lighter, then extended it to her. He got up from his seat and slowly headed for the door. He paused. "I don't care about getting in trouble, McBride. I'm just worried about you."

"I'll be fine," she said, and smiled.

"Take care of yourself."

On the radio, Etta James was ordering one for her baby and one for the road.

When Johnson left, she gazed out the window. Edinburgh breathed on as it had done for hundreds of years. The rain was beating hard against the cobbled streets; the wind carried it around the rooftops, creating a curtain of liquid silver. Even in the rainy mist—especially then—the soul of the city strolled proudly through the streets and you could feel ghostly apparitions hovering above the towers and roofs, hear their footsteps echoing along the corridors and stone archways. They weren't sinister, hostile ghosts, dragging something heavy across the cobbled alleys and spiral staircases; they were ghosts of absence and loss, and the glow that illuminated their form was merely borrowed, visible only as long as you could will it into visibility with your mind, like Dr. T. J. Eckleburg's eyes. That was what made the residents of this city so lucky; and they didn't even know it. The students laughing their way back to their digs, the punters bumming a fag, the ragged homeless man sitting at the foot of the Playfair Steps—none realized the treasure they had breathing next to them.

Her glance faltered back into the flat for a second. She eyed the folders, wondering if she could resist. A cigarette pack rested on the living room table.

Damn it, Guy. The one thing you shouldn't leave in my flat.

She considered it: the prospect seemed irresistible. She picked up the folders, tried to focus; she kept sneaking peeks at the pack. Finally she grabbed a piece of paper and copied an address from the folders. She picked up the pack and headed downstairs.

Walking downhill from St. Andrew Square, she paused outside the entrance to Princes Street Gardens. The mist still lingered. A few people walked past Jenners and the shops. A brave couple was sitting on one of the benches, the man complaining to his wife that there were no pigeons or Canadian squirrels to feed crumbs to. Another person was reading the Thursday paper.

Who was this Whitman character, anyway? And how did he fit into all this?

The castle reared above everything, its flag flying briskly in the breeze. The Gothic tower of the Scott Monument pointed believers in the "right" direction. A family was trying to snap pictures of it; never mind what the monument stood for, as long as the picture was taken with an expensive camera. So much time spent milling around, only to miss the underlying essence. These days, there was more to the locale than tartan and shortbread, whisky and castles. Had they caught wind of the news on the missing girl? Could they surmise that a serial killer was on the loose? Even the CID hadn't figured that one out.

She took the crumpled note out of her pocket, smoothed it out. Raindrops pattered on the piece of paper, leaving spots of liquid velvet. She glared at the address.

34 Thirlestane Road, Marchmont.

She would go and find this Alex Whitman. Today. Before the CID got to him.

23

Everything was there in the film, crying out to be seen. Sekuler had recorded it all so intricately, down to the tiniest of details.

"I can't believe this works," Charlie said. Before, he had been complaining about the smell of Whitman's fridge leftovers. Now he seemed oblivious to it, transfixed in the moment. "I mean, the trick doesn't really work, but . . . my God, it's incredible."

"It was supposed to work."

"How's that?"

"Film is made possible by the observer's persistence of vision: many single frames, photographic images played one after the other, appear as if they're moving. Before twenty-four frames per second became the de facto standard, frame rate was variable. The projector could catch on fire; the distributor might have to attach notes for the projectionist, giving them the speed the reels had to be played at."

"Like Griffith's instructions for *Home Sweet Home*," Charlie said, "recommending different frame rates for each reel."

"Eighteen frames per second is one-eighteenth of a second, or 55.55 milliseconds."

"At 55.55 milliseconds, you still perceive it," Charlie said.

"At twenty-four frames per second, the duration of each frame would be even shorter, but still within perceptual limits."

Charlie stretched his shoulders and arms, looking away from the footage on the screen. Outside, the breeze was turning into a wind.

"I don't get it. Doesn't this mean that it's impossible to present an image beyond a human's perception in film?"

Charlie caught Whitman smiling that dry grin again and shaking his head.

"Look at what he did. In a fast visual, looking at two images, T_1 and T_2, occurring between two hundred and five hundred milliseconds of one another, you can't see T_2. Show T_2 at below two hundred milliseconds or above five hundred milliseconds and you'll see it."

"So Sekuler placed four blank frames one after another," Charlie said, playing with Whitman's lighter on the corner of the desk, "totaling two-hundred-plus-something milliseconds."

"And when he placed a single image directly after those frames, it remained . . ."

"Hidden," Whitman said.

They were silent for a second, taking in the genius of the French inventor.

"But in the world of twenty-four frames per second, each frame is projected for 41.66 milliseconds."

"Four frames would total something over 160 milliseconds, well within the perceptual window."

"So it wouldn't work; you wouldn't be able to hide something in it. That's the case here; the media player on this computer projects in standard NTSC video, twenty-four frames every second."

With a stunned look in his eyes, Charlie turned to his friend.

"What?"

"Do you think there are more hidden images in there?"

Whitman had been so caught up in the idea of subliminal frames that he had not even considered what else might be there.

Another hour of tinkering with the footage followed; sixteen more images had been embedded. They printed every frame in the film, allowing them to have easy access to a hard copy of the material.

"The first film ever recorded and it's filled with subliminal imagery. Amazing." Charlie ran his hand through his beard. "What do you think it means?"

"It looks like some kind of trick, a 'look what I can do' type of thing. Victorian books, like *Alice in Wonderland,* contained little puzzles within the text, so maybe Augustin thought it would be innovative to incorporate that into his invention."

Charlie pointed at the wooden board frames preceding every hidden image. "What about this? It's weird. You think it's of any significance? They look like domino pieces."

Whitman took the pack of Old Holborn out of his pocket and fished for his rolling papers, his eyes never leaving the screen. The frame image looked like a series of hundreds of dominoes strewn next to one another. He shook his head. "Hardly seems so. It looks like some sort of Victorian clapperboard or bookmark." His hand found the rolling papers, and, holding them, he made a slow karate-chop-like gesture culminating in midair. As in *The hidden stuff starts here.*

They needed coffee. There was a long road ahead of them. Valdano would have to wait.

Whitman headed for the kitchen, passing a nest of tables alongside the wall.

Some households are arranged so beautifully and with such precision that even changing the slightest of details will make it seem off. This was not the case with the Whitman household. Yet the nest of tables was different. Three round tables, each sporting a solid oak cross-frame with a chrome finish, were arranged in a nest. He and Kate had bought them from a department store in St. James mall in an attempt to soften the contemporary feel of the place. Kate always wanted them in a specific arrangement. She used to call them her "OCD tables."

"So why do you think Sekuler hid all this in here?" Charlie asked.

Whitman didn't reply. He could only stare at the tables, the way they were slightly angled out from the corner instead of lying flat against the wall as they usually were.

"Alex? Are you there?"

Whitman wouldn't shift his eyes from the tables. "Something's not right here. Did you move this?" Whitman asked, tapping the wooden frames and feeling the back compartments of the tables. He found nothing suspicious.

"I don't think so."

Whitman looked around. The window was closed. He ran his finger along the frame of the bookcase and examined the thick dust on his finger, thinking, talking to himself.

"Someone's been in here."

Whitman was opening drawers, checking the furniture, even examining the ashtrays in case any cigarette brands other than his own had been stubbed in them.

He found nothing.

The kitchen seemed untouched, too. In his bedroom, all the projectors and film paraphernalia were stacked the way they had been for the past ten years. The picture of Mr. Pabst on the wall seemed angled right, the work desk undisturbed.

He opened the door to Ellie's bedroom.

A man was lying on the bed. Whitman recognized him despite the modifications someone had inflicted on his face and body. The first thing he noticed was the lips: they had been left twisted into a grim smile, as if he was leering at Whitman. Then, the smell. The odor was mixed with something coming off his own body: fear.

He coughed, leaning over with a muffled sound, hoping to deter what wanted to come out of him.

Oblivious to the adjacent room's new occupant, Charlie was still working on the film. Whitman limped to the table and poured himself a drink. His legs were shaky.

"Find anything?" Charlie asked, focused on his work.

Whitman downed the glass. "It's funny you should mention that." He finished swallowing and pointed to the bedroom. "There's a dead body in there."

"A dead body," Charlie repeated, hypnotized by the sheer effort of cutting the frames in the right place.

"Yes. A dead body. In my daughter's bedroom."

"I don't see what's funny about that, Alex."

Whitman motioned him to go see for himself.

Charlie stopped outside Ellie's bedroom and peered in.

It was Nestor, the film restoration expert from the Archive.

He was on the bed, partially clothed, his shirt cut open like a robe, showing powdery white skin and a wisp of black hair leading down to what used to be his genitals. The feet were nearest the door, the head turned slightly to the right and pointing toward the room's projector. The right leg was bent at the knee, splayed open, the left jutting at an angle. His eyes were in a wide stare. There was something protruding from his mouth; Charlie realized it was part of the man's genitalia. Holding his hand over his mouth, he ran to the bathroom, barely making it in time.

Over the sounds coming from his friend, Whitman poured another glass of Chivas.

"I think the fuckup fairy has visited us again," he said.

"We've been working on the film for the past few hours," Whitman said, "with a dead body lying in the next room. Oh, this is great. Just great."

The phone rang. He picked up.

"Hello?" he breathed into the receiver.

"Get out of the house." A woman's voice. Scottish accent. "Now. You're in danger." The line went dead.

He brushed the living room curtains aside and peeked out the window. A police car was parked next to the main door of the building. Within seconds, another police car pulled up in the middle of the road directly opposite the tenement. Two uniformed officers came out of the first car and went straight for the main door of the building. Even before Whitman heard the buzzer ringing in his flat, he knew they were coming for him.

"But wait a minute," he said. "Wait a minute, you ain't heard nothin' yet!"

"Who's buzzing?"

"The police," Whitman said.

"It can't be the police," Charlie said. "We have a dead body in there."

"At least they're fast," Whitman said, lighting a cigarette.

The buzzer rang again.

"Are we going to answer that?"

"Let's think about this," Whitman said, exhaling a cloud of smoke. "The last person who slept on that bed was you, and that was last night."

"Right."

"As I'm sure you own a well-proportioned brain, you would have noticed if there was a dead body gathering flies next to you."

The buzzer rang again.

"We left for the Archive just before four in the morning. When we got there, Nestor was nowhere to be seen. It seems logical that at that point he was already dead and probably not inside the building. So the only answer, since neither you nor I could have murdered him, is that someone moved the body here while we were at the Archive."

"Someone really wants this film."

"No shit, Sherlock."

"Why do they want to set us up, then?"

"I don't know, Jabba. This is a whole new kind of weirdness."

The buzzer echoed throughout the flat for a fourth time.

"You think we should let them in?"

"You crazy? It's like a scene from *Eyes Without a Face* in there!" Charlie went to the living room table as Whitman gathered Valdano's files and stubbed his cigarette in the ashtray.

"What do we do now? How do we escape?" Charlie said, the laptop case slung around his arm.

"Through the front door, of course."

"But they'll see us. We're going to get pinched."

"I didn't say otherwise, Chubs. Observe."

Whitman opened the door of their flat. The tenement building consisted of four floors, each accessible by a central stone staircase. They heard buzzers ringing in the other flat on the same floor. Charlie had started down the stairs when Whitman grabbed him by the arm. He pointed the other way, up to the fourth floor. "That way."

They trudged up. From downstairs, the sound of a buzzer and a lock giving in. The main door had opened.

Footsteps echoed throughout the building.

The fourth floor consisted of two flats. Charlie and Whitman waited between the two doors silently.

The footsteps headed up the stairs, accompanied by the cackle of a radio. They stopped one floor below them.

"Mr. Whitman? It's the police." They were knocking on the door. And after a beat: "Open up."

Just wait it out.

They were banging now. "Open up."

No response.

Whitman put his finger over his own lips, motioning his friend to remain silent.

"Mr. Whitman?"

Whitman heard them talking.

It became apparent they didn't have a warrant.

After a few more knocks, the uniforms gave up. Whitman heard footsteps heading downstairs.

24

Elliot stood in front of his neighbor's door for a long time.

In the end, he threw the dice, so to speak—perhaps he wanted to tempt fate with the chance to stop him.

The door opened, and before he knew it, she was standing in front of him. Those velvety legs, the delicate hands, the tangles of soft hair outlining a shadow on her brittle neck—all of these features like snapshots braided in a spiral, and at its center an apparition that irrevocably seized his thoughts.

Something in her silence was haunting and hit close to home. But it was impossible to further acknowledge this, because by the time the realization had hit him, he had been ushered in her smell, in her ways, and in everything wicked she summoned inside him, a flickering charge of elated fervors and carnal desires registering too fast for him to catch up, in the blackness of her hair, her emerald eyes the only source of light, tongue tracing the contours of her lips—first the bottom, then the top— her pale skin emitting surges of warmth barely contained by her shirt, thighs brushing against the insides of her robe swishing the way a jungle will do in the wake of a tropical thunderstorm and one glimpse just one glimpse at the ambiguity of those eyes and he would be flying with her, speeding along a highway at night, leaving all the collapsed buildings and broken cars behind them, wind scoring their faces, their freedom informed by something deeper and unknown, holding on to th—

The woman asked whether she could be of help.

For a second he considered telling her it was a mistake. A part of him just wanted to go home and forget all about this. As he hesitated, the woman almost smiled at him. He surveyed her hallway and saw it was empty. He then knew it was his chance.

His face changed, his brow furrowed. He looked worried. "I'm your neighbor from across the hall," he said and the woman's expression indicated she recognized him. He made a movement with his head, as if by way of apology. He knew his face was turning red, but he couldn't help it. He couldn't even look her in the eye, just kept staring down as if he were talking to the ground. Yet for a moment he thought she had smiled at him.

"My daughter," he finally said, pointing back to his own flat. "She's having a severe asthma attack."

"Oh, my God! Do you want me to call someone? An ambulance!"

"No, no," he said, shaking his head, "I've done that already. Just need someone to stay with her while I get everything ready."

"Oh, of course." She seemed to recollect herself, grabbed her handbag and keys from the stand, and then thought of something. She darted to the living room.

Elliot heard her speak to her daughter: "Mommy will be next door, darling. I'll just be a few minutes, okay?" He smiled like a hungry wolf.

"What's her name?" she asked while shutting and locking the door to her flat. She placed her keys in her pocket and joined him in the hallway.

He could feel her breathing next to him, and he enjoyed that. He wanted to inhale her breathing and let it slide inside him. He wanted to inhale it and quench this irreparable need. He wanted to devour it and feel it run through his body as if this very act could fix him, put him back together. Make him what he should be. He wanted that lively, luscious breath that permeated her long black hair running to the base of her spine, the breath that pumped those green eyes—the kind that change color depending on the amount of sunlight; the breath that escaped from the pores of her pale white skin and her thick, blood-red lips. He looked at her clothes—the blue jeans and the skirt over them and the slippers—and he got the feeling that whatever she might wear would look oversize on her frail body.

Make me what I should be.

Seeing her face, Elliot realized a reply was expected. He did a double take. Then, upon understanding what she meant:

"Amanda. My daughter's name is Amanda."

"That's a beautiful name," she said.

"I took her for a tea today at this beautiful café on Drummond Street. She loved it so much . . . but I think the excitement and the walk back knocked the wind out of her."

"Oh, I know the one you're talking about . . . I go there all the time. It's called Black Med—"

She must have realized he was standing too close to her, because she moved. But it was too late. The knife was out of his pocket.

She was so surprised she didn't even make a sound. Everything seemed to be happening in slow motion. He pressed the knife against her spine and pushed her forward. He urged her down the steps, humming his little melody.

He finally got her inside the vault, then he jerked closed the door, got in, ensured she was still in place, and shut the doors. She was his now, and this was exciting. Her face was plain white—she was a sight for sore eyes, really. Her eyes were pleading and afraid. On some level it was funny. She just stared at him, waiting.

Everything was so quiet down there, like the dry summer afternoons in the shade of a tree. She started bawling and shaking so hard she could barely walk. He lowered his hand off her shoulder to grasp the upper part of her arm, holding her up. They were still walking, but she couldn't feel her legs.

She turned to run, but he grabbed the back of her hair, spun her around to face him, and pulled her up by the hair until her toes grazed the ground. The pain was excruciating. All she could do was try to kick and pound her fists on his arm. She screamed as loud as she could.

He slapped his free hand over her mouth and said, "Down here no one can hear us." He got a pad from his pocket and flung it right across her mouth and nose. He thought he could smell fumes, even though there was no fire. She struggled like a small animal. But she was too weak, such a small thing.

She clung to the arm that held her and tried to hoist her body up, to take away the pressure from her scalp. He lowered his arm slowly until her feet touched the ground. One of her slippers had fallen off when she tried to kick him, so she was off-balance and stumbled backwards. The step hit the back of her knees, and she landed on her rear end at the foot of the stairs. She sat there and stared out at him as the chloroform took effect, shaking so hard her teeth chattered. The horror took over only when she realized he had seen her put her house keys in her pocket and her daughter, Lily, was all alone in there. From her vantage point at the foot of the stairs, the light was bright behind his head, turning his face dark and outlining him in light.

He whispered into the darkness:

"Have you ever seen a fire, my love?"

25

The place stunk of voodoo.

They were sitting in a popular student haunt on the corner of Nicolson Street and Drummond Street. It was a brooding, totem-poled coffee shop, where they sometimes misspelled "cappuccino" on the menu board behind the bar. The ethnic decoration was packed with carved, tree-trunk-like benches uncomfortable to a man's behind, but the interior was warm and cozy, playing off the ergonomic driftwood theme of quirky au naturel chairs and tables.

Whitman and Charlie were sequestered in a little corner, sheltering from the rain. Whitman looked at his friend; his eyes were bloodshot, teeth chattering, tremors slowly quivering his limbs.

"What do we do now?" he kept saying.

Whitman remained silent.

A beeping sound from Whitman's phone interrupted them. He looked at the screen, expecting to see Valdano's number, but it was an 0131 number: local. He answered.

A male voice asked whether it was speaking to Mr. Alex Whitman.

"Who is this?"

"My client's name is Kasper Gutman."

"I don't suppose he wants me to find a missing bird for him?"

"You have something in your possession he is very interested in."

"Wouldn't be my good looks, now, would it?"

"The film, Mr. Whitman."

"I don't know what you're talking about."

"The film. My client can offer information about the film that would be particularly important for your . . . research."

"What research would that be?"

"I surmise you have already figured out there are hidden frames inside the film?"

Whitman didn't reply.

"Surely you are aware the film is incomplete," the caller said.

"How do you mean?"

"The last five frames are missing. I have them here with me. Pictures of a little girl. She might even remind you of someone."

Whitman silently breathed into the telephone. He realized the man was not talking about a client anymore; it was "I," and "me."

"How do you know about the last frames?"

"The copy you have?"

"Yes?"

"I left it there for you. Are you still there, Mr. Whitman?"

"I'm listening."

"I understand you have a deal with a quite prosperous client. In exchange for the voiding of this deal, I can provide the remaining frames and a hefty six-figure sum. Needless to say, I will hold on to the original paper film."

"I don't suppose you have anything to do with the dead Catalan."

"Excuse me?"

"What do you need me for?"

"I need help with deciphering the codes."

"What's in it for you?" Whitman said. *Codes?* he thought. *What codes?*

"That should not concern you."

Whitman weighed his options.

"Clock's ticking," the man said.

"Name a place."

. . .

"He said something about a code. That he needs help."

"Who cares about that?" Charlie asked. "Nestor's body is in your house!"

"You can bail if you want to. I need to stay and figure this out."

"Curiosity killed the cat, Alex. I think we have to watch our backs." He was still shaking.

Whitman tried to laugh it away, hoping his relaxed demeanor would calm his friend.

Charlie nodded in return. "Want me to come with?"

"No, I'll call you when I finish."

Outside, students with tired eyes just out of Old College; skate kids with baggy trousers newly purchased from Flip; cheap-food aficionados with their bellies full from the Chinese buffet up the road; a blind man waiting on the traffic light. Whitman watched the light turn red and heard the beeping sound echo, an acoustical guidance tag to help those with loss of sight. The blind man began to cross the street, his cane moving left to right, feeling the way. The frequency of the guidance sound increased and then ceased, giving the man enough time to get across to the other sidewalk.

Whitman got up from his seat, almost spilling his mug of coffee. "We need to get to a library. Now."

"You got a sudden craving for reading?"

"Remember the clapperboard? The 'dominoes'?"

"Yes."

"It's not what we thought."

"What is it?"

"It's braille," Whitman said. "The son of a bitch put braille code inside the frames."

They crossed the road, turning onto Chambers Street; at the end of the road they turned right onto George IV Bridge and stopped in front of the National Library of Scotland.

Three crows were perched side by side on the pavilion roof of the Edinburgh Public Library; a further two flew in circles around the octagonal Caenesque lantern, all below an ashen sky.

Whitman and Charlie sat at a computer on the library's ground floor.

Charlie hauled a few books from a shelf. It turned out they just needed one; it was called *Braille in Brief,* by an author named Kyoko Toshiego.

Whitman pulled out a piece of paper. From their printed material, they aligned the image of the first "domino frame" and began their trials. Two words formed.

DEAR FRIEND

They looked at each other, their gut instincts confirmed.

It took them the better part of an hour to decipher the code. Whitman held the paper in front of him. Augustin Sekuler was talking to them.

Dear friend, I have experienced the most horrendous of times these past months. I found solace in the animated pictures. Although it gave me comfort, I eventually encountered the demons that sleep within that medium. I am surrounded by shadows and closely watched by hungry eyes, who aspire to my demise. And you, dear friend? Are you truthful to my values?

I have thought greatly over this matter in search of a vessel for my secret, a way to protect it against the burning of memory and the oblivion of time. I have found no such vessel greater than the moving picture. Its frames have the capacity to embody the truth of man, even in its most abstruse form.

My name is Augustin Louis Sekuler and I importune neither confidence nor conviction. Primarily so in the series of events I am about to embark on, where perception scorns reason and observation impugns perspicacity. I have been inspired by this city and its ancestors, whose works will stand after a thousand years. It is in this city I have hidden my greatest secret and I invite you to find it. I regard this city as an entity; its soul has survived until today and it has been my companion in struggle. I have used it to devise a series of riddles which mask my great secret. Their solution can unveil my true words. You must prove yourself a lover of this city and its beauty, so that I will know your intentions are honourable. Should you accomplish this, the city itself will reveal the answers to you.

The first clue is among you, for all to see. 'Tis a house that argues

with its neighbours and it speaks; yet only the mirror can see the secret
it keeps.

PESPECTOIRESUMRAHDIECRASTIBIVITAEMRTALIUM
CRIGITURCRASMIHIUTTULINGUAETUAESICEGMEARAU
RIUALTERACNSTANTI

The smell of honeysuckle and an image of a little girl riding a bicycle
along the path of an Edinburgh park.

That girl in the hidden image was Ellie. He knew it.

The film was made a hundred years ago. Ellie's dead.

"A secret?" Charlie said. He looked at the letter, then up at Whitman
in amazement. "Like what? A treasure?"

"I want to try something else," Whitman said. He typed the braille
code from the dominoes of the second hidden frame.

A set of nonsensical words ran across the lines of the paper.

"It's gibberish."

"Of course it is," Charlie said. "Don't you see? It's a sequence of codes."

Whitman nodded.

"I'll transcribe the whole thing; but we'll need the code word for the
next riddle in order to make sense of it." Charlie took the paper. "Why
do you think he did this? What's the secret?"

"Maybe our mysterious friend will have more answers. I'm meeting
him in twenty minutes."

26

The rendezvous point Whitman had chosen was outside the McEwan Hall in Bristo Square. Making contact near his flat could have proved dangerous; the police were probably watching, and there was always the question of the caller's intentions. The mystery man had called asking about the possibility of striking a deal involving the missing frames. It was unclear how he fit into all this.

Whitman turned around and looked at the building behind him. McEwan Hall, Whitman thought, with its decorative Italian Renaissance style, was much more beautiful than the flat-topped, copper-clad, domed Usher Hall. The intricate structure was a grandiose creation, extravagant in both its internal and external finishes. It was now a venue for graduation ceremonies and other academic events. Kate's graduation had taken place in there.

Students passed him on their way to the medical school, Teviot Place, and Potterrow. A homeless man sat on the other side of the street, reading a *Metro*. A young girl his daughter's age was missing, the headline said. A kidnapper was on the loose. Whitman tried not to think about it: one foot into the big four-oh and at the end all one had to show was a busted marriage and a missing—or dead—daughter.

At the foot of the lofty building, he lit a cigarette and leaned against the wall, watching the traffic go by and listening to the soft drizzle tap on the pavement.

His contact didn't keep him waiting. At the designated time, a white Chrysler limousine veered out of the traffic coming from Teviot Place and slowed to a halt at the curbside. The uniformed driver looked at him, wondering if he was the right person. Whitman opened the rear door and got in.

"Mister Whitman?" the driver asked. He had a unibrow on his pointed forehead. Whitman nodded.

The car accelerated along Lauriston Place and turned into Lothian Road, heading north. Whitman watched the city center flash by. The weather had started to clear by the time they reached the outlying area of the city. Roadside pubs flew by, mirrored on his glasses, followed by Victorian buildings, until there was just the wood and shrub of Dean Village.

Whitman retreated into his thoughts. His business was chasing facts, not dreams. Yet somehow, a malevolent force from the cupboard of nightmares had sneaked into the world and into his life and his daughter's disappearance. The hidden frames worried him; logic dictated that this girl was not Ellie, but to him it felt as if she was.

He thought about his mysterious caller: Kasper Gutman. Whitman knew Kasper Gutman. But it couldn't be the same guy. The Kasper Gutman he knew was from *The Maltese Falcon*. Sydney Greenstreet; Kasper Gutman was the villain's name. Whitman knew Kasper Gutman. How ridiculous. And why did he live in Dean Village? Who the hell lives in Dean Village, anyway?

The caller had asked for Whitman to bring the memory stick with his copy of the film so that he could be satisfied there had been "no omissions." How did he know Valdano had contracted Whitman to find it? All he would have to do was to help decipher some codes. Not a bad way to make an extra six figures. But something didn't feel right; that sensation in his gut was growing stronger.

He had taken precautions. If this was a diversion, they wouldn't know where to find Charlie, who had an extra copy of the film on him. They could target the house, but they would find nothing. They could have followed Charlie . . . but no plan was foolproof. Maybe he was just paranoid.

The limousine slowed down. Perhaps they'd arrived. A single house sat in front of them, surrounded by trees and thick bushes.

The car paused in front of a garage and the door opened. The driver eased the car slowly in.

Whitman was reaching for his backpack when the driver pressed a button on the overhead control panel. The central locking system clunked to engage. There was a whirring noise, and a thick glass partition glided up, blocking Whitman off from the driver.

"Hey," he said, rapping the glass. "Are we here? I'm talking to you."

The driver switched off the ignition and the headlights went out. The garage door rolled back down, rendering the place pitch-black. The driver opened the door and a light came on inside the car. Whitman glanced at the partition between them: it looked like reinforced steel panes embedded within the glass.

"Hey!"

The driver quietly got out and slammed the door shut, and the interior was sunk again in darkness. A quivering beam of flashlight jiggled as the man rummaged through the garage, searching for something in the tool rack.

Whitman pounded on the glass partition. The only thing he could see was the glimmer of the beam of light, bouncing from side to side. The driver found what he was looking for. Whitman couldn't see what the object was, but it looked long, like a rope.

He fumbled about in his compartment for a way out. The man drew closer to the car. Whitman tried the locks again; he knew it was pointless. He knew the door would soon fly open, revealing the driver with a gun in his hand.

To his surprise, the man walked past and around to the back of the car. Still carrying the object, he bent down, the back of the vehicle obscuring him from Whitman's view.

There was a noise and the man rose again, heading back toward the driver's seat. He opened the door and reached inside, snaking the black object into a hole connected to Whitman's backseat compartment. In the internal light of the car, Whitman saw it was a rubber hose.

Then the man reached for the keys. As he worked them into the ignition, the tense silence was interrupted by the loud, shuddering sound of
the car's exhaust. With a cough and the splutter of the exhaust pipes, the
engine started.

No way out.

Death within minutes.

The man waved goodbye to Whitman with a grim smile and closed
the door, dipping him again into darkness. He left through another door
in the garage, leading into the main house.

Whitman's eyes were adjusted to the dark by now. As the carbon monoxide filled the car, his eyes and throat started to feel irritated. He glanced
at the window beside him; it was blurring from condensation.

His head ached, throbbing to the beat of his racing heart. He looked
down at the hole connecting to the rubber hose.

When a man is about to die a senseless death, common sense will
often desert him. Whitman took out a pen and tried to detach the hose
from the hole. No luck. He even tried one of his shoes—a shoe, for
Christ's sake.

It took him another minute to figure out that even if he could move
the hose, it would still remain inside the locked vehicle, pumping carbon
monoxide all over the place.

He was a dead man.

His lungs felt as though they were condensing.

Water drops the size of queen bees were forming on the glass windows.

There had to be a way out.

The daze was overtaking him. He hesitated, then started beating on
the glass again, then punching it, punching it until his palms were red
and his knuckles were bloody.

He looked out the window, as if the answers lay in the darkness
beyond. But no answers came. There were boxes and tools sprawled on
the floor: a hammer, a blowtorch, things that could get him out if only
he could get to them.

He thought of Ellie and his wife, and for some reason he thought
of the hidden frames. Only now, in the grip of imminent death, did he
realize the girl in the hidden picture—an almost spitting image of his
daughter—was none other than Zoe Sekuler, the mysterious inventor's

daughter, who had also disappeared. It was a coincidence of some obscure significance he couldn't put his finger on, but it was there, and it had to mean something.

The oxygen in the compartment was so depleted that he could feel the pressure on his temples. He could breathe only through his mouth.

His eyelids became heavy. He tried to force them open; were he to succumb, there would be no coming back from that kind of sleep.

There was the thunderclap sound of collision.

He cringed and moved away from the left window.

The car shook once more.

Another collision. Something was out there.

Another crash. The car's pane began to give way toward the inside. He crouched down. He could barely keep his eyelids open.

The voice from outside was muffled, unfamiliar.

"Whitman? You in there?"

It was a woman's voice. He couldn't work out whether he knew the person calling out. Not that it mattered; things were starting to slip now, slowly and slowly condensing and slipping away slowly and slipping away and slipping away and slowly slipping away and slipping away slowly slipping away slipping away slowly slipping away slipping away slowly slipping away slipping away slowly slipping away slipping away slowly slipping away slipping away slowly slipping away slipping away slowly slipping away slipping away slowly slipping away slipping away slowly slipping away slipping away slowly slipping away slipping away slowly slipping away slipping away slowly slipping away slipping away slowly slipping away

"Get me out of here," he whispered. Ellie was the last thing he saw.

The woman had found the steel hammer in the tool rack. She brought it up and swung with all her might at the window.

The reinforced glass spiderwebbed but did not give.

Inside, the atmosphere was stifling. Water started pouring out of the hose.

Frustrated, McBride threw the hammer to the back of the garage.

She tried the driver's door.

"Way to go, Detective Sergeant," she said to herself with a snort. "Open the whole time." She climbed inside.

She banged on the glass partition dividing her from Whitman. There was no response. He must have lost consciousness. There was no way to tell; the glass was ridden with soot and she couldn't see him anymore.

She looked around the driver's compartment. She began pressing buttons frantically, hoping something would happen. Nothing did.

She found another button and pressed it.

The lock shifted to disengage.

She rushed out of the car and opened the back door. Whitman was unconscious.

She grabbed him by the arms and carried him onto the garage floor.

He was breathing. She reached down to perform CPR. Her lips were an inch away from his mouth when his eyes opened.

He tried to sit up. Halfway up, he realized the pain was excruciating and leaned back down again. He rubbed his aching head. "Who the *fuck* are you?"

She threw him a look. "You're welcome."

He gave no reply. His eyes were watery and he was shaking.

"Let's take you out of here," she said.

The wind whistled at Whitman through the crack in the car window. McBride's Volvo was accelerating along Queensferry Road, out of Dean Village.

"My name's Georgina McBride," she said in the silence. Whitman didn't answer. He just wanted to get to the city and find Charlie, find a place for the night.

Without looking at him, McBride reached into her coat with one hand and produced her badge. "I'm a detective sergeant with the Lothian and Borders Police." She could sense him fiddling in his seat.

"And what were you doing back there?"

She snorted. "Apart from saving your arse?"

He was silent.

"We'll talk about this later. I'll chum ya to the Royal Infirmary first. You need to see a doctor."

"No hospitals. Just drop me off anywhere. Here should be good," he said, gesturing to nowhere in particular and reaching for the door. McBride pressed a button and the doors locked into place. "What's the matter? Afraid I'll pinch you?"

He laughed it off. "I don't know what you thought you saw back there . . ."

"I know what I saw, Alex," she said.

She knew his name.

She put the car in third gear, taking advantage of the green lights— a rare blessing at this time of day—and made the turn into Lothian Road.

Whitman took out a packet of Rizlas, slid out a paper, and tore off part of the packet, twisting and rolling it into a roach. His hands were trembling. "Okay, I'll bite: What's your story?"

"In case you haven't heard, we've got a perp out there who's kidnapping little girls."

Whitman plucked some tobacco from his pouch. McBride glanced at him spreading it, pinching it all the while across the paper. The smell reached her nostrils and she had to look away.

"And what do you want me to do?" Whitman said. "Castrate him?"

"I want you to help me find him."

He shook his head. "How would I do that? I find films, memorabilia, posters—you know, those kinds of things. Not children."

"There's some connection between my case and yours." She eyed Whitman. His tongue darted out, licking the gum, sealing the paper with the air of a job well done; he had wound a perfect tube. He ran two fingers across the roll-up, top to bottom, in a swishing motion.

"I don't understand," he said.

"Why did you come back here, Alex?"

"The sunny weather?"

"You haven't been back here in ten years."

"You've been checking up on me. What a treat."

"You don't seem to have any friends left here. And I've spoken to people who know you; they say you're a vulture."

He placed the cigarette between his lips. "If I had a penny for every time I heard that."

She turned and glanced at him. "It has to do with that film, doesn't it? That's why that guy was trying to kill you."

Whitman blinked, Zippo frozen in one hand, cigarette dangling unlit from his lower lip.

"Yes, I know about the film," McBride said. "We managed to recover a fraction of it from the hard drive of the computer at the Archive." She eyed the cigarette. "You think you should be doing that after almost dying of asphyxiation?"

He laughed. "We're great lovers, me and nicotine. I take her in sweetly; she kills me slowly." He sighed. "I found it. This is my film. Someone tried to take it. Don't ask me why; I have no idea."

"What's in the film, Alex?"

"You've seen it?"

"Fragments. And our perp has paid homage to one of the hidden sections."

"When was this?"

"Long before the business at the Archive."

He frowned, eyes widening with every word. "It can't be. I have—had—the only copy."

"Apparently not."

He sat staring at the license plate of the car in front of them.

"We're going to have to trust each other," McBride said. "I could have brought you in the moment I had you on the floor back there."

"You're kidding, right?"

"But then I saw your daughter's name. She's one of the girls who disappeared. And then it hit me: You're still looking; you've been looking this whole time."

"My daughter's dead. I came here to find a film."

"You found the film, Alex."

"Some films refuse to stay on the screen where they belong, Serpico."

"Unless you help me out, I have no other option but to take you in."

"Blackmail: a great way to start a new collaboration." He sighed and his expression changed to one of resignation. "Okay. You got me. Let's get a coffee and talk this whole thing over."

She nodded, satisfied with herself.

"I just need to do something first," he said. He gestured at an ATM booth coming up on their left.

"I can't park here."

"Next one up, Chuckles."

Earl Grey Street's wide boulevard was packed with shops, beginning to recover from a long period of decline. Goldbergs had built their new store there, with its merry-go-round, but that was now gone, as was Jenny's Wardrobe and the imposing St. Cuthbert's complex. The latter had been replaced by a five-star hotel with majestic corridors and luxury interior decor, not far from St. Cuthbert's Co-op where Sean Connery used to work as a milkman. But times had changed; the Palais de Dance was now Bingo, and there was no doorman outside.

She turned the car left into Lauriston Place and brought it to a stop. He got out.

She thought for a minute, then opened her own door.

He gave her a glance.

"Thought you might need some company. Three minutes," she said, right before he entered the booth. She tapped a finger below her left eye. "I'm watching you."

Whitman grinned. He was holding his sarcastic comeback for his own pleasure.

Cars were halted at the traffic light on the main road. She hesitated, then got out and searched in her pockets for a lighter. She had quit many times in the past. Every time she gave in, it felt worse.

She exhaled the smoke, reveling in the pleasure of nicotine hitting the receptors in her brain.

She looked back at the booth. Whitman had his back to her.

Students waited for the bus on the way to classes. A shabby man in his wheelchair, obviously homeless, cowered on the side of the walkway, half-asleep. A few people headed up the street to catch a concert at the cap-domed Usher Hall. A man with a large beard led a group of tourists on a ghost tour.

The tourists enjoyed the macabre spirit of the city, the hundreds-of-years-old murders and body snatching. It was concise and effective; it shifted their attention from the true horrors in life. Had they heard of the stabbings in Royston or the gang vandalism in Niddrie? How about the prossies in Leith or the junkies in West Pilton? Major Weir and Deacon Brodie made sure these people didn't get wind of anything more up to date.

A man stopped next to her and asked her for a light. She obliged. He thanked her and continued on his way.

She turned toward the booth.

It was empty.

She saw Whitman running down Lothian Road and turning into East Fountainbridge.

"Oh, sod it," she said, throwing the cigarette to the ground.

Whitman took East Fountainbridge farther east, running through the road junction known as the Pubic Triangle; there, young lads lured in by tacky fairy lights and thumping music entered the den of sirens proclaiming private dances. It was strange how they were all part of the same local area, elements of different standing working together to improve and entertain the city: the lap-dancing pub a stone's throw from a four-star hotel; the establishment of naked waitresses neighboring an antiquarian bookstore; the body-entertainment people and the book people, focusing on different aspects of customer delight.

He had now slowed to a fast walk, glancing over his shoulder every few steps. No sight of El Porco. By the time she realized he was gone it would be too late. He crossed over to the West Port, past more bookshops, toward the Grassmarket. The castle's rear end appeared over the open space.

He glanced at the pubs to his left, close to where the last public hanging in Scotland had been carried out. The condemned man had been granted one last drink right here, in the pub known as the Last Drop.

He needed a beer. But now was not the time. He had to find Charlie.

At the end of the paved street, he climbed Candlemaker Row. He felt in his pocket for his cell phone; it was switched off. He looked at the device, focused, still walking.

Then his face exploded.

A punch.

The pain soared through the whole of his face, centering on the septum of his nose. His eyes watered and closed shut, tears oozing from the sealed red sockets. It took five seconds for him to open them again. His face felt numb and his ears were buzzing. He dropped his palms from his face and saw them covered in blood. He looked up and, through soggy eyes, saw Georgina McBride standing in front of him, grinning.

"You almost broke my nose!"

"Quit acting like a child," she said. She pulled a pack of tissues from her pocket. "Here," she said. "You look like shit."

He opened the pack and used one tissue to wipe his hands and two more for his face. The last he kept over his nose, making his voice muffled.

"You're dangerous."

"And you're in need of a nose job. Come on, criminal, let's plunk yerself down and get that drink."

27

They met with Charlie at West Nicolson Street, inside an eighteenth-century pub named after the two sturdy trees that had been planted in front of the edifice.

There was smoke all around. Cigarettes burned between yellowed fingers, which in turn were clutching pint glasses. A projection screen was mounted on the wall on one side of the bar area, but the sounds of the football game being broadcast were drowned out by the music.

McBride was lost. "So are you going to tell me how this film fits into the whole story?" she asked.

"You tell me, Serpico," Whitman said, drawing on his cigarette. "You show up out of nowhere, talking about a murder I know nothing about, when I've been minding my own business."

"We're going to have to trust each other, Alex."

"Three heads are better than one," Charlie said, looking at Whitman.

"There are hidden frames in the film, pictures that don't make any sense."

"The one I saw with the girl." She noticed the expression on Charlie's face and took a few minutes to explain how she had made the connection between the serial kidnapper's video of the girl in the mirrors and the almost identical frame from Sekuler's film, as found in the Archive's computer.

"But there's other stuff, too," Charlie said. "Codes."

"Codes?"

"Some of the frames are coded in braille. It's a letter. Written by Augustin Sekuler, the man who invented the moving pictures." Whitman pushed the piece of paper with their notes toward her. "The end of the letter is a code, its solution being the key word to decipher the next coded frame."

She read the letter. "So each code presumably leads to another location in the city."

Whitman nodded. "That's what we think."

"What's it all for?"

"We don't know yet," Charlie said. "Sekuler talks about a secret, something he had to conceal in the frames of 'Séance Infernale.'"

"But the film is incomplete—on purpose," Whitman cut in. "Which means the missing frames, wherever they might be, are hiding something."

She studied the letter and the notes. "Well, whatever it is, it has to do with the city."

"He talks about it like it's a real live person," Charlie said.

"Doesn't surprise me," McBride said. "There is magic in this city, Charlie. It escapes words, but it recognizes greatness. Like it did with Dickens."

"Dickens?"

McBride nodded. "He was in Edinburgh," she said, "for a series of lectures. He was wandering the city, killing time before his talk, when he visited the Canongate Kirk graveyard. On one of the tombstones he saw a memorial slab that read, EBENEZER LENNOX SCROGGIE—MEAL MAN; it belonged to some man from Kirkcaldy who was a corn merchant—a meal man. But Dickens misread it as 'mean man.' He was shocked by the description, and two years later he used it as inspiration for *A Christmas Carol*, which featured Ebenezer Scrooge, a 'mean man' erroneously based on Ebenezer Scroggie."

Whitman cut in and said, "Wait a second." He pointed his finger at McBride. "I still don't get what's in all this for you. How could a film shot a century ago have any bearing on a modern murder?"

She fidgeted on the leather chair. "Like I said, our perp has paid homage to one of the fragments hidden in 'Séance Infernale.' You found a copy in Sekuler's old workshop and you thought it was the only copy. But it's not. The footage the perp sent as a videocassette back in the 1980s is similar to the one we found a few days ago at the Archive. So . . ."

"So your perp has seen the frames in 'Séance,' " Charlie said.

"Exactly. How many places could Sekuler have stashed his work in Edinburgh? His workshop and his house are prime candidates. You searched his workshop, where you found the film. That leaves his house. You said you don't know its location, but the perp obviously does. It's been almost a century since the film was made, and a lot of things can happen in that time. Sekuler's property may have changed hands from one person to another until . . ."

"Until the killer got to it."

McBride nodded. "Maybe it's the place the perp happens to live, or where he works; maybe it's an abandoned warehouse or tunnel that only he knows about. With this"—she gestured at the notes on the table—"we have a shot at finding the place. If we follow the frames, we find where the other copy is stashed . . ."

"And we also find your perp," Whitman said. "And the missing girl—Amanda Pearson, was it?"

She nodded. "Indeed. So you find your inventor's treasure—or whatever he's hiding—and you help save a little girl's life, at the same time clearing your name. Not too bad from just a movie."

"Sounds like an adventure—right out of *The Goonies*," Charlie said, raising his pint.

McBride laughed at this. And then she straightened the notes and pointed to the first riddle. "I'll tell you what, though: It is so true about the house that speaks. That is exactly what my grandmother used to call some houses when I was a little girl."

"How do you mean?"

"Speaking houses. If you observe them carefully, the façades of most houses in Edinburgh bear inscriptions. Usually it's the name of the person who built it, or the owner's; sometimes it's the year it was erected. Other times, though, there are little pieces of wisdom, scattered in the city for all to see. Especially the one I'm thinking of. They call it the Speaking House."

Charlie stared with wide eyes. "Where is this house?"

28

It was one of those treasure boxes dotting the city, a maze of historic rooms crammed full of iconic objects from the capital's past. Huntly House was a typical sixteenth-century edifice, with triple gables over the lower stories. Charlie, McBride, and Whitman stood on the Canongate, facing the building once known as the Speaking House. Some of its windows were open, but no one was watching them; in museums, nobody looks out the windows.

Inside, informative displays told the history of the city, from prehistoric times through to the nineteenth century. Visitors could see collections of colorful shop signs, pottery, and silver and glass. But Whitman and his companions were not interested in the inside; in Edinburgh, the buildings themselves are often the real attractions. Sometimes, if you listen closely, they speak; and their stories whisper of their past.

People were moving by them, not paying attention to the three figures looking up at a sixteenth-century house with alabaster inscriptions on its stone walls.

Do they know? Whitman wondered. *As they head to their jobs and schools and colleges and meetings and lunches, does anyone pay attention to these bizarre words hovering over their heads?* A couple of tourists were waiting for the bus, resting their backpacks against the Speaking House's walls; a man was gazing at the Ouija boards and alchemical jewelry in the Wyrd Shop's window. Across the street, the Doric-columned portico of the Canongate Kirkyard stood as it had since the seventeenth century, inviting the world to explore the necropolis unraveling beyond its black iron fence. The few rays of light coming through the clouds gleamed on the stone clock of the Old Tolbooth, once a toll-collecting gate, at another time a prison for Covenanters. A few hundred years ago, across the street, a lord justice clerk had reputedly once succeeded in raising the devil in his backyard.

"You see?" Charlie said.

"See what?"

"The inscriptions." He took out his notes. He had been scribbling in his notebook from the moment McBride gave him the clue he needed. McBride and Whitman huddled around him. Charlie had written down four inscriptions, followed by their literal translations. "Some were added during the 1930s. I've only written down the ones that existed in Sekuler's time."

HODIE MIHI CRAS TIBI CVR IGITVR CVRAS—Today to me, tomorrow to thee; why therefore takest thou thought? (I am a happy man today; your turn may come)

VT TV LINGVAE SIC EGO MEAR(VM) AVRIM(M) DOMINVS SVM—As thou of thy tongue, so I of my ears, am lord (As you are master of your tongue, so am I master of my ears)

CONSTANTI PECTORI RES MORTALIVM VMBRA—Mortal affairs are a shadow to a steadfast heart (To the constant heart, things of the mortal world are but a shadow)

SPES ALTERA VITAE—There is another hope of life

"The builder incorporated the inscriptions into the walls," McBride said. "Evidently, many of the neighbors didn't want the house to be built and took their frustrations out on the builder. So he carved these inscriptions; it's like a dialogue with the annoyed neighbors. But as long as the house stands, only the builder's side of the dialogue remains."

"Nice little story," Whitman said. "What's the point?"

"The inscriptions," Charlie said again. "Compare them to the last part of Sekuler's letter."

Whitman's eyes widened in recognition as he scanned through Sekuler's words, shifting his gaze back and forth between the message and the house's inscriptions.

Charlie was right: the alabaster inscriptions looked alarmingly similar to the letters from Sekuler's frames.

"They're identical?"

"Almost," Charlie said. "Some letters are missing. Guess what happens when you write the letters down."

"A word?"

Charlie nodded. "The code was simple—if you knew about the house."

"So what's the word?"

Charlie showed him, but he placed his hand over the rest of the notes, holding back another surprise.

SOROBORUO

"What the hell is that?" Whitman said.

"Beats me."

McBride scratched her head. "So that's the key word?"

"I've already tried it," Charlie said. "It's not."

"Then you're wrong."

"Already ahead of you. Don't forget," Charlie said, "there's the last part of the message: 'Only the mirror can see the secret it keeps.'"

"So," McBride said, "if you read the letters in reverse, you get the word we're after?"

Charlie nodded and slid his hand down another line, revealing the word in reverse:

OUROBOROS

"In true mirror reverse, the R, for example, would look like Я, but it would still signify the same letter," he explained.

"Sounds like . . . something. Any idea what it is?"

"No. But it is a real word. And I know this because it works." He handed his notebook to Whitman, who proceeded to read it under the light of the moon. It was another letter by Augustin Sekuler. As he read, his gaze strayed to the street across from them. A man was sitting on one of the benches outside the kirkyard, doing a bad job at pretending to read a newspaper by moonlight. Whitman could see right through him: silk shirt, tobacco-stained smile, gold rings adorning his fingers.

"Stay calm," he said. "I think we have a spectator."

"What?"

"Don't look. Guy on the bench across the street, reading the paper."

They pretended to idle in front of the building for a few minutes, then slowly retreated toward McBride's car, which was parked about fifty yards away, outside the People's Story museum.

Whitman scanned the reflections in the shop windows; he noticed the man had stood up from the bench and was following them.

They picked up the pace.

When they were just a few feet away from McBride's car, they saw the second man. He was hanging around under the arches, near the sign proclaiming gifts that made a difference, looking into the windows of their car. The man hadn't seen them yet; he was smoking a cigarette and flicking the ash on the tray top of the garbage can next to him. Whitman recognized the man as the unibrow limo driver who had tried to murder him.

"Is that . . ."

"Yup. There's two of them."

"What do we do?" Charlie said.

"Keep a calm sooch," McBride said. "Let's get in the car."

Unibrow finally saw them and turned to face them. He was a bear of a man. He stood, blocking access to the driver's door. In the distance behind him, Whitman saw there was a third man, standing on the cobbled footpath a good fifteen yards away.

Charlie stepped behind Whitman and McBride, avoiding eye contact with anyone. The limo-driver guy had almost caught up with them; he stood on the opposite side, a stone's throw behind them, another human barrier ensuring they wouldn't make a run for it.

Unibrow stared at Whitman. "Do you know who we are?" American accent, McBride noticed.

"Sure," Whitman said. "You're the Three Stooges: Moe, Curly, and"—he gestured at the third man far behind them—"I always forget the other guy."

"Maybe you'll remember this." The man brushed aside the tails of his overcoat, revealing a semiautomatic in a nylon holster under his left arm. "Mr. Valdano would like his film back. The memory stick."

"What if I don't want to give it back?"

McBride quickly read what was about to happen. She saw the man's eyes; he would not hesitate to harm, even to kill, Whitman on the spot.

"I've got it," she said. "I have the memory stick."

The man granted her a glance for the first time.

McBride fished in her coat pockets.

Whitman was dumbfounded. He shot her a *What the hell are you doing?* glance, but she didn't see it.

From a pocket, she produced a set of keys. Whitman couldn't see a memory stick anywhere, and that puzzled him even more. The keys were mounted on a ring, and the ring was mounted on a stainless-steel handle.

McBride's hand closed tightly around the base of one of the serrated keys. She swung it across Unibrow's face, in a fast, slashing motion, like she was trying to split the air in two. Blood spurted, spraying across Unibrow's cheeks, across everybody's shirts, and across the wall to their side. Unibrow felt the blood with the tips of his fingers. He barely made a sound, crumpling to the ground almost instantly.

Nobody believed it at first; they stood over him, sucking in the cold air, the key in McBride's hand resting by her side following the sweeping movement, blood still dripping on the cobbles.

McBride made for the car door, but Whitman grabbed her and pointed down. She gasped; one of the Volvo's front tires lay flat; someone had slashed it.

By now Unibrow had recovered consciousness and was trying to get up.

McBride acted quickly. "Follow me. When I give you the signal, leg it like hell."

Whitman and Charlie gave each other a look. They followed her as she darted forward, away from the car, straight onto the Canongate, toward the bridges. Toward the third man. He was baffled at first, seeing his victims sprinting toward him, but he quickly moved toward them, too.

On McBride's signal, the trio broke into a run. People around them made way, staring. "Over here," McBride said, and signaled Whitman and Charlie to take a right, on a cobblestoned path that led into the Calton Tunnel.

They heard shouts behind them. Two of the thugs were after them.

"Nice going, Serpico," Whitman said, already out of breath. "Two guys in one day. You must be proud. I don't suppose I should wait for a third one anytime soon?"

"Three's my lucky number," McBride said, grinning through gritted teeth.

"Stop or we shoot," one of the men behind them shouted.

But Whitman and his companions kept going, bulling their way through the street, their shoes flapping on the cobbled stone.

Thunder rumbled overhead. Rain began to pour down.

Whitman heard short wheezing sounds from behind him: Charlie was panting already. A man his size . . . maybe this hadn't been such a great idea.

A few hundred paces farther and they were entering the tunnel, taking them into the bowels of Calton Hill.

Whitman could hear the thugs behind him. How long could he keep this up? A stitch began to nag on his right side.

"Come on, come on, get them, get them!"

They entered the tunnel. Running frantically, Whitman felt his way along its wall, desperately trying to find a door, an exit, a way out of this mad chase.

Behind them, the other goons had been joined by Unibrow; he didn't seem happy.

Whitman swung his arms level with his shoulders to keep his balance. His breath whooshed from his lungs in the chilly Edinburgh air, billowing and twirling before his face. His chest heaved as the oxygen supply shortened and the lactic acid ran in high concentration through his lower limbs.

By far the most physically active of the three, McBride had broken into a full sprint and was yards ahead, turning her head and urging Charlie and Whitman to go faster, warning them that the bad guys were catching up.

My legs are going to give out any minute, Whitman thought, *and they're*

*going to catch us and kill us and it's not going to make a difference because I
have failed you again, Ellie.*

"Stop or we'll shoot!"

McBride heard one of them say her name, telling the others to watch
it, in case "the bitch is strapped, too."

"Come on, come on, we're safe," she called to Whitman. "Don't
worry, they'll never shoot."

The men started shooting.

"You were saying?" Whitman said between his teeth, even though he
knew McBride couldn't hear him.

One of the bullets flew past them and shattered a glass window. Charlie let out a whimper.

"At least they're crap at shooting," Whitman said.

He had thought that once they were inside the tunnel they would be
safe, but it was a no-win situation.

The men were right behind them; they had almost caught up.

In a matter of seconds they're going to get to Charlie, Whitman thought,
*and then you're going to have to stay behind. Unless you're too much of a
chickenshit to help your friend. You didn't even help your family—how the
fuck do you call yourself a human being?*

He stumbled over a stone and fell to the ground, and his teeth sank
into his tongue. He got up and kept running, tasting the blood in his
mouth. A fragment of his trousers had been torn off at knee level.

He had to go faster.

He could hear them now. Their guns were out; they were within
range. He heard Charlie crying out and urged him to go faster.

As the bullets erupted behind him, Whitman dived again, sliding out
of control across the cobbles and crashing in a heap against some railings
in an alcove on the stone wall.

Accompanying the roar of the gun, he felt a sensation he had never
experienced in his life: the peculiar feeling of a bullet sweeping past his
flesh. There was a hissing sound, like the backlash of a whip, and the
bullet clanged deep in the cobbles with a flurry of dirt. Blood surging,
Whitman heaved his body the rest of the way and got up. Aching and
depleted, he broke into a loping run.

He didn't get to run for long.

There was a gunshot and then a large thud on the ground.

One less set of footsteps flapping on the cobbles.

He turned around and saw Charlie lying on the ground.

There was blood.

Whitman stopped running. He was staring at his friend lying there; it was as if his brain was screaming at him inside his own head, screaming, "Run!" but the message wasn't getting through—there was something else in the way, something else holding him back with Charlie inside that tunnel.

He heard McBride cry out and could see her reaching toward him, trying to pull him away. But it was too late. The men were mere feet away. It was all over.

They pointed their guns at Whitman and McBride. Other than Unibrow's blood-painted face—that dirty grin spattered with russety spots—nothing registered with Whitman. One of the men began to say something, but Whitman couldn't understand.

He heard the sound before he saw it coming.

The screeching of tires.

Out of the corner of his eye, a brown car, tinted windows, sped inside the tunnel, colliding with one of the men, hauling him down to the ground, and spinning round to face the others.

The two remaining thugs were at a loss; they clenched their guns tightly.

The car revved its engine, roaring.

Unibrow made a movement to raise his gun, and the car revved again, inching forward just a bit. The sound was hard, deep, guttural, as if inviting a game of chicken.

The toughies dropped their guns slowly.

McBride glared at the car. It seemed to be waiting for them to make a getaway.

Seizing the opportunity, she grabbed Whitman by the arm and they both helped Charlie up. He had lost some blood, but he was miraculously hanging on to consciousness.

McBride went to the car and tried the passenger door; it was locked. The back door was locked, too. The mysterious driver was keen on helping them, but not willing to take them out of there.

Whitman looked at the driver's window. A woman was sitting in it. Medium-length black hair. He recognized the blood-red nails gripping the steering wheel.

With Charlie's arms around their shoulders, they headed up Calton Road, the revving engine still blaring at the three thugs behind them. They kept going. Minutes passed.

Looking back, they saw the standing goons tending to the fallen one. The car was still there, an insurmountable boundary, its engine warning.

Once they reached the Royal Mile, they looked back again: there was no one on their trail. They entered one of the desolate closes and set Charlie down, his back against the stone wall.

"Was there really a car?" Charlie asked, unsure. McBride nodded and told him to keep quiet.

She tore off Charlie's sleeve and examined the wound. Whitman lit a cigarette. He knelt down, ruffled his friend's hair, and told him everything would be all right. But would it?

He reached into Charlie's pocket, searched for the decoded letter.

Kneeling in the dimly lit alley, he held it up and read Sekuler's words.

Now that you have found your path to my second entry, faithful friend, you might begin to understand the essence of my secret. For centuries the alchemists have strived to procure the *elixir vitae*. I regret to say I have encountered it.

Its messenger appeared to me on a tempestuous Edinburgh night. I remember that night with entire distinctness. I had concluded my moving picture experiments and was walking alone in the Gardens. Bells rang in the distance, distracting me. I paused to count the chimes. By the last toll, I had lost count.

For a moment, all was still and silent, save the voice of the bell. The sound of the last toll was echoing in the air when at length there broke in upon my awareness a successive breathing, intermingled with many low moanings.

At once I was vigilant. Its sounds were concurrently human and inhuman. In dismay, I saw a statue that I was certain I had never seen before. I looked into its mask of a face and at once I felt enshrouded in its shadow; its breathing pierced through me, coursing through my body. I shivered. For a moment I was one of those stiff-frozen statues of the city, too. This fiend before me was not of this world. I could hear it whispering, calling my name. I gasped and struggled at each call, I shrunk at its every whisper, such as I might had it arisen out of hell. Before the ringing of that last bell had utterly sunk into silence—a still present auditory mirror image—the fiend dragged me with it into the darkness. Deadly terror gripped my bones as I heard what it was whispering. When I saw his pipe burning in the dark, I already knew.

I wanted to scream, but at that moment the dark silhouette took off the mask concealing its face. And then I knew what it looked like, even though evil always bears the same face.

It was Carlyle Eistrowe; that fiend who had once been my family's friend.

"Your daughter," he whispered. "Your daughter is mine now."

Mary Rex has lost her precious jewel; descend to Walker's to the place of the cold and cruel, ascend it once and twice again, behind the close where Allan once lived, look for the bells, the bells that never ring: ornate bells whose knells make the angels sing.

The close was deserted and narrow—a rusty nail in the city's skin. The moonlight cast tapered glimmers of silver-gray on its dirt-ridden cobbles. A maze of small courts led off into the shadows, crossed by other closes equally uninviting in the dim light. Above them, the walls of the houses seemed to lean in, nearly touching one another.

"You have to tell me who's trying to kill you," McBride said, still examining Charlie's wound.

"He knew," Whitman said. "The bastard who hired me. He was watching me the whole time, making sure I didn't screw with him."

"Is that what this is, Alex? Does he just want the film?"

"He's got the film. He killed one of our mutual acquaintances to get it."

"The Basque guy at the Archive?"

"Catalan. He had the guy's penis severed and stuck in his mouth."

"The good news," McBride told Charlie, "is the bullet just grazed your arm. You're going to be okay."

"Are you sure? It feels like I'm dying."

"You're going to need stitches."

Charlie winced. "I was kind of hoping that was the bad news."

McBride shook her head. "The bad news is we have nowhere to go." She turned to Whitman. "Any ideas?"

Whitman gave her a blank stare. For a moment, they listened to the wind whispering its secrets to the close's walls.

"We can't go to yours," McBride said. "And those men knew my name. They'll be watching my flat."

"I know a place," Whitman said, helping Charlie up.

"Are you sure this is going to be okay?" Charlie asked, pointing at the blood on his arm. "You're not, like, hiding something from me, are you? Am I dying?"

"If only you were a few hundred pounds lighter, Goodyear, this would never have happened," Whitman said.

"Where is this place?" McBride asked.

"You wouldn't believe me if I told you."

29

The air was cool, and there was a hint of a breeze. Around them, crowds were heading for the pubs on the Grassmarket, an alcoholic parade under an amber-colored sky.

The three of them walked quickly until they sighted an arcade of shadows on the foot of the West Bow, opposite the well—the short, and sole, stretch of the Bow that remained. The bleak, imposing buildings seemed to curve in on themselves like briars of stone against the gloomy lights.

Whitman went up to a wooden door. It had been red but was blackened by age; it looked as if it had been shut for centuries. It was considerably smaller than a modern door, suitable for a time when locals were of challenged dimension.

The scarlet brass door knocker was shaped like Medusa's head. Whitman knocked four times. In his daze, Charlie expected the ground to shift; it seemed more probable than the antediluvian door should open.

As they waited, Whitman looked toward the top of the steep street.

The glow from the streetlamps filtered through the mist in oblique streaks before settling down and licking the ground.

Just when it seemed there would be no response, there was the jingling of keys. The door rattled as a tumult of padlocks and latches were unlocked, one after the other. The door creaked halfway open, as if muttering a curse, and air was sucked in and blown out from the inside. A tall, frail man with a stern gaze peered at them from within. His face was almost entirely hidden behind a thick cotton-candy beard hanging to his waist. He stared at them as if they weren't there; he did not seem to recognize Whitman.

"And our password will be?" the man asked.

Whitman cleared his throat. "Llanfairpwllgwyngyllgogerychwyrndrobwllllantysiliogogogoch."

McBride glared at them, frowning.

Charlie thought for a second. "*Barbarella*?" he asked Whitman.

"The prodigal son is back," the old man said. "But, lo and behold, he comes in the company of friends." The man was like a ghost. He turned to face them slowly, his lips curled into a quivering grin. His eyes navigated the emptiness, his pupils faint dots of white. McBride gasped; he was blind.

"I wouldn't stretch the 'friend' bit too far. She's police," Whitman said, pointing at McBride.

The old man's face hardened for a second. "Even you know better than to bring the law into this establishment, Alex."

"I don't have a choice, Henri. We need help."

No sooner had they stepped across the threshold than the old man swung the door shut. He engaged the bolts and fastened more latches than they could count. A heavy-duty deadbolt scraped into place, slamming against its holder. He rattled a steel chain, twisting it around the bolts. Finally, he grabbed a gas lamp from the wall and raised it to Whitman's face. "You sound like shit."

"You should hear the other guy," Whitman said, looking at McBride.

They followed the man through a corridor leading into a round hall, some kind of reception room that couldn't look less receptive. It was a dark, damp place that smelled of vinegar.

Henri told them to watch their step. "Into the belly of the beast we go."

A grandiose stone staircase wound down into blackness, seemingly inviting them into the bowels of the earth. Shadows populated both sides of the balustrade: a terra-cotta army of statues was looking down on them.

"I thought there was a hostel or a sandwich bar in here," McBride said. "Where are we?"

"Underneath that," Whitman said in a whisper.

"What is this place?" Charlie asked, and when Whitman didn't answer: "Am I hallucinating or is that a statue of Sam Peckinpah?"

The old man smiled behind his thick beard. His expression managed to look both cheerful and demented.

They advanced further through the building's innards until there appeared in front of them a brass entrance door.

"Here we are, then," Henri said, swinging it open, inviting them onto what looked like a balcony lined with rails.

The mysterious keeper stopped and stepped aside. He raised the gas lamp in the air, put his chin up in theatrical fashion, and widened his eyes. "Welcome to the Keepers of the Frame."

They grabbed the rails, looking down at the sight before them.

It was a series of immense, monumental labyrinths of film archives, each containing further labyrinths of smaller scope but rivaling complexity, labyrinths of rows and corridors and alleys outlined by shelving anchored in damp earth. Paths veered away onto other levels, following their own perilous course: hidden crevices, furtive corners, and fissures blacker than the night, where forsaken winters had gnawed at the sunless stone.

"I love the smell of nitrate in the morning," Whitman said.

This behemoth of a structure was suspended over a sea of pale mist; it was as if they had been anchored on a veil of velvet. Gaslights were scattered like moths in the confusion, their rays glimmering into the Gothic. Amid the glow was movement, shadowy figures strewn throughout the corridors and walking the platforms.

Henri, holding the lamp, led the climb down the balcony staircase to the labyrinth below; they followed, all the while staring at the sight, mouths agape. Above them, incredible towering ceilings stretched forever high—easily the tallest they had ever seen. A huge blue glass vault presided over all, but no shafts of light passed through it, being blocked by the foundations and floor of the edifices above them.

They continued, immersing themselves in the depths of the labyrinthine structure, an omphalos of intersecting passages and bridges of
mind-boggling proportions.

Charlie still wasn't certain of what he was seeing. Maybe it was the
loss of blood that was messing with his head. Nevertheless, he found it
difficult to keep his mouth closed. "Eat your heart out, Eastman House,"
he managed to whisper. He glanced toward the immensity of the maze,
the pain from his injury gnawing at his mind.

"How do you index such a thing?" McBride asked, helping Charlie
along.

"It has been a work in progress for many, many years. We are helped
by the orphans," Henri said, gesturing to the shadowy figures scattered in
the labyrinth. Charlie squinted through the haze of the mist: he thought
he saw children, somewhere between seven and twelve years old, brows-
ing reels of endless wisdom.

"How come you never . . ." Charlie began.

Whitman gave a soft laugh.

"A long time ago, he did try," Henri said. "I could see through his
tactics. I knew he wanted to relieve us of anything of value. He convinced
a projectionist who frequented this place to show him around. When the
others saw him stealing, his pockets packed with so much material that
he looked like the Michelin Man, all hell broke loose. Film people are
normally placid, unless you threaten that which they most treasure. Then
God help you. My friend Lotte wanted to take his head."

They were approaching the other side of the labyrinth. Staring into
the void, Henri said, "The projector, my dear, the projector." A split second later, McBride had struck her foot on the lamp housing of the Elmo
projector lying on the floor. She cursed at it, then at its mother.

"How does he do it?" she asked Whitman. "Is he really blind or what?"

Whitman broke into laughter.

Charlie held his arm around McBride—the pain was still searing—
and urged Henri to carry on with his story.

"Several of my colleagues had been alerted to his behavior and had
encircled him with threatening intentions. I approached the scene, and
they explained the situation to me. I decided a Jean Valjean moment
would be the best solution. I answered that I had granted Whitman the
right to take any films he wanted for a brief period of time, provided he

would return them. It was for a very serious purpose, I explained, one which was so personal I could not divulge it. 'You forgot that Murnau picture,' I told him in front of the lynch mob. Which one was it, now? Ah, yes, the one that people still think has only three minutes surviving, that's the one. The next morning, every film was back in its place. After that he spent his time here in peace. He is a good kid. He has just been sidetracked, searching for substitutes for that which he cannot find."

"This is where I got the idea for the shop," Whitman told Charlie. "This was my inspiration for the Crypt."

"But how? Why? When?" Charlie had so many questions.

"These are matters best discussed with one's glass full," the old man said with a mysterious smile, motioning the group into a room in the periphery of the circular archive.

30

Henri listened to their story, stroking his candy floss beard.

"Remarkable. Truly remarkable. Who would have thought Sekuler was making movies when everyone else couldn't even construct a working camera?"

The room was a mess of projectors, reels, books. Henri and Whitman were sitting at a large wooden table. Charlie was plopped on an upholstered sofa, which took up one corner of the room. McBride was kneeling next to him, tending to his injury.

"Do you make anything of the last bit?" Whitman said.

"Some kind of riddle or code, no doubt. Doesn't look too complicated. Not like proper encryption methods. Sometimes things are more complex, of course. Like the Blitz ciphers—ever heard of them?"

They shook their heads.

"Pages concealed in the wall of an East London cellar within a wooden box, discovered only because of a German bombing during the Second World War. No one's ever deciphered them, not even the modern prodigies of cryptography."

"What about this *elixir vitae*?" McBride asked. She opened the first-aid kit Henri had offered them and applied a handful of disinfectant solution on Charlie's oval-shaped wound, soaking it completely. Charlie winced in pain; she gently blew on the wound.

"The philosopher's stone."

"Transforming metals into gold?"

"That's the part everyone knows," he said. "But it wasn't just some medieval cooking recipe. What they were really after was the elixir of life."

"Which was?" She turned to Charlie again—"Don't look"—and inserted the needle downward through the subdermal layer of his skin, leveling it off until it reached the wall of the wound. When Charlie winced again, she said, "It's going to leave a cool scar," and winked at him.

"Immortality, of course," Henri said. "The whole 'transforming' of metals and the idea of gold were merely metaphors. Even though they had their share of charlatans and madmen, some were astronomers and philosophers and chemists. They made world-changing discoveries, even if it was through trial and error. Alchemy and the sciences began to diverge only about a century before this film was made. Those quacks invented many of the procedures and much of the equipment we still use to this day. Hell, even gunpowder, metallurgy, nuclear transmutation. Name John Napier ring any bells?"

"There's a university here named after him."

"A Scotsman. He gave us natural logarithms and decimal notation. He was also an alchemist."

"So what is it? What are we looking for? A stone?"

Henri fished a hardcover book the size of an encyclopedia from a shelf. "Listen here," he said, tracing sentences with his index finger, his white pupils fixed on Whitman. Charlie was dumbfounded; the blind man remembered every sentence from the book, word for word:

> The philosopher's stone is the most ancient Stone, the most apocryphal
> of secrets; it is incomprehensible in earthly properties, it is celestial,
> blessed, sacred. It is the supreme and unalterable Reason; to be able to
> find the Absolute in the Infinite, in the Indefinite, and in the Finite,
> this is the Magnum Opus, the Great Work of the Sages, which Hermes

Trismegistus called the Work of the Sun. It is the perfect equilibrium
of all elements, the materia prima. It is the catholicon of all ailings,
the most precious of treasures, the greatest possession in all of nature.
He who has this Stone has all, and needs no other help.

He shut the book. "*Arcanum Alchemicum,* 1728."

"Captain Fantastic," Whitman said. "I didn't understand a single
word. How can a rock be all of this?"

"The alchemists," Henri said, "looked at crystals growing and vol-
canoes erupting and they believed minerals were alive. Minerals were
thought to grow from seeds, deep in the earth, maturing as they rose
up. Knowing the secrets to the perfect mineral gold would allow one to
understand perfection in the world."

He turned to McBride. "Stones were also believed to be sexual, my
dear." He smiled approvingly. "If you don't believe me, go visit a store
selling diamond rings."

McBride laughed. "A woman's best friend."

"Indeed so," Henri said. "Alchemists started from goldsmiths and sil-
versmiths and welders and enamelers, based in Sumeria, ancient Egypt
and Greece, and the Near East. They were mixing metals, producing
compounds, amalgams of minerals. Hence the sexual component and
the concept of fertility: you mix two different things and create a third
thing, something new. It's what they called a 'holy wedding.' Listen to
this." He opened the old thick volume and located his place without
looking; it was a description of the alchemical operation of making the
stone:

Marriage, increase, pregnancy, birth and nourishment are necessary
to you in the conduct of this operation. For when the conjunction
has been achieved, immaterial conception shall follow; and pregnancy
arises from conception, and birth follows pregnancy.

"They married silver with gold, did their tricks, and ended up with
more silver and gold than before. You understand?"

"Midas's touch," Whitman said. "Getting something out of nothing."

"Also, being careful about what you wish for. Remember, some of
them were deeply religious men. Alchemy for them was about harnessing

divine energies. You had to destroy in order to create. There's marriage, passion, death, and resurrection."

"Sounds like a soap opera."

"Only they talk of killing monsters, hanging men, hunting demons. They created arcane inscriptions and macabre engravings—you've seen the crazy pictures in this type of book. Sometimes they depict the stone as a virgin or a child, sometimes as Christ or a phoenix. And the process of producing it was one of purification and redemption. Your original component persists after destruction, but there's something new out of it, something born out of the ashes. You see?"

"I suppose so. But I still don't understand: What is it? Is it a stone? A powder? Liquid?"

"Hell if I know. Here, this is just to show you how big your list is." He flipped a few pages, then rested the book on the table, turning it around so they could see. It was unbelievable; he was on the correct page. "Abraham's wife said it's something from the tomb of Hermes. Nicolas Flamel wrote it's a powder. Other sources say it's a serpent. Fire. Vitriol. A dead body. The blood of saints. It's the Americas. It's chaos, a toad, an adder—you name it. It can be anything in the world."

"Great. So Sekuler might have hidden a toad. Was he nuts? Maybe from all the fumes from the mineral burning?" Whitman said.

"Maybe. Maybe it's something . . . ineffable."

"This doesn't exactly help us."

Henri placed the book back on the shelf with uncanny precision.

"Perhaps it's whatever you want it to be. Each era carries its own little forbidden fruit. Wealth, riches, sex, success, immortality. Look at what they're doing now: virgin births, women having babies without ever having been impregnated by a man . . . They always said they could do without us; now I guess they've gone for broke."

McBride smiled. "What about this ouroboros? Is that a snake?"

"Ah, yes, the ουροβόρος όφις. It's an ancient symbol, usually a snake or a dragon that devours its own tail. It's often used in alchemical and religious writings to represent self-reflexivity or cyclicality; especially so in the sense of something constantly re-creating itself, the eternal return, and other things perceived as cycles that begin anew as soon as they end. In alchemy, it was also associated with the circular nature of the alchemist's opus."

"The perfection of a circle."

"But life doesn't work that way," Whitman said. "In life things are far from perfect."

Henri nodded. "Well, let's consider this idea of imperfection. Think of a person who is ill and near the end of his life. Experience and historical precedent have told him he cannot escape death; we are but the most fortunate of species to know from our birth that we will die. Think about this person: What can he do to extend his being?"

"Receive some kind of treatment for his illness?"

"Of course, but there is only so much modern medicine can do. We cannot escape death for long. How do you live on?"

"Through your children."

Henri nodded. "Reproduction. That's why a brilliant Oxford man called our genes 'selfish.' You have a natural tendency and desire to find a mate—preferably one with healthy and desirable traits—so you can pass part of your genetic code to your offspring."

"I call that 'Friday-night clubbing,'" Charlie said in a daze.

"So consider this process of passing your DNA to your children. This is essentially replicating, or rather transferring, as what is part of you now also becomes part of someone else."

"Something out of nothing. So Sekuler's talking about reproduction?"

Henri stroked his endless beard. "I believe he's talking about something akin to that. How do you transfer yourself into something else which will outlive you?"

"Pictures?"

Henri nodded again. "That's what I thought. A moment in time has been captured on a piece of glossy paper. However, this lacks a vital characteristic of life: motion. And that, my friends," he said, pointing at some reels at the side of the room, "you get through film."

"Which is essentially a series of pictures shown sequentially."

Whitman shook his head. "I don't buy it. I mean, it's ridiculous to think you can achieve immortality through film. Sure, I see Humphrey Bogart on the screen every day; that doesn't mean he's still out there. Pictures may look like they're moving, but they're really not. They're just that: representations, results of the observer's persistence of vision. Even when you pool the pictures together and roll them through a projector,

they're still not alive, whether they look like they are or not. If you perceive that they are moving, it's an illusion; if you believe it, it's a delusion."

"Of course," Henri said. "But this type of delusion has kept many
people going for years." His white pupils drilled into Whitman. "Fur-
thermore, we don't have the whole picture here. You say there are more
codes?"

"Riddles," Charlie said. He struggled to the corner of the table, joining them. He tapped on his notebook. "But we need to figure out the
next answer if we want to continue."

"The first thing I noticed about this riddle," McBride said, "is that it
contains clear instructions: 'descend,' 'ascend,' 'behind,' and so on. He's
giving us directions to find our way."

"But you need to start from somewhere if you want to follow them.
Some kind of a starting point," Charlie said.

"How about this: 'Mary Rex has lost her precious jewel.'"

"Jewel could be the elixir—the stone or whatever it is."

"*Rex* means 'king' in Latin, right?"

"Could he be talking about Mary, Queen of Scots?" McBride asked.
"Something related to the Palace of Holyrood?"

"'A cold and cruel place,' huh? Where does she fit into all this?" Charlie said.

"Terrible taste in husbands and losing her head on the chopper. I don't
buy the connection," Whitman said.

McBride looked at Henri. "Any ideas?"

Henri stroked his beard. "I'm not sure."

"You don't think he's referring to Queen Mary?"

"Perhaps he is, incidentally. But I'm looking at something else."

They all stared at him.

"Figure of speech," he replied with a grin.

"What is it?"

"The other names: Walker's, Allan."

"Tell you anything?"

He fished another book from the shelf. It was a Victorian map of
Edinburgh. He placed his finger near the Royal Mile and traced it near
the bridges, toward some alleys (*closes*) with obscure names piercing the
Mile on either side.

"How the hell does he do that?" Charlie whispered to Whitman.

"Allan's Close," the old man said.

"Let me see that," McBride said. "The close where Allan once lived." There was another close, called Walker's, nearby.

"He's giving us directions on how to go through these closes, toward his next clue," Henri said.

"But what does Mary, Queen of Scots, have to do with this?" McBride asked.

"She doesn't," Whitman said. "*Rex*, in Latin, means 'king': Mary King. He's talking about another close?"

"A very important and famous close, in fact," Henri said. "During the modernization of the town—seventeenth century, mind you—they built the administrative building of the City Chambers on top of some streets. Mary King's was one of them."

"There was an article in the paper about that place about a year ago," McBride said. "It said that some company's bought it and they're renovating it, turning it into a tourist attraction—hauntings and ghosts and the usual."

"We have to get into that close," Whitman said. "Tonight."

"You're going to need something to force the doors open," Henri said, looking at Whitman. "And flashlights. After all, it's dark down there. Hidden things usually are."

"Hidden?" Charlie asked.

"Of course, young man. Mary King's Close exists only underground," Henri said. "It's hidden below the city."

Part V

December 6

31

There she was.

When D.I. Guy Johnson had started trailing her, he could not have expected this.

Crouched in the shadows, he watched his partner walking on George IV Bridge alongside the two men, both suspects in the fire-and-missing-person investigation at the Archive. She didn't appear threatened by them, and this alarmed Johnson. For a fleeting instant, he wondered if they could be allies with McBride in some shady business.

He pulled out his mobile phone and dialed her number. Instantly, he saw McBride fish her mobile out of her pocket. She glanced at the caller ID, then pushed a button. The voicemail broke in on his end.

Something weird was going on. He had bombarded her with calls and messages, asking her what was wrong, but she hadn't responded.

Then there were the three men. He had seen them trailing McBride and the others for some time now. The sudden dread in his soul made it hard to stay still. But he forced himself to; it was not yet time. He would move when he had figured out what the situation was. And that was going to be soon. He decided to stay there in the darkness and watch their every move. Keep trailing until the right moment.

His partner was in great danger. He could feel it.

A long wooden spiral carried them down into solid rock. As they cork-screwed deeper and deeper into the vertical tunnel, the sounds from the world outside faded away to nothingness. After a while, the staircase ended; a level passageway snaked off into the darkness. There was only one way to go. The only sound was their echoing footsteps and the drip of water. The smooth, rounded walls of the tunnel structure were high enough for them to walk upright.

Without warning, the tunnel reached a sharp bend, and for a moment Whitman thought they'd come to a dead end. But then he felt something stirring his hair, a cool breeze coming from their left. McBride raised the flashlight. There was a passage with more steps climbing down.

Nothing Alex Whitman had heard about this place prepared him for the sight of it. Facing increasing commercial competition from the hand-some and spacious New Town, the authorities in 1753 had decided to build their own bang-up-to-date Georgian commercial center, the Royal Exchange. The problem was they built it over Mary King's Close as well as other alleys. Those streets became the foundation for the building and ended up being a sealed-up time capsule.

The colossal subterranean hollow stood before Whitman largely unchanged; crumbling walls and small houses lined the sides of the cave-like structure.

The air smelled lifeless. An awkward grid of narrow walkways wound between the decaying rooms. Like columns of dust, countless pillars of unexcavated earth rose up, supporting a dirt sky, which hung high above them.

City of the dead, he thought, in a mélange of fascination and dread. They continued deeper along the winding passages.

Once, he stumbled on a sheet of broken rock and had to grab hold of McBride's arm. "You all right?" she asked, but he kept quiet. His unease grew.

He fished the bottle of codeine pills from his pocket and swallowed two in one gulp, waiting for the cold sweat and the trembling of his hands to stop. It could not be any other way. He was going to find the clues. Find his daughter.

They were deep inside the tunnel now, surrounded on all sides by thousands of tons of solid rock supporting a convoluted maze of timber scaffolding. On their feet, tidemarks from old puddles of water. In the distance, the tunnel ingested the sounds of rats gnawing and scraping at rock.

"This is it," McBride said. Whitman looked ahead. Mary King's Close. The passageway stretched out indefinitely in a steep decline into the darkness, doors to further passages lining one side. On the other, rusted pipework laced the walls all the way down into the blackness. Signs of renovation lay everywhere: bags of cement, scaffolding, pails and shovels. The passageway was wide enough to accommodate a four-wheel drive. The dim light hovered around them, but the corridor surrendered into the darkness farther ahead. A dank breeze rustled out of the blackness—a disquieting memento of being deep below the ground. Whitman could feel the weight of the soil and stone suspended over his head.

"We're right below Cockburn Street," McBride said.

The uneven passages were narrow and dark, with floors of packed earth and walls lined by tiny unlit oil lamps. They peered through a window: The room was vaulted, with whitewashed walls anchored to an earthen floor. There were blunt objects everywhere. Iron hooks suspended from the ceiling. Saws hung from the walls.

Charlie almost let out a whimper.

"Grow up," McBride said. "Probably a butcher shop."

"Are you sure?"

She shook her head.

"Henri said that when the plague ravaged the city, they sealed up the close with all the people inside and set fire to it."

"Sounds too macabre to be true," McBride said.

Whitman cringed at the mere possibility of people having been burned alive in there. Either way, frightened, sorrowful wails had once pierced this air, victims falling to the dreaded plague around the serpentine passageways. Chilling figures in birdlike masks, dressed in heavy leather cloaks, tending to the sores and boils of bedridden children while their mothers lay alongside them, their skin covered in black patches. Bodies already succumbed to the plague awaiting collection from the "foul clengers," the cleanup crew. The plague had immobilized Edinburgh and claimed more than half of its population.

"According to Henri's map, we should take a right . . . here."

"Be on the lookout," Whitman said.

"So we're looking for . . . bells, I suppose?"

"Bells that never ring, whose knells make the . . . whatever the rest of it was."

"Sounds ritualistic. Something from a church or a place of burial."

They entered the rooms. Shelves, ladders, and stairs. Glass glittered. Dust abounded. Sections of the crumbling walls were papered, three-hundred-year-old floral and other displays stenciled on the lavatory closets. Astragals on the oval windows also remained, surrounded by flat fillets and topped by jambs or worked stone; a number of moldings and tapestries adorned the hallways. Around everything, the remains of fireplaces and built-in cupboards. The carved oak paneling had rotted away.

Charlie ran his fingers over the plaster. "Original. Nice."

McBride inspected it closely. "Yeah. They used to make these out of human ash."

"Fucking hell."

"What about this hole in the ground? What was it for?"

"Guess."

"Oh, shit."

She nodded. " 'Oh, shit' is right."

"He said 'behind Allan's Close,' right? It's in there."

They made for the threshold and then stopped. What had once been Allan's Close was now a shambles roofed over by the toppled building; mounds of dense rubble, worn into a grotesquery of angles, and stone. Hard, dense, solid whinstone, sheathed in a film of dirt. Compacted. Impenetrable. Failure was staring them straight in the eyes.

Whitman placed his palm against the solid mass. Pushed. It was immovable. He closed his eyes.

"We have to get in there. There has to be a way around this," McBride said.

Whitman slowly shook his head, eyes still closed. "Not unless you're packing a diamond drill." And then: "Look at the map. This is the only way in there. And there's nothing here. Absolutely nothing."

"We can't give up," McBride said. "We can find something, someone. Some help. I can call someone who knows construction; maybe we can get some excavation equipment down here."

Whitman scowled at her, shaking his head. "No dice, Serpico. What do you think is going to happen when they figure out that someone's broken into this fucking place? New locks, security, you name it. We're screwed, underground style."

He walked out of the room with his hands on his head. He hadn't visualized the possibility of defeat. Not like this. Not when they were so close.

He ran his hand through his hair as he considered his options. Surrender to the police? That was out of the question. They wouldn't stand a chance. Take the ferry to Zeebrugge? Thoughts of possible extradition crossed his mind, and he tried to wave them away. They had to escape. Ditch the cop; get out of this fucking place.

A stab of nausea ran through him. He steadied himself, his hand against the plastered wall.

God, he was tired.

How do I get out of this? he thought. *How do I get Charlie out of this?* Once more he was failing his daughter.

On the other side of the room, McBride stood thinking. Charlie was sitting on the ground. "What do we do?" he whispered.

"I don't know, Charlie."

Whitman took his hand off the plaster, the dust flying in all directions. He felt the urge to sneeze, and positioned his hand closer to his mouth. He realized he wasn't going to sneeze after all. And he saw that a dust imprint had come off on his palm. It was the imprint of the floral pattern from the wall.

The flower.

A bluebell.

A bell that never rings.

"Motherfucker," he said.

"Dust is bloody awful down here," McBride said.

He shook his head, smiling. "No, no, dust is beautiful, Serpico. I'm telling you, it's beautiful."

McBride and Charlie edged closer to him. He showed them his palm. "What?"

"Don't you see? They're bluebells. Goddamn bluebells. Flowers."

"Bells that never ring," Charlie said. "Damn it, Alex, you're a genius."

"What does this mean?" McBride asked. "Assuming you're right."

"It means that our next key word is fucking 'bluebells.'" Whitman snapped his finger. "Let's work our magic, Jabba."

Charlie had already opened his folder and was scribbling furiously. His injury seemed long in the past, and his hand was working across the lines of the notebook without a hint of tremor. Sekuler would whisper to them again.

My dear viewer, you will soon encounter the burden that I have hidden. I am terrified by the notion of those who wish to take my invention away and claim credit for themselves; in such situations, alliances between the greedy and the evil are formed easily. I plan to board a train, but I am unsure whether it will reach its destination. In the event it does not, this moving picture will be irrefutable evidence of what occurred.

I still remember that forsaken night. After having been seized by the evil itself, I awakened to the darkness, restrained, unable to move. But as my eyes adjusted to the dark of the room, a circumstance of frightening nature attracted my attention. I was in my own workshop. Before me was my sweet, beautiful daughter, restrained in a chair. Carlyle Eistrowe stood next to her. But a man, dressed entirely in black, was next to them where none had been perceptible before. In my confusion I mistook him for a priest. He had a boyish face and bloodshot blue eyes and a head crowned with snow-white hair falling over his forehead. The man conferred with Eistrowe in hushed tones and I realised that the both of them had conspired in my demise. They had kidnapped my Zoe. Eistrowe motioned him to advance as he wished. The man then proceeded to extract an object from the table and place it into his bag. I realised that the object was one of my projectors! And as the man turned, his face entered the light. It was Thomas Edison himself. He was stealing my work—my cameras, my projectors. He nodded at me familiarly, a greeting from his strong chin, an acknowledgement from his dark eyes—and I realised the two men had perpetrated this act as part of an agreement: Edison desired my invention and Carlyle could provide it by betraying me. I demanded at once that they release me and my daughter. Edison laughed. My Zoe was crying.

Zoe's small, delicate feet were gleaming in the glass across from her. Carlyle was smiling. He left his pipe aside on the floor—he was always smoking it incessantly—so that his hands were rendered free, and took seating next to her. One of my cameras stood next to me, recording the terrible ordeal.

There was a rabid frenzy in my thoughts—a hideous and insatiable clamour. In the darkness I saw that the whole structure had been re-laid before my eyes: they were both seated in front of a small assembled chamber. I realised what they were facing inside was not a window; it was a mirror. I reasoned it was a transparent mirror, one that allowed you to see through it. Another mirror had been positioned at the wall of the chamber so it was directly facing them and the first mirror. I had come to know those mirrors, as Carlyle had previously relayed to me their mystical properties; he had purchased them from a warlock residing on Candlemaker Row, and he claimed that the materials used for their construction had been taken from the staff of Major Thomas Weir himself. Weir was a retired soldier, a serious man of grim countenance, who always carried a black staff and led prayers with a fervour that inspired much awe in the community. He was attending a religious service when he suddenly stood up and began to confess to being in the service of the Devil and to an incestuous relationship with his unmarried sister. Eventually he was sentenced to be strangled and burnt. His staff was taken from him, for they claimed that he had been given it by none other than the Devil himself, and it was an instrument of terrible power.

Edison seemed as terrified as I. He gathered my inventions and finally exited the basement, leaving my daughter and me at the mercy of the fiend. The camera next to me was still capturing the ordeal.

Carlyle was whispering in a language I could not understand. His voice grew tender and low—yet I would not wish to dwell upon the feral sense of the softly whispered words. My mind staggered, entranced, as I became aware of a refrain more than mortal—of longings and passions which the living had never before known. Then,

Zoe appeared to be fainting and gradually closed her eyes, and Carlyle closed his eyes in turn.

I knew what he was planning to do. I knew, my friend! I could not believe it. Not that the contour of each hurried reflection failed, at any time, to imprint its own idiosyncratic outline upon the fiendish mirror—but that mirror, un-mirrorlike, retained more than the vestige of the reflection, as each departed into infinite alcoves of further reflections, stretching into infinity. And at its heart, at the heart of the infinite reflection: the unity of an exchange.

My daughter stirred—and now more strenuously than hitherto, although arising from an integration more atrocious in its absolute nature than any other. And as she slowly opened her eyes, through the adversity of horror and of dread, I saw these were not the eyes of my daughter—and an undeniable helplessness, fostered by horror, charged every fibre of my being.

Its eyes! Its eyes, my dear friend! They were blacker than the coal chambers of midnight! She smiled at me and I recognised that smile! It was Carlyle's!

Minutes elapsed before any event appeared to throw light upon this anomaly. My daughter finally rose from the chair, picked up the pipe from the floor, and placed it in her mouth. She smiled again at me, and I was certain beyond any doubt that she was not my daughter, that the man who had been standing next to her had taken residence inside her. It may have been her skin and her body, but that was not her. She— it—immediately ran out of the cellar, and I never saw it again.

Carlyle opened his eyes and was staring inside the mirror, lost, seemingly unable to fathom what had happened. I then realised I had been watching, with feelings half of disquiet, half of terror, the workings of my daughter's countenance. As it came to my rescue, untying my hands and feet, and crying, crying endlessly, I understood.

"Now at last," I cried, "I am certain—more certain than I breathe— that these are the brimming, and the blue, and the innocent eyes of my own daughter; of my Zoe Sekuler!"

I have tried to make sense of the unspeakable horrors of that night and I cannot.

In the following days, I would look at the fiend's eyes, and I would see that my daughter was in that body. I knew she would never return from this dreaded purgatory, the result of this "Séance Infernale." I asked around if anyone had seen a little girl with a sardonic smile, but to no avail. On occasions I have heard laughter echoing in the dark closes, and that is when I fear most for my life. I have no choice over what I shall do next.

Thus I have tried to cover my secret, embed it within these frames, unperturbed by the passage of time and, alas, by the burning of memory. I implore you, my dear friend, to be careful. Perhaps Edison and his men will come to realise the evidence that has been left behind in the form of moving pictures. They can make sure I am no more. You will hear no more of me after this riddle, which will lead you to the location of the remaining moving images and the irrefutable proof which they hold.

From Alexander Seton it started
I found it, hid it where dead men guard it
though Time slips in the hourglass of life
men of wisdom know not when they must die
but if you so wish to find my secret
you must count the grains remaining in it
they forgot in time what you must not
find the secret knot

George Mackenzie. Alexander Sterling, Esq Elizabeth Moncrieff William Boswell Esq X – Christine Gilbert. George Joseph Donaldson Margaret Reid Jane Bennet

Standing in front of the jaws of a murky opening that seemed to corkscrew deeper into the ground, Whitman hesitated, looking behind them. He couldn't be sure, but he thought there had been movement in the darkness.

Silence.

"Sounds like your filmmaker friend was seriously deranged," McBride said.

"Maybe."

"What do you mean 'maybe'? The guy thought his daughter switched bodies with another person. And what about that sentence near the end?

'I have no choice over what I shall do next.' It sounds like he killed his daughter in the end."

Whitman felt his forehead. "What do you care, Serpico?" he finally said. So it had been a case of betrayal all along—Sekuler's friend, the occultist Carlyle Eistrowe, had forged a deal with the inventor Thomas Edison. "The girl you're after is getting her freak on with your perp."

"You don't believe what he wrote in that letter is true, do you?"

Whitman turned and looked behind them again. This time he could swear he'd seen movement.

There was a sound. Charlie and McBride turned, and Whitman knew he wasn't imagining things.

Whitman felt his blood drain. He was ready to dart into the tunnel, to flee like an animal.

The figure walked into the dim light and drew its hood back, revealing its face.

32

Elena Genhagger stared at them, as if giving them time to take in the surprise. Exactly what she was doing in underground Edinburgh or how she had ended up there from the French part of Switzerland was unclear. "That hardly matters," she said. "You know you're being followed."

"Who?"

"You know who."

"Who is she?" Charlie asked.

"Swiss chick." Whitman quickly explained how he had found the Lausanne address to Sekuler's last known descendant; how Elena Genhagger had proved to be Sekuler's great-granddaughter; the circumstances under which Whitman had found her unconscious.

Whitman brushed past Elena into what had once been the door of a close. He listened. Noise suddenly amplified in the underground space, somewhere in the far distance behind them. He crept around the corner, watching. He could hear footsteps, and voices echoing. He tiptoed down a wooden ramp until, crouching low, he could see silhouettes in the distance heading toward him.

"How did you know they were coming for us?" he said.

"I followed them here."

"You followed us, too." Whitman stared at her in the dim light. Her face was expressionless.

"Who is this?" McBride asked.

Charlie moved forward, farther into the tunnel, but Elena stopped him. "It's a dead end. You'll be trapped before you know it."

"Okay, I'll bite," Whitman said. "What do we do?"

"We don't have much time."

Elena moved forward into the alcoves before them. Whitman and McBride looked at each other.

"When did she become leader?" Charlie said.

McBride flicked her flashlight on. Whitman and Charlie followed, trailing a few feet after her. The light dimmed behind them, giving in to blackness. The effect was uncanny, Charlie thought, as if the tunnel were alive. In the darkness behind them, the voices were drawing nearer.

Shining the way ahead, Elena led them through the passageways toward a large cylindrical rock standing on its edge against the wall. "This way."

"Behind that?" McBride asked. "They're going to pass right in front of us!"

"C'est ça," Elena said. "It's hollow inside."

Whitman gave Charlie a look. Charlie raised his shoulders. The voices from behind were almost upon them.

Grunting with effort, they rolled the stone back through a groove cut in the stone wall. McBride lost her footing and fell. "I'm all right," she told Charlie, who offered her a hand up. She rose and dusted herself off.

As the stone turned back on itself with a grating sound, the cold air rushed out of the chamber.

The rock covered the entrance to a short tunnel. Through the mouth of the cave, they could see only darkness.

"What is it? A passageway?"

"Another dead end, I'm afraid," Elena said.

What if she's in on it? Whitman thought.

They rolled the stone back, leaving just enough space for them to squeeze out if necessary.

McBride clicked the flashlight off. "We're right below the City Chambers," she whispered.

The cavity was like a sensory-deprivation chamber, a dark, barren confine in a stone-walled burrow. They listened.

Faint voices, rolling echoes taking form in the stillness.

Approaching footsteps.

Boots stomped past the opening. Then stopped.

McBride heard distinct voices.

The silhouettes of the men loomed like exaggerated specters against the wall.

They were right there. Inches away.

The four stayed crouched on the ground of the hollow, holding their breath.

Then the sound of a match being struck, and the soft burning of the tip of a cigarette.

McBride's right hand felt for her mobile—she had to make sure it was on silent mode—but she only touched the emptiness of her pocket. Her eyes widened. She gave Whitman a look; he had seen her mobile was missing.

She was tempted to rise. She could remain crouched, waiting for the voices to resume or leave. But she suspected she knew where her mobile lay.

She made a movement toward the opening. Whitman shook his head, eyebrows slightly raised.

She crouched toward the opening, trying not to make a sound. At last, as the muscles in her thighs and calves began to cramp, she eased up to the gap and carefully peeked out. She half-expected the men to be lurking there, guns ready.

Only one of the men was still there, smoking his cigarette, his back turned to her under a blue haze. The other two were out of sight; presumably they had gone further into the darkness in search of them. She looked at the ground.

The mobile was there.

It was inches away from her. Within reaching distance.

It would take only a slight turn of his head for the man to see it.

Was there a signal down there? What if someone called her? Was the phone on silent mode?

She half-glimpsed the goon's shadow turning around, and she pulled herself back and tried to shrink into the darkness. Her muscles flared from adrenaline. Had he seen them? Had he seen the phone?

The others stared at McBride. They had surmised what had happened. Their breath remained in their lungs. Silence swamped the passage.

With her heart in her throat, she sneaked another look through the opening. The man was still there, back turned to them.

She stretched out her hand, groping for the mobile; she only touched the stone floor.

She reached out again.

Just a little too short.

Again. The only sound was the pounding of her heart, each beat coming after each realization of a miss.

Miss. Beat. Her fingers barely nicked the phone.

She moved forward and stretched her arm again.

Beat.

She hit a loose rock resting atop another.

In slow motion

she felt the rock

slide out of place.

The rock

fell

on

the

stone

floor,

its

echo

swallowed

up

he

in

the

bowels

of

the

tunnel.

And that was when the sound of her heart and the adrenaline rushed back into her eardrums. The whole thing came away, crashing into her brain on the inside of her ears. She grabbed the rock and ran toward the man, who by then had half turned around.

She drove the blunt end of the rock into his face and heard the bone of his nose break. His hands covered his face, and that was when she delivered a careful kick to his knee. His kneecap moved. The man fell down, cowering, screaming in pain.

She turned around and ran to the others. They had fled their hiding place for the corridor that led to the City Chambers.

"Told you: three's my lucky number," she said to Whitman as they ran.

In the distance they heard the voices of the other men, calling their comrade's name from afar. She turned around and saw only darkness. They were nowhere in sight; groans and curses were swallowed by the tunnel.

McBride thought they were safe.

Streetlamps flickered and a flash of lightning bathed the buildings in a sudden white. They had cascaded through the Upper Bow and Victoria Steps and rushed as far away as their energy permitted. There wasn't a soul to be seen on the streets. They took refuge in a gallery under a series of arches. The fog had been scattered across the four winds, but the rumble of the storm could be felt through the city walls, through the arches, getting closer.

"I think we're safe for now," Whitman said, catching his breath.

McBride looked around, surveying the grounds. "We should head back. Lick our wounds and regroup."

Whitman shook his head. "There's no time."

Charlie had already fished out his notes. He motioned them to examine the second line of the riddle: " 'I've hid it where dead men guard it,' " he said. "That's easy, right? Where do you find dead people? Graveyards."

"Hold on," Whitman said, pointing at Elena. "Aren't we going to talk about what just happened? How Ida Lupino here's been following us, and why?"

"Remember," Elena told Charlie, ignoring Whitman, "you're in Edinburgh. Dead men are everywhere. Churches, tombs—*putain!*—even below the street we walk on."

"And who is this Alexander Seton?"

"*Un alchimiste.*" She placed her finger on Charlie's notes. "We must look at the names. They have something in common."

"And I suppose you just happened to know this? Where from?" Whitman said.

"I'm helping you."

"For some reason, it doesn't feel that way."

Elena shrugged.

Whitman shifted his glare toward the notebook. "What about the names? What do the names tell us?"

"I've never heard of them before," Charlie said.

"Me neither," McBride said. "Except this guy." She pointed at the first name. "George Mackenzie. He was a hanging judge. He persecuted thousands during the Restoration. He was so relentless in his pursuit that he was given the nickname 'Bluidy Mackenzie.' "

"Joy."

There was a roaring sound; they stared out at the curtain of white lightning traced across the sky.

"Is his grave around?"

"In Greyfriars."

Whitman seemed to consider this, nodding, stroking his beard. "What about the rest of them? There must be a pattern. What do they have in common?"

"Are they all dead? I guess they have to be, by now."

Whitman nodded. "Are they all Scottish?"

"Mackenzie was. He was famous. The rest I don't know. They all sound like Scottish names. If they were all born in Scotland . . ."

"Does that mean they died in Scotland?"

"Maybe they're all buried here, in Edinburgh."

"All those people are buried at Greyfriars Kirkyard," Elena said.

Whitman glared at her. She knew more than she was letting on.

"Wild guess," she said.

"Soon you're going to tell us what you know," Whitman said.

"Soon?"

33

The madness of a Gothic moon loomed overhead, shining on rows of uneven gravestones. Greyfriars Kirkyard was eerie, the kind of place nightmares are made of—the kind of place you encounter when you break into church grounds with a crowbar in the late hours of December's darkness. There were wooden benches around the church and a low, shedlike shop of a structure at one end. Ragged trees and ferns were scattered around hundreds of gravestones and vaults. Naked branches formed a tracery that perplexed the eyes and clasped the heart. There was a rush of wings as a group of crows rose into the air as one.

Charlie had been nervous about the cemetery. He had imagined smells and vandalism and eeriness. And that was all there; but there was also mossy stone and the soft tapping noises of the trees. A wonderland of the dead.

The sounds of the graveyard itself filled the silence: the squish of their shoe soles on the path; the whisper of the wind in the trees; light traffic up and down the hill; the chirps of insects; Charlie's overcoat flapping behind him.

"We'll get through this more quickly if we split up," Whitman said.

"What are we looking for?"

"Dead people. A pattern: family, dates, anything. I'll take the south end; Serpico gets the division adjoining this; Charlie will be over at the north side; and you"—he pointed at Elena—"you stay out of fucking trouble. West end." They parted ways, four shadows scouring tombstones in the dead of night.

Whitman used his flashlight to cover ground faster. There was a half-moon, but the lofty branches above him made the night raven-black. He switched off his flashlight and listened. He was pleased to be in the cemetery.

He found Alexander Sterling's tomb; it was the family grave of an Edinburgh merchant. He also traced the relic of Elizabeth Moncrieff, a reverend's daughter. He took note of anything that might be of interest: the type of grave, the letters on the tombstones, their birth dates, death dates, their occupations, their families' names.

He decided to move to Mackenzie's tomb, a well-documented tourist site. Through the bars of the iron gate, there stood the Covenanters' Prison, where Bluidy Mackenzie was buried; it was a terrain of slaughter. As he busted the lock open with the crowbar, he wondered if the Covenanters were pissed off that a mutt on four legs had stolen their thunder in fame.

The mausoleum was an octagonal, Corinthian-columned, domed neoclassic. The massive door featured a bas-relief of a pelican feeding her young with her own blood, a symbol of the Resurrection.

With a crack, the lock busted open. He stood on the threshold of the gloomy structure. Dust had accumulated in the corners of the circular space. The coffin was lead-lined, for aboveground burial. Behind him, the wind continued to whisper in the trees.

A twig snapped. Something was breathing in the dark directly behind him. He started to spin. The cold muzzle of a gun kissed the base of his head. Even before he turned, he knew who the gun belonged to.

34

Angela was unsure how long she had stayed restrained in the stuffy crypt-basement. It was a hateful, primitive place where the walls squeezed in on her and she kept listening for the man, all the while getting used to the silence and the always of waiting.

By that time power had become real for her. The door bore no keyhole. It was not meant to open from her end. Every night she wished the door would open and that her restraints would magically vanish and she would rush at him and beat him senseless and escape into the light of day.

And then the door with no keyhole opened. He walked in and untied her. He propped her over his shoulder and carried her out of that horrible place and into the flat proper.

The first thing she did was cry.

She was grateful to be alive. She was a coward and she didn't want to die. She never knew before how much she wanted to live. *I don't care what he does,* she thought, *as long as he keeps my daughter alive.*

No sooner was the man standing over her than she remembered

wanting to be sick and afraid of choking under the gag. And then being sick.

When he came into the room, he just stood there looking gawky, and then at once, seeing him in the half-light of the still open door, she recognized who he was. Her neighbor. As if knowing what she was thinking, he went red. Blushing, Angela would find out, was a frequent occurrence for Elliot.

Tall, skinny—gangly, more like it—with hands so pink and white you'd think they were a boy's. Blank face, dull hair, receding hairline. All bland and meh. Even his speech was awkward, marred by the kind of words that require additional justification for oneself—"sorry" succeeding every sentence. He had been secretly following her for a long time, watching her and her daughter.

The first thing he told her was that her daughter was safe. She was asleep. If she behaved herself, he would allow Angela to see her.

And then she remembered the knock on the door, the man luring her out of her apartment by lying about his daughter's asthma attack . . .

Will anyone know if I die?

He, on the other hand, was exhilarated at the capture of his prey, the beginning of the Grand Plan . . .

Angela looked weak, flushed, but she seemed to know where she was all right and who Elliot was, her eye following him all the while around the room quite normally—that appeased Elliot. He thought the worst was past, the first obstacle. Acceptance and all that.

She turned and squinted with the one eye that wasn't swollen shut. She took in the room, dimly lit by an open fireplace. It could have been the spare room of an ordinary flat: tall-backed upholstered chairs stood in two corners, and table lamps rested on each side of a canopied bed.

A tripod with an old wooden projector faced the fireplace.

She looked quite the sight, almost out of it, like she was sleepy, with Elliot's shirt too big for her, one shoulder exposed, her hair falling to one side. Nothing filthy, nothing like that. It got Elliot excited seeing her like that. Like she knew who her master was. It gave him ideas.

She spoke in a low, hoarse voice. She said she was cold. Elliot got her jacket. He pulled it over her shoulders, smoothed it, and let it drop. As he did so, he gently touched her arms, and that sent shivers up both their spines.

He applied the restraints. She did not protest. He said he would stay with her and that he would look after her from now on.

She began to cry again. It wasn't like ordinary crying; she just lay there expressionless, her eyes brimming with tears, as if she didn't know she was crying. Then she said, "Please don't kill me," and Elliot said, "I'm not going to kill you." He smiled at her.

"Don't be silly," he said. "You are my soul mate. We are destined to live long and be happy together."

"I won't tell anyone please let me go please I won't tell anyone."

No reply.

"Please don't kill me," and then again: "Please don't kill me." And another time, and each time Elliot told her to stop saying that, but she didn't seem to hear.

She didn't understand.

It seemed like the right moment, so he set up the old projector with the ancient movies he had found in the crypt.

"I have a present for you," he said. It took him a few attempts, but in the end he did it—the lights were dim, the projector chattered. Motes of dust danced in the light beam that swept through the darkness; like Dr. Frankenstein, the shaft of light touched the blank canvas of the wall and the screen sprang to life. Elliot hummed the *duun-dun-dun-dun-dun-dun-duuun* theme of the 20th Century–Fox fanfare. As the paper film clicked into action, the place transformed from bedroom to the Kingdom of Shadows.

What a marvel it was, seeing the shadows on the wall, just being there, almost as alive as they had been at the time of its recording.

"Have you ever seen anything so beautiful?" he asked.

She started to move a bit, and finally saw the projections on the wall. They were grainy, as if they were projected on grains of sand, and they were slow, as if they, too, had been kidnapped and brutally forced to stay up there, constantly moving in spite of their own will.

Angela was confused. On the wall, a little girl sat in front of a set of mirrors, watching herself, an expression of silent horror on her face. There was a man with a mustache sitting next to her, also looking into the mirrors. The girl looked frightened out of her mind; either she was a great actress or this was not a movie at all.

What the hell is this?

After a moment the girl went quiet, and both she and the man closed their eyes. Within seconds they opened them again. The girl looked fine now. The man seemed disoriented but quiet.

Another man appeared in view. He was dressed all in black and looked young, with a boyish face. The man in black untied the girl. The girl then smiled as if this had been her plan all along and left the room to go out into the night. The man in black also left, leaving the mustached man alone. This was all very confusing.

Another person appeared on the screen. He still had restraints on his hands, suggesting he had been tied up somewhere offscreen. He knelt down to the man with the mustache. They were both crying. The screen faded to black.

Elliot stopped the projector and carefully took out the movie reel—it was as soft as paper. Something old and pure like that. It was the perfect opportunity. He stooped down next to her as if he was holding an engagement ring.

"It is for you. Feel how warm it is, my love."

She looked confused. *But beauty does that to people,* Elliot thought.

She whispered, "Thank you" and closed her eyes. Elliot placed the reel in her jacket pocket. It would be a token of their love and all the great things to come.

The doorbell rang, echoing from one side of the hallway into the barred windows of their room, forcing its way into the darkened flat. Elliot's heart caught in his throat and he almost jumped.

He should have known it was coming.

He had mentally rehearsed what he would do in this event. He was ready for it.

What he didn't expect was Angela's response.

Her eye sprang open and she suddenly lurched up from the chair. Her strength got her only to the point of managing to drop on the floor. Mustering all her strength, she began to crawl to the door, but she was so slow, the whole movement seemed comical. It was a kind of uninterrupted fright in slow motion.

Her right foot swung into the fireplace, kicking a burning log out of the hearth and onto the carpet.

Elliot grabbed her shoulders and pulled her out. He could smell the burning on her clothes, and that made his heart beat faster. She turned and tried to claw at him, but she barely managed to tug at his shirt.

He propped her back up on her seat, pulled her arms behind her back, and tied them to the bars at the back of the chair. The restraints sliced into her wrists.

As soon as she saw him grabbing the gag, she shook her head, pleading for mercy. She cried that she couldn't breathe with the gag.

He didn't understand what all the fuss was about. After all, the hidey place was well aired, as was the rest of the house.

The gag went on, and her throat constricted. Her scream became a whimper.

Her head hung back, and Elliot imagined how, if it wasn't for the gag, her throat would gape like a second mouth, caught in a silent, dark red scream. But it, too, would soon be silent.

He kept listening for the door. And watching the log on the carpet—it was smoldering heavily, and it filled him with all kinds of nasty desires. Smoke was filling up the room.

The loud tone echoed around the flat but fell silent. Only a slight breeze from underneath the building's main door stirred the wind chimes he had left hanging above his door so that he would know when Angela and her daughter had returned. He realized he would not need those anymore.

When the doorbell rang again, he considered the possibility that whoever was on the other side of the door was not about to leave until he made them.

As soon as he sensed her energy dwindle, he let her out of his sight and put the fire out with water from a bucket. He didn't want to, of course, as the sight was stirring his insides with all the vile, unspeakable things he would do to her.

He tiptoed through the hall and leaned forward to the peephole. On the other side was the unfamiliar face of a man holding a briefcase. He had a dimple on his right cheek, Elliot could see. The man had moved on and was rapping his knuckles for good measure on the door of the flat across the hall. There would be no reply, of course; neither Angela nor her daughter was there.

After a couple of unsuccessful attempts, the man with the dimple let out a grunt and began to ascend the stairs in search of other customers.

Eye pressed to the peephole, Elliot smiled. They were safe. The man was not looking for them. Elliot turned back to the room where Angela was held.

After he was done beating her, she said, "Kill me." She had the gag on, of course; but even if he had heard it, Elliot would have known she didn't really mean it. They were destined to be together. He would be as gentle with her body as he had been with her heart. Even if that meant they should die together.

35

Heart pounding, Whitman drew back from the man who had hired him to find Sekuler's film in the first place. Valdano's eyes looked sunken and evil in the receding haze hovering around the tombstones.

"Hello, Mr. Whitman." With his free hand, Valdano frisked Whitman's pockets, relieving him of his mobile phone.

Five figures stepped through the iron entrance of the Covenanters' Prison. First, Charlie and Elena, then Unibrow, and finally McBride and the second goon. Broken Nose was MIA; maybe a busted kneecap had been enough to make him quit.

For a moment, no one said anything.

Valdano shattered the silence. "Toss the notebook, McBride." A sharp taunt.

Whitman saw McBride's eyes flicking sideways. Valdano noticed it, too.

"Don't even think about it, Detective McBride." Simmering.

Out of the corner of his eye, Whitman could see Valdano's finger caressing the edge of the trigger. The air reeked of cleaning oil and gunpowder.

"The cops will be here any minute," McBride lied.

Valdano laughed. "Then we're going to have to finish this off, aren't we?" Words boiling under the surface.

"You'll never get away with this, Valdano."

The cold bore of the gun dug into Whitman's jaw. "Let's see you bet your friend's life on it." Whitman felt his blood throbbing against the core of cold steel.

"The fucking notes!" Valdano sputtered the words like rapid gunfire.

"Why don't we all just calm down." McBride held the notebook by its spine, then tossed it in Valdano's direction.

"Slowly," he said, ramming his fist on Whitman's ribs.

Whitman bent and picked up the notebook. As he handed it over to Valdano he could smell sandalwood and cologne mixed with musty sweat. Valdano took the notebook.

"Mr. Ericsson," he ordered the unibrowed limo driver. "The rope."

Ericsson did as he was told.

"Now the mobile, Detective McBride."

McBride tossed her phone. It landed between Whitman's feet. Again Whitman was made to pick it up and hand it to Valdano, who placed it in his jacket pocket. Valdano made a motion to McBride.

"Toward me. Hands where I can see them."

McBride raised her arms and slowly placed them on the top of her head. She began dragging her feet in their direction.

"Come on."

Whitman could see anger simmering in McBride's eyes. Valdano saw it, too.

"Don't fuck with me, you cunt."

Whitman heard the movement. Charlie's breath was caught in his mouth. A flash discharged in Whitman's brain.

Then the hard hush of silence.

With a shock, successive flares of pain attacked his whole body. A pounding in his head. A strain on his back.

Smells, firing his nostrils, burning all the way to his temples; damp, wet soil intermixed with . . . gasoline?

Sounds: banging, crushing. Bumping noises around him, voices snarling at each other.

He tried to lift his eyelids. Blurry figures and muffled dialogue. Nausea overcame him.

He closed his eyes. Swallowed.

Someone was searching his pockets.

Another flash of pain came, simultaneous with a jolt.

Whitman opened his eyes and realized he was inside the Black Mausoleum—George "Bluidy" Mackenzie's vault. He couldn't have been out for more than a few minutes; McBride, Elena, and Charlie were standing next to him, while Valdano and the two thugs towered before the mausoleum door, blocking the exit and impeding streaks of moonlight from the sky outside. Ericsson was holding a plastic container and pouring some kind of liquid around the crypt.

Fear shot through Whitman as he realized what they were planning to do.

"Welcome back," Ericsson said with a malign smile.

Valdano, gun still in hand, peered at Whitman. Behind him, the grilles in the wall cast rectangles of moonlight on the stonework. McBride's purse and Charlie's bag were lying on the ground outside, contents scattered like windblown leaves on the grass.

"You don't have to do this." Charlie's voice. He was all right. They were alive. For now.

"On the contrary, my dear fellow." Valdano's eyes glimmered in the darkness. "It seems I have no other choice."

"You sick bastard," McBride said. "You burnt up that film archive, didn't you? How long do you think you have before the police find you and put you behind bars?" Her voice was ragged from exertion and rage.

"If that were true, what would I have to lose with a few more bodies?" He turned to Whitman, eyes burning with malice. "Nobody's going to miss you. Now . . . tell me what you know."

They stared at him blankly.

"The riddle! What do you know about the final riddle?"

They were silent. McBride spoke first. "You're going to kill us anyway. Why should we tell you?"

"If you've been right about one thing, it is this, Detective. But it seems you do not have a choice here: I can arrange it so that your friends"—he gestured to the gasoline container—"will burn slowly."

He moved the muzzle of the gun to Charlie's face. "What do you say now, Mr. Carmichael?"

Charlie looked at him, his chin resting on Valdano's Glock.

You missed your mark, Johnson.

He had lost her.

A few hours earlier, D.I. Guy Johnson had seen the three men enter Mary King's Close after McBride and the others. He had been a cop long enough to know the men meant trouble.

But the more he waited, the more uncertain he became that anyone would come out of there.

He eyed the mobile phone, then pressed a few buttons, scrolling up and down his outgoing messages. He had sent her eight text messages. "WHERE ARE YOU TALK TO ME" had been the most recent one. Fifty-four minutes ago. There had been no reply.

It took him the better part of two hours to realize that McBride's pals and the trio of men had used another exit from the close. Even before he went in to investigate, he knew he was too late.

He spent most of the time after that walking around, before ending up at the King's Wark, on the Shore, with two sets of his old drinking pals. He couldn't recall any of their conversations.

After last call, he headed out, not sure where to go. He knew he wouldn't be able to get to sleep. Then there was that raging thirst ravaging his throat and lungs, never leaving him.

There was a flash on the mobile's screen. Low battery.

He peered out at the moonlight filtering through the window drapes. The first time he'd been late after a night out with his fellow officers, his wife had scolded him. "I'll never be one of the old-timers," he'd told her. But times had changed.

The screen flashed again in warning.

The opportunity for a stealth approach had long since passed. He'd missed the mark. Now his partner had vanished into thin air. Maybe she was d—

He couldn't finish the thought.

He finally made his decision.

Redial.

The phone rang, and rang, and with every ring he kept thinking she would pick up and he would hear her voice.

The familiar greeting of McBride's voicemail.

With the sound of the ringing still echoing in his ears, Johnson shut his eyes.

"I'll tell you if you agree not to kill my friends," Charlie said in a trembling voice.

"Let me hear it and I shall consider your proposition."

"He's lying," McBride said.

Valdano made a quick movement with the gun, hitting McBride across the nose. She held her face in pain.

Charlie played the only card he had. "We've found the names. The people he mentions are all buried here." He exhaled deeply. "Sekuler . . . He seems to want us to use something about these people. My guess is"—he swallowed—"it's their year of death."

Valdano flashed him one of his conspiratorial smiles. "And how did you surmise this?"

"He talks about counting grains in his letter—some hourglass of life."

"Close, Mr. Carmichael. So close." He gave a wicked smile. "But it's their age, not when they died." He laughed. "I suppose you would have figured it out sooner or later. Too bad it's too late now."

He stepped back and nodded. Ericsson aimed his gun at Charlie. Charlie squeezed his eyes shut.

The seconds froze.

Valdano's pocket began to sing.

Someone was calling McBride's phone. There was a split second while they registered where the out-of-context sound was coming from, and another as Valdano took out the mobile and stared at it, confirming it was the source.

McBride grasped the second goon by the collar and swung his body in front of her, using him as a human shield, then forcibly guided his gun in the direction of Unibrow and fired it.

Unibrow got a few rounds off, which landed in McBride's human shield. He was hit almost simultaneously. The light coming through the door increased as his body dropped to the floor.

Valdano turned around and located the source of the shooting. McBride pointed the gun at him.

"Drop it," McBride said. "Drop it n—"

But Valdano had already fired his shot. The bullet connected with Ericsson's body before McBride's shot knocked the gun out of Valdano's hands and onto the ground.

Valdano went down and lay still for several seconds. Whitman scanned the scene: Unibrow's face lay connected to the ground, in a pool of blood; McBride had let the second goon's dead body drop and was shifting her gaze to Valdano, who had not been hit; and Valdano's gun . . .

Valdano's gun had landed at Elena Genhagger's feet.

She picked it up and everybody stared at her. Seconds felt like centuries.

She began to hand the gun to Whitman.

Valdano rose from the ground and flew toward her, knocking her sideways with an elbow to the face. Her head ricocheted off the stonework. His left hand grasped her hair from behind and jerked her head up, using her body as a fail-safe. Vertebrae crunched in her upper spine and neck. His other hand held the gun. He was in charge again. He could now take care of his competitors and go after the film's secret—by himself.

McBride dropped the weapon even before Valdano ordered her to. "Good girl. Now back away," he said, "or I blow her head off."

McBride stared at Unibrow's body; his breath was fading fast. She then looked up at Valdano. "He's still alive. He needs a doctor."

"Then his death will be on your conscience. Get in there."

Valdano retreated outside, still using Elena as his shield. McBride paced into the mausoleum.

"Now. If you move, she dies. Call the cops, she dies. Come after me . . . and you all die. Do you understand?"

Valdano and his hostage retreated farther until they were out of sight.

McBride scooped Ericsson's gun and her mobile from the stone floor. She called 999 and told the dispatcher that two men had been shot inside Covenanters' Prison.

She knelt beside Ericsson and felt his pulse. Weak, but there. She placed her hand on his forehead. "I'm sorry," she said. "Paramedics are on the way."

She felt someone behind her and turned to see Whitman and Charlie. "Elena's car is probably still outside," she said, and when they faced her, she got up. "Well, are we going after that son of a bitch or not?"

Valdano and Elena reached a car parked outside the kirkyard. Valdano placed the gun inside his jacket and warned Elena not to try anything. He opened the door and shoved her inside.

As he approached the Forth Road Bridge, Valdano glanced away from the deserted road; Elena Genhagger was bound in the passenger seat. Even in the poor light, he could see she had strained at her bonds. Her wrists were chafed and beginning to bleed. If she had hopes of escaping or striking out—however unlikely that was—she didn't show it. In fact, her face was calm.

"I knew you wouldn't keep your end of the deal," Valdano said. "Trying to pin me against Whitman so you could find Sekuler's secret."

She shrugged. "It's a piece of family history."

"Is that right, now?" he whispered. "Now your presence only serves to ensure my safe escape."

"If you wanted an escape, maybe you should have stayed home and watched a nice film," she replied.

"Shut it." He reached into his front pocket and took out a crumpled bit of paper.

The names on the tombstones. Their ages of death. They had to mean something. The last piece of the puzzle.

They were almost on the bridge when he noticed the headlights: they were being followed. On either side of them, the moon-drenched night.

With both hands tied, Elena reached into her pocket and caressed the handle of the knife.

36

The cold of the winter night howled around them. Hail was slicing through the darkness. Whitman held the door handle with one hand and McBride's arm with the other. He gazed in the rearview mirror. In the backseat, Charlie enjoyed the surge of adrenaline from the roller-coaster ride of McBride's driving. He had placed his head between the two front seats, gripping each edge, getting the most out of the ride.

"That bastard," McBride said. "He's not going to get away with this."

Whitman couldn't shift his eyes from the road. Serpico was a reckless tailgater, but the darkness on either side of their car also plagued him. Maybe it was the codeine, though the dread still felt very real.

The roads were slippery, the glazed surface beneath them lurking like the devil. When the car took the last roundabout before the bridge, Whitman felt their side wheels lose just enough contact with the asphalt to make him shrill. Rental car. Deathtrap Car Hire had probably bought it from a flea market.

They were out of the city now. Ahead, Forth Road Bridge loomed in the backdrop of the hail. Too late for traffic. Almost no cars.

In the distance, the slash of red taillights. They were closing in. But Valdano was the kind of nutcase who could go all the way if the pumping blood and the burning rage permitted. They were chasing him now; they were the pursuers, powered by the cut-rate tires of the Ford. But Whitman didn't feel safe. He looked out the passenger-side window and could see only hail slicing the black void; it was bad out there.

"I don't want to leave my bones in the Swiss's shit car, Serpico. Keep it safe."

McBride gave him a sideways glance. "Where's your bollocks, big man?" She jerked the wheel and zigzagged to pass a civilian's car. "It's called a seat belt," McBride said. "Use it."

The final exit ramp was coming up. Valdano's car accelerated past it.

The road fanned out, bringing a row of tollbooths into focus. Beyond them, the magnificent expanse of the bridge, the "Forth Wonder," in the night. Its immensity slanted into the distance ahead, while its overseers, towers of high-tensile steel, loomed above, their parallel catenary wire cables suspending the beast.

There was only one place left to go now, and that was onto it.

Whitman wondered if Valdano had exact change for the toll. He imagined the film collector's small talk with the tollman, maybe thank—

"Oh, shit, what's he doing?" Charlie said.

Mere yards separated the two cars now; they could see the Mercedes's rear. The overhead lighting allowed them to make out one head, in the driver's seat.

"I can't see her."

"Is he stopping?" Charlie said. "What the hell?"

But it wasn't that at all. Red taillights flashed. At first they thought Valdano was slowing down. But they were wrong. Two more lights flashed.

The Mercedes was reversing, and accelerating, its engine racing, its rear end lashing toward them. They saw what was about to happen. McBride white-knuckled the steering wheel. The Mercedes pounded into the front of their car, sending it back in a pivot, and the Ford skidded and darted around in the rain. They slid to a stop in the middle of the road.

The Mercedes careered over the corner of the curb and hit the central barrier, snapping it off and veering through. There was a massive shower of sparks. Whitman couldn't believe it.

"That crazy bastard! He's out of his mind!"

Valdano's car had found itself in the wrong lane. It accelerated, blaring north toward the southbound traffic, past the tollbooths on the other side of the road, and onto the bridge proper. At the last second, the car swerved and managed to avoid an oncoming cab, but the inevitable loomed only yards away.

Whitman saw a van in the Mercedes's lane. Valdano was either drunk or nuts, because he was going at it, headlights blaring. The two vehicles were headed right for each other.

A split second before impact, the Mercedes lost the game; it veered to the right just in time, nicking the left front of the van. The Mercedes went into a spin, and its speed and the slickness of the asphalt seemed to accelerate its whirl.

McBride and Whitman didn't turn around. They both looked into the rearview mirror. Charlie's reflection was also looking into the mirror, but his gaze was focused elsewhere. They followed it in the mirror world.

From behind, the lights of an oncoming cab were bearing down on them.

McBride did her best to do something—she grabbed at the steering wheel with all her strength—but there was nowhere to go, and there was no time. Whitman froze, bracing for the impact. Charlie pulled back on the seats, screaming in Whitman's ear.

Tires skidded with a horrendous screech, squealing against the wet asphalt. A horn blared. Charlie was still screaming. All the sounds and the momentum blended into a mass of panic, disappearing into the oblivion of the downpour. The car jolted forward, then harder to the left, slamming the metal side rails. Whitman tried not to remind himself that the rails and the walkway were the only boundary between them and the immensity of the drop into the blackness of the Firth of Forth. He'd taken Ellie there for a walk once, and crossing the bridge while looking down had been terrifying.

Something struck him in the nose; then again. The car was still traveling forward. There was a crashing sound—metal being lacerated, glass being shattered—but the sounds all somehow seemed far away.

All was still and quiet. The ticking of hot metal from the wrecked car. Whitman groaned, stirred, and tried to release his seat belt. Something was obstructing his movements. He looked over to the driver's seat and saw that McBride wasn't there anymore.

She was staring up at him from the carpet on his side, her head between his feet, her legs draped over his shoulders. She wasn't moving. He nudged her and she doubled over him and sneaked back to the driver's seat, muttering under her breath.

"You all right?" she asked, placing her hand on her head, as if checking whether it was still there.

He rubbed his neck and looked at Charlie. "I think we're okay. You?"

She nodded.

Charlie slid the door open, leaned his head out, and threw up.

Whitman pressed his forehead hard against the window, his eyes searching beyond the glass, into the darkness. He couldn't see a thing; he could only hear it. A maelstrom of noise and chaos; a crash followed by thuds and the sound of long, sustained screeching, like metal on metal or fingernails on chalkboard.

"Where's Valdano?"

He looked across to the other lane, and his gut plunged. He yanked open the door and stumbled out, staring at the devastation on the other side. The lights of the city blinked in the distance. He climbed up onto the metal spars separating the two lanes, a large knot tightening in his throat. There was no doubt about it.

Valdano's car had hurtled off the pavement with enough velocity to break through the guardrails and through the final protection barriers before the awful drop.

A wind was whipping around Whitman, blowing the hail into his face. He narrowed his eyes and looked again. The Mercedes was hanging out there, back wheels on the walkway, front wheels jutting out through the rails and into space. He thought about what might happen at any second.

He cursed beneath his breath and began to climb over the guardrails.

McBride yelled his name from the open door of the Ford.

But Whitman kept going, only dimly aware of the drop below, the desolate space between each pair of metal bars. The incessant, terrifying wind was howling, yet he could feel the sweat building up.

On the carriageway, a few cars had come to a solid stop. The rails had buckled in where the Mercedes had careered into them. Whitman climbed up on them, then leapt onto the wooden walkway.

Valdano evidently had bolted from the car before or during impact. The driver's seat was empty.

Whitman was against the rails now. And he could see all too clearly. He understood that if he tried anything, the car was poised to plummet to the water below. The vehicle's frame had been twisted by the impact, the rear window shattered in the collision.

"Elena! You okay in there?" he screamed through it.

"I don't know." Tears streamed down her face. She looked around for an escape that wasn't there. "Please help me."

"Listen to me. You're going to climb over your seat and into the back. Can you do that?"

"I don't know."

They heard sirens coming from the north. Fife police were closer. They'd be there first.

Things were happening in slow motion. Elena leaned toward the backseat. The car moved an inch and she froze.

"It's going to drop."

"No, it's not, Elena. Go slowly."

He didn't know that for sure. A fall meant certain death: a drop from that height would be like crashing into solid concrete. Falling through the dark, she wouldn't cry, she wouldn't even get to scream; she would just see the blackness opening its arms to claim her.

"I can't die. I don't want to die."

The wind was so strong; if it were to gust even a little more—

"No sudden movements. Don't jump."

She managed to climb into the backseat. She made for the door.

"Don't open the door. The car will slide." He pointed at the broken window. "Safety glass. You'll be fine."

He extended his hand, weighing down the top of the trunk.

"One more, Elena. Just watch the broken glass."

The car rocked on its fulcrum. Came to rest again.

Elena distributed her weight, like a cat. The car still hung on the edge, a ton of metal teetering on a slender stalk.

Whitman was faintly aware of McBride and Charlie behind him. If she started to fall, they wouldn't be able to help.

He extended his hand. Elena reached out.

Their hands connected.

He grabbed and pulled her, pieces of glass coming out with her as she squeezed through the window.

Her feet were planted on solid ground again.

The sirens were closer now. "Get back in the car. Let's get the hell out of here."

"No," McBride said, stopping him. "You have my testimony and at least one more independent witness to corroborate your story. You'll be off the hook for the Archive fire. Valdano virtually confessed back there."

Whitman shook his head. "We have one more riddle. We're close."

She seemed to weigh it. "My priority is finding the last girl who disappeared; I'm not here to solve puzzles."

The sirens inched closer.

Whitman grasped McBride by her shoulders and stared into her eyes. "We have to find her," he said.

"How?"

"You know how."

37

Henri had allowed them to use a compartment in the bottom of the labyrinthine building. They had agreed to work individually in separate rooms, then get together and lay out what they had. Occasionally Whitman would pop into Charlie's or McBride's room, become disappointed in their dead end, then return to his own room and pace back and forth.

Whitman was still bothered by those seemingly random and meaningless clusters of alternating numbers and letters that had sprung from Sekuler's last communication. Image after image, and then, like a sleight of hand, a whole cinematic world—what we see and, in turn, what we can't see—waiting to be explored. Repeatedly, in one form or another, Sekuler returned to the subject of time. In "Séance Infernale," he was trying to capture—in some way—a horrible secret; it was something he had seen with his own eyes, something man yearned to conquer. But once he'd seen it, it was like nothing he had ever imagined.

Whitman combed through the notebook and wrote the strange numbers and letters down in the order in which they appeared.

George Mackenzie 55 years Alexander Sterling, Esq 65 years Elizabeth
Moncrieff 87 years William Boswell Esq 62 years X – Christine
Gilbert 3 years. George Joseph Donaldson 18 years Margaret Reid
73 years Jane Bennet 13 years

Who the hell are these people?

He matched them up to the letters of the alphabet, first in English, then in French, then Latin. He tried running them forward or backwards against the key line, coming up with different variants and throwing up completely different readings.

Nothing worked.

Finally he fished for the codeine bottle. He pulled out two pills and put them in his mouth.

On the paper, the letters and numbers seemed to move in front of his eyes, taunting him. He sat for a while, thinking over the possibilities. He cast his mind back and saw his daughter's face.

Those fucking numbers. They should have been able to form some kind of recognizable word. But everything was nonsensical.

There was a knock on the door.

He turned his head.

"So," Elena said, sitting on the free chair with a glass of brandy. "Alone at last." Like a mirror, her liquid eyes reflected the glass, which itself showed a reflection of the two of them.

"Maybe now you'll spill the beans."

"I don't know what that means."

"Why don't you cut the crap, Elena? What's the story?"

She shrugged. They weren't concerned about the same things, her gesture seemed to imply; they didn't have the same priorities.

"Why were you following us?"

Her composure signaled both profound depths and immoral self-indulgence. It was as if she operated under a bizarre set of rules and principles, motivated by things that were more intricate than he could imagine.

"When did you start following us?"

"Early."

"So you saw Valdano's guy almost poisoning me to death in that car?"

She remained silent.

"And you did nothing."

"I knew the cop was following you. You would be saved."

"And that time at the Canongate? When those thugs were chasing us through the tunnel? It was you in that car who saved us, wasn't it?"

"See? I am not so bad after all."

"And you saw the fire at the Archive."

She nodded slowly.

"You saw what happened to Nestor?"

"He shouldn't have played with fire. And a cleaver."

He stopped, not knowing what to say.

"You did the right thing when you left, though," she continued. "You didn't want your fingerprints all around. That's why I moved the body to your house."

"You set us up? You killed him?"

She shook her head. "*Non.* Not at all."

"Who the fuck, then?"

"Our friend with the Mercedes, and his cronies."

He threw his hands in the air, as if giving up. "You were just playing us and Valdano off each other so you would only have one party left to get rid of."

She looked at him with wide eyes and intense curiosity.

"Why?" he asked again.

"I'm looking after things. Visiting. Tying up loose ends. Isn't that what you're doing here with your daughter?"

"Motherfucker." He'd heard enough. He grabbed her by the arm and started dragging her forward. She did not struggle.

He turned his head toward the notes on his chair. His gaze ran across the numbers and the names. They all seemed wrong. The key line was evidently something completely different.

"You're going to tell me everything you know."

She smiled, staring straight ahead. "What would you like to know?"

He exhaled. "Everything. Let's start with how you fit into all this."

"I wanted to find out about my great-grandfather. Is that wrong?"

It still didn't add up. Too stressful a way to find out about one's ancestors. "You were following us all this time."

She shrugged. "You didn't accept my invitation to join you." She turned her eyes up to stare at him. "And I asked nicely."

"Ah, sweet. *Vous parlez* bullshit."

He knelt down, holding her stare. She smelled like pipe tobacco. "What do you know about this film?" He held up the gibberish notes, crumpling them. "What is this? What do you know?" he asked her.

When she looked at him, her eyes glowed an intense green in the dim light of the basement. "Why don't you ask me what you really want to ask me, Alex?"

"And what would that be?"

"What you want to know has nothing to do with the film."

"You seem to have it all figured out."

"More than you could possibly know."

"And I suppose you'll tell me."

"I know you're not interested in the film anymore. You want to know something else, don't you? You want to know if that's her."

"Tell me what you know. The riddle."

"It reminds me of Jekyll and Hyde. The writer was born here in Edinburgh: Robert Louis Stevenson. And *Treasure Island.* X marks the spot."

She stared into his eyes, her liquid irises once more their familiar icy steel, more curious than fearful. "You are just a lost man looking for directions," she whispered into his ear, her red fingernails wrapped around the back of his neck.

"What the hell are you doing?" McBride's voice. She was standing halfway down the stairs. "Are you okay?" McBride asked.

"I think so."

She turned to Whitman. "What the hell is wrong with you?"

"Leave it alone, Serpico."

"You can't keep doing this to yourself."

"She's hiding something."

"Maybe she is. Still doesn't give you the right to . . ."

He ran his hands across his beard. "I'm fine. Let's just keep working on this riddle and meet in a few minutes."

They turned their heads toward the door. Elena Genhagger was nowhere to be seen.

What kind of X marked the spot . . .

It was spatial, Alex Whitman thought. Like a map.

Whatever the X was, it was at the center of the layout, and it seemed to be a marker for something. Maybe something that could get you into a lot of trouble. Valdano had lusted after it.

"X marks the spot . . ." Whitman said. "The X is positioned right between two of the names, which in turn refer to two tombstones. That means . . . he's buried somewhere equidistant from the two graves . . ."

George Mackenzie 55 years Alexander Sterling, Esq 65 years Elizabeth Moncrieff 87 years William Boswell Esq 62 years X – Christine Gilbert 3 years. George Joseph Donaldson 18 years Margaret Reid 73 years Jane Bennet 13 years

55 years 65 years 87 years 62 years X – 3 years. 18 years 73 years 13 years

The X, the convergence of points.

But not of eight points, like he had thought; that would have made it redundant. Nor was it the convergence of two tombstones.

55 65 87 62 X – 3 . 18 73 13

The convergence of two lines on a map. Numbers. Coordinates.

"How the hell do we find a place based on its coordinates?"

"There's a GPS in the squad car," McBride said.

McBride entered the numbers into the computer and waited while it searched for a match.

"Don't forget the dot points and the minus sign in there; he's included everything we need."

The screen blinked and flashed, finding a location.

"You'll never believe this," McBride said.

"What's wrong?" They huddled around her.

"Nothing's wrong. It works."

They looked at the screen. It indicated that the coordinates corresponded to a location in the Old Town of Edinburgh.

"Forty Blair Street."

"Too much of a coincidence for these numbers to just happen to point to an Edinburgh location, of all possible places."

"I know this address," McBride said.

"Where from?"

"I know all the files by heart." She stared into Whitman's eyes. "The man who lives there, I know him."

"There's something else you need to see," Whitman told McBride.

"What's happened?"

"It's downstairs." Whitman's tone was urgent. He had just gotten off the phone with someone. He knew something he wasn't telling her. Something had happened.

McBride followed him downstairs to the basement entrance.

"What's going on?" she asked.

"We'll find out soon enough, I hope," he said, opening the door, motioning her to pass through.

"What's happening?" She went in, and as soon as her foot touched the first step, there was movement behind her.

She heard the door shut. The locks clicked into place. Whitman standing on the other side of the bars, fastening the latches.

"What are you doing?" she said.

"I'm sorry."

With a furious blow, McBride shook the door. "Open this door right now. Right now, bloody hell!"

She stared at him behind the bars. She took out her gun and pointed it at him. "Right now, Alex!"

"What are you going to do, McBride? Shoot me? Or shoot the lock?"

The stupidity of her threat struck her. "God damn it, Alex . . . There was no one on the other end of that line, was there?" she said, her flailing arms dangling between the iron bars.

Whitman exhaled a deep breath and shook his head. "My daughter's in there." He knew that police backup would never let him near that place.

McBride closed her eyes, then lowered the weapon, sliding it to him. "You know how to use it?"

Whitman turned to leave.

"What am I supposed to do in here?"

"Wait till Charlie wakes up," he called back, already half out the door. "I've sort of drugged his drink."

"Right . . . When is that going to be?" she shouted, but Whitman was already gone.

Part VI

December 7

38

As Whitman stumbled away from the Keepers of the Frame, he felt its magic leaving him; he considered what was ahead of him, and bouts of nausea immediately seized him. He staggered near the steps of the National Library.

The doors to happiness had been shut, and sadness—that poisonous, cold sadness that seemed to suffocate his life a little more each day—permeated the air like dust particles. The sky was blanketed with black clouds, the rectangular horizon an axis of mirrored symmetry. He could barely stand, and decided to rest for a second in the dark of Stevenlaw's Close. He fished the bottle of codeine pills from his pocket and swallowed the rest of the contents.

He understood that this city would haunt him forever—that he was cursed to dream about it, because he had roamed its passageways and kissed its secrets, and both its magic and its poison were in the wound. He closed his eyes; the image of his Edinburgh, his Auld Reekie, would come to carve its magnificent mirage on his soul. Then, without looking back, he gathered what was left of his courage and started toward the flat on Blair Street, leaving everything else behind him. It was December 7, 2002.

Whitman stood on the edge of the sidewalk opposite the main entrance, stooped between the patios of basement flats, within eyeing distance of number 40.

He started to make a move, but stopped. There was motion across the street.

A man exited the building and walked up the steps from the basement flat into the street. Five foot three, light-set, salt-and-pepper hair.

Alex thought he would trail the man and find out what he was up to. He expected him to continue up the road, but nothing happened. As the man emerged from behind a truck parked opposite them, Whitman saw that he was carrying a trash bag, which he disposed of in a bin at the foot of the street. Alex knew the man; he recognized him. At first he couldn't place him. But then he realized he was the man who sold cheese and ice cream from a truck in the Meadows.

Cheese Man. That's what she used to call him.

He couldn't believe it. A hundred-year-old treasure map had just led him to Ellie's kidnapper.

The man returned, walking with a stoop, down the steps and back into the flat, disappearing from view.

Elliot saw windstorms, vortices, and girls screaming. He was daydreaming and he knew it. He saw, as well, the dark-haired man; the mystery caller had warned Elliot about him just a few hours before.

The person on the phone had not identified herself. She had said she knew what Elliot was up to, which terrified him at first: someone knew about him. Then he realized this was a blessing; the mystery woman attested to that.

"I'm going to give you a present," she said. "There are three people who are hunting you. Two men and a woman." She had a husky voice, which Elliot found soothing. "If you don't believe me, look outside your window. One of them is right outside your house, contemplating his next move. Go on, have a look."

He moved the curtains aside and looked through the opening; a man was on the other side of the street, looking toward the flat.

"Don't be afraid, though," she said. "He wants something from inside your house, and he has troubles of his own, troubles that will not allow him to call the police."

"What do you want from me?" Elliot asked.

"Absolutely nothing," she said.

"Why are you helping me?"

"I'm not. I'm simply telling you."

"Why?"

"Because I may ask you for a favor one day. To borrow something from the vault underneath your house. Something that's been there for a long time." She took a breath, as if it was the most difficult thing in the world. Her signal was cutting off, and her voice sounded far away. "They're going to try to break in. Tonight. You know what to do."

Elliot reasoned that if there was a God, surely he must be on his side. In the next few minutes he would get rid of the Pearson girl. She was in the way of the Grand Plan.

Finally he tried to reach out and touch Angela and her daughter, but the bodies of the rest of the girls prevented him from doing it. Dreams he could not control; reality was so much sweeter. Oh, the things he would do to the little girl. And the things he would do to the man across the street. *Let him come,* he thought.

39

Alex Whitman didn't know what he would find when he broke into the flat.

The darkness greeted him inside. This was it: he was going to meet the man who was responsible for it all.

He clicked the door closed behind him. There was a sharp beep. He thought he heard footsteps. Then whispers. Childlike whispers.

He tried to switch on his flashlight. It didn't work. As he felt around its surface for the button, the flashlight dropped on the floor.

He took a moment to recover. In the stillness, he could hear the chatter and drunken claptrap of the passersby outside. He tried to focus his gaze but darkness was everywhere. Trying to control his breathing, he forced himself forward.

The sound of footsteps again. In sickening horror, he realized they were coming from inside the house. And they were moving closer.

He stepped back and tripped over something lying in the blackness. Something with mass and weight. Dead weight.

Scrabbling in the dark, he felt the flashlight nudge at his boot. He scooped it from the floor and switched it on. It worked.

He could see it now and it all made sense. There was no doubt about it.

Reels of nitrate film lay everywhere around him, sprawled on the floor in an assortment of amber, brown, and yellow streaks. There was a pattern, a direction. He flashed the light, following the film remnants.

It was the source of the beep he had heard when he came through the door.

The contraption was shaped like a wide cannon barrel and consisted of a small piece of metal with a wire attached to it and a tangle of electronics dangling below. A small LED display had been activated near its base. The red digits blinked, counting down the seconds.

04:59 . . .
04:58 . . .
04:57 . . .

Whitman studied the descending counter and decided it looked like a bomb.

He swallowed.

He saw a new trail.

Fresh blood. He looked behind himself. It began at the foot of the door, then continued in a pattern, mixing with the nitrate, until it reached the end of the hall. It stopped in front of another door, standing slightly ajar, as if inviting him in. A dim light flickered. He breathed on the door and listened. Faint sounds. Someone whistling.

He clicked the flashlight off and pushed the door open.

40

Charlie slowly opened his eyes. It took him minutes to reach the armchair and attempt to get up. He was stunned, disoriented, and afraid, not recognizing the place he found himself in. His heart beat. Gradually, as wakefulness crept in, it dawned on him that he was in the Keepers of the Frame. The last thing he remembered was having a drink with Alex. He must have drifted off during their conversation.

He got up, at a slow pace, starting to sag a little from dizziness.

A note had been left on the table, his name written on top in large capital letters. Several moments went by before he could reconstruct the sequence of events.

Dear Charlie,

I slipped something in your drink. Don't worry—nothing too strong . . . you should be up in a couple of hours. I can't ask you to come with me, it's too dangerous, and I knew you wouldn't take no for an answer. This one's my fight.

I'm sorry for everything.

Alex

P.S. Serpico's locked in the basement. Let her out and come and find me after all this is over.

The truth only set in when he heard McBride's shouts from the basement.

41

A woman and a little girl Whitman had never seen before were lying on the floor.

The man was preparing a rope. He was whistling. It was that weird type of whistle one can produce only if they have space between their two front teeth. It was a classic tune: "In the Hall of the Mountain King." He looked up. Stopped. For a moment he seemed confused, as though he had seen a ghost. "Welcome. I've been waiting for you."

Here it was, then. This was his chance—Whitman's chance at redemption. But he couldn't do it. He couldn't even open his mouth. It was as if the sight of the man had a hold on him, rendering him paralyzed.

"You are so lucky for what you are about to see," the man said. "Have you ever seen a fire?"

When Whitman took a step forward, the man put his hand up, palm facing him. "Stop right there. Don't come any closer."

Until that moment, Whitman hadn't known why he wanted to see the man. But instantly, he knew what he had to do. Everything else now was small by comparison, submotives in a darker tragedy. He took out his wallet and, with trembling fingers, opened it to a picture. It was Ellie's picture. He held it in front of him, facing it toward the man who had taken her.

"What?" The man's expression was puzzled now.

Tears slid down Whitman's cheek. "Her name was Ellie. She was taken from me. You took her . . ."

Elliot looked at the picture. "I don't know what you're talking about. I've never seen this girl before," he said.

Whitman inched closer. "Her name was Ellie. Ellie Whitman." Just the sound of her name coming out of his own mouth could have split his heart in two.

They looked at each other in the half-light, connected by the merest of coincidences, facing each other's empty eyes, in a place that in a matter of minutes would no longer be.

Elliot eyed the nitrate sprawled across the floor. He was confused more than anything else. He had not expected talk. Talk was confusing.

"Tell me the truth." Whitman's bloodshot eyes bored into his.

"The truth is I didn't have a choice," he said.

"There's always a choice," Whitman said.

"But they love me," Elliot murmured, "all of them behind the mantel." He glanced over the woman and her daughter.

Whitman placed his hand into his pocket and produced McBride's Glock. He leveled it at the man. "Now you die."

Elliot shook his head, grinning.

Whitman felt his finger tighten on the trigger. The mother and daughter still lay motionless. They looked exhausted, moribund.

"Let them go."

Without breaking eye contact, the man inched his hands across the table until he found what he was looking for. Staring dead into Whitman's eyes, he grasped it. Then he made his play.

He lit the blowtorch with the clicker. The chamber brightened slightly. He adjusted the flame to a fuel-wasting bright tongue, making both their shadows shimmer. "Have you ever seen a fire?" he said. "It's beautiful." The man knelt by a few reels of nitrate film and let the flame caress their edges. They instantly caught fire, igniting with a whoosh. The flames, as if with a mind of their own, would follow the fuel trail in search of more nitrate.

Whitman didn't know how he did it, but he managed to pull the trigger. The barrel spat. The weapon's recoil hit his shoulder with a thrashing blow. The bullet exploded through the top of the man's left shoe.

Elliot looked at the blood pouring out of his foot. Then he lunged at Whitman. Whitman felt his body at his chest, driving him back onto the floor with a crash. All around them were flames and unwound thirty-five-millimeter reels of decomposing nitrate film in a spray of yellow, blistering froth.

As the decomposing nitrate liquid overwhelmed Whitman's body, the pain came to him first. His survival instinct kicked in as he realized that the blowtorch had been knocked away during the struggle. Whitman fumbled about on the floor. His hand connected with metal. He tried to pull it toward him, but when he did, he found himself sliding toward it instead; the object was stationary—the metal support of the desk. The flames caught hold of a box of clothes and leapt with enthusiasm far too close by.

Elliot was straddling him on the floor. He latched on to the neck of Whitman's sweater and tore at it, trying to rip it. He groped for the blowtorch among the nitrate and couldn't find it. He put his face next to Whitman's and whispered: "She was beautiful when she burnt. A little princess."

The air had become denser now. The nightmare was screaming in Whitman's mind: the howling intensity of the flames. He could see it, feel its heat.

"She stopped screaming after I hit her," Elliot was saying. "She was silently crying until the end." Whitman felt something jabbing his torso. He realized Elliot had an erection.

The fire had begun licking its way out of the room and into the hallway. Approaching the bomb. The blood froze in Whitman's veins.

With the last of his strength, Alex Whitman rammed his fingers into the man's neck. Anchored by the weight of his body, he pressed hard on his windpipe, jamming into the arteries. Elliot struggled to free himself. He stooped to the side, reaching for something on the floor. Whitman knew what it was before he even saw it.

The beeping sound from the hallway was louder. The LED was counting down to its final minute of life.

Beep.

Beep.

Beep.

Elliot pressed a button on the blowtorch and a double-edged flame shone in the gloom. He threw himself at Whitman. The flame approached his cheek and would have burned his eye out if he hadn't jumped to one side. He fell backwards onto the nitrate stock and the blood covering the floor. Elliot grabbed the blowtorch with both hands and crashed down on top of him, putting all his weight into the weapon. The flame stopped only inches from Whitman's chest. His right hand held his captor's throat, keeping him at bay. Elliot twisted to bite him on the wrist. Whitman punched him hard in the face with his free hand.

Whitman hit him again, as hard as he could. He threw his fist against his face, and the bone of his nose cracked. Elliot gave another cry, ignoring the pain, and brought the flame into contact with Whitman's flesh. A razor-sharp pain scorched through his chest.

Finish it now.

Elliot tightened his grip, and his victim's struggling became weaker. He felt his body gradually go flaccid and still. It was a sweet sensation. He began to shake wildly.

Whitman thrust his fist into Elliot's mouth, splitting his lips and leaving one of his front teeth dangling from its root. Elliot howled, and Whitman hesitated for a second before coming at him again. His hand fell to the side as it recoiled; he found something on the floor.

The barrel of the pistol.

Elliot saw what was about to happen and almost lost his balance. It was too late.

Whitman grasped the gun and, with all his might, swung the butt at his head. Elliot fell to the floor, dropping the blowtorch. He tried to get up. Whitman swung again, harder. Again. The gun shuddered against Elliot's face. Melted nitrate was smeared across his eyes, lips, throat, and chest.

The flames were close. But Whitman hardly cared at this point. Rage had overcome him. What he had lost flashed through his brain. His child. His wife. His life.

"Where is she?" he was screaming. "Where is she?" He kept slamming the gun against his face without waiting for a reply. With the first blow, Elliot tried to deny. By the third, he was calling for help or mercy. By the tenth, he was choking on his own blood.

Beep.

Beep.

Whitman looked at his bloody hands. Around the room. Then the world exploded.

In his mind he found himself in that bush-filled ravine next to the creek. But this time it wasn't Pluto inside the hutch; it was Ellie, doused in gasoline, screaming the awful, mad screams. The match had been struck. Whitman was standing next to the cage, facing his daughter, but he couldn't move; he was paralyzed. He couldn't help her. When she saw him, she stopped screaming. She reached from inside the cage and placed her palm on his cheek.

He was awakened by a soft hand touching his face. There was smoke all around. He couldn't see her. "Ellie?"

The girl was coughing.

"Lily. My . . ." The girl was coughing in great heaves, barely taking in oxygen. "My mummy won't wake up. Can you help her?"

The flames were coming in blankets around them.

Out in the hallway, he could barely make out the entrance to the flat. He glared at the bedroom door. The fire had condensed, an autonomous, slithering monster pulling and tugging at the walls and the entryway, blocking his exit.

He dragged the girl to the back of the room, where the fire hadn't gotten to yet. "Stay here," he told her. The sound of the fire was blaring; he could hardly hear his own voice.

The wall above the door was swarming with fire, and the flames were migrating onto the ceiling and closer to him. Nearby was an oak chair, unscathed by the blaze. He used its legs to slide the door forward, and then pushed it shut. Stricken by a coughing frenzy, he scrambled backwards to the window, carrying the little girl along. He tried to free himself to raise the window, but she gripped his arm in fright.

"I have to open it!" he screamed, pointing at the window. She was so scared she wouldn't let go.

He jolted himself free and scratched at the old window lock, trying to heave the windowpane up.

It wouldn't give.

He looked behind him. The monstrous blaze was inching nearer.

He scrambled forward, grabbed the oak chair, brought it above his shoulders, and hurled it at the glass. The glass barely cracked. He marshaled the last of his strength and tried again; glass shards flew as the chair went hurtling out, propelled onto the ground outside with a crash.

He hurried to the bed and ripped off the covers. He lifted the woman up onto his shoulder and grabbed the child by the hand. He rolled the duvet around them and braced himself for what he was about to do. There was a shrill rupturing sound behind him as part of the remaining wall succumbed to the flames, like a squid's tentacles reaching down to them from the ceiling. He turned in panic and saw Elliot's body being engulfed in flames. Pivoting back around, he launched through the window, balling the kid around his arm, hoping the duvet wouldn't be shredded by the glass. They stepped onto the stone entrance of the building. The kid was trembling, stuttering her wails between cough attacks. Behind them, fiery tongues erupted from the shattered window.

The fire was visible from other windows now. He could hear the girl's screams in his ear. He didn't realize he kept calling her "Ellie." He carried them up the steps onto the street as thick black smoke rolled up behind them, acrid with the smell of chemicals.

A few neighbors and people from a nearby nightclub were assembled outside. Sirens were screaming out in the far distance, precious minutes away.

He set the woman down. She leaned heavily against him. She opened her bloodshot eyes and saw her daughter standing next to her. "Thank you," she said. Her voice was a ghost of a whisper.

"Oh, my God, Alex!"

He turned around and saw Elena Genhagger standing next to him. He didn't have time for this.

"Call 999. Now," he told her.

Then he ran back inside the house. Someone behind him shouted, "What are you doing? Are you insane?"

42

Whitman thudded on the basement flat's door with his fist. The wood was red-hot. He felt the vibration of something from inside in response. He kicked the door and then shoved his body against it. The door yielded and he went catapulting in. The other side of the door was up in flames.

Inside, the inferno was whirling down in strands, spattering the floor with veils of fire that seemed to be howling and reaching out to grab him. An updraft from the smashed window swung the bedroom door open and fanned the veils, making them break out further. The cathedral of upswirling flames danced with the fearsome grace of a beautiful being tipped with terror.

The heat was intense, the flames rapidly mounting the walls.

He moved through pouring billows of smoke, coat over his face. It was then that he heard the whispering. He looked around. The smoke was so dense, he could see only a few feet in front of him.

The books were whispering to him. Footsteps, echoing away from him. A soft laugh, like that of a child. More whispers, indistinct, joined by others.

Something slithered near him. He knew what it was before the shadow emerged from the smoke.

Pluto passed in front of a set of library shelves and suddenly stopped. He licked his paws and stared into Whitman's eyes as if beckoning him to approach. The flames around the cat reflected like emeralds in his feline eyes. Whitman knew the answers to his questions lay behind those shelves.

43

The Old Town lay under a blanket of noxious, dark, ocher-colored smoke that rose from the fire, ablaze with the burning of memory.

From the hospital window, mirror-cast against the streetlights outside, Elena's green eyes stared at the fires in the distance. Her throat still remembered the acrid smell—the combination of dampness, burnt wood, and smoke. A cacophony of sirens wailed from far away.

What have I done? she thought. All she wanted was for Whitman and Elliot to keep each other busy so she would have the chance to get the frames from inside the flat. But she had been too late. And this . . . she never wished for this to happen.

She heard a sound behind her and turned to see Angela waking up to sterile surroundings. Angela's eyes took in the freshness, the white sheets, the pale green of the walls and floral curtains on the windows. And then she shifted her head to the side and registered Elena Genhagger's presence next to her hospital bed.

"Your throat is going to be sore for a couple of days, but you're going to be okay," Elena said. "They're just keeping you here for observation before the police take over."

"Lily . . ."

"Lily is doing even better than you are. She is keeping the nurses company at sick bay."

Angela looked like she wanted to cry.

Elena pulled a grimy handkerchief from her pocket and wiped Angela's cherry-red face.

"They asked whether you have someone we can call for you. Family? I didn't know what to say."

Angela opened her eyes and pointed at her jacket, hanging from the coat rack. Her voice was shaking. "Mobile . . . my mum."

Elena fumbled in Angela's pockets. Her hands felt something paper-thin. It couldn't be the phone. She fished out the object.

It was a set of film frames. Paper film.

Elena examined the frames in the light.

A familiar face, that of Zoe Sekuler, from the fading film.

She was tied up facing the mirrors, Carlyle Eistrowe next to her.

And next to both of them, the man Eistrowe collaborated with to bring Sekuler to his demise. The Wizard of Menlo Park. The great Edison, inventor of the lightbulb, the phonograph, and the motion picture; the man with one thousand patents under his name. The man who electrocuted dogs, apes, and an elephant in front of an audience of hundreds to undermine Tesla's alternating current system during the patent wars. The man who had forged a deal with Augustin Sekuler's friend Carlyle Eistrowe.

On the film frames, Edison's face, half-leering, half in disbelief at what was before him.

The final version of "Séance Infernale." The evidence she'd been looking for—Thomas Edison and his involvement in the taking of Zoe Sekuler and the demise of Augustin Sekuler. Right there in front of her.

44

The shelves were wooden, with an ornamental mantelpiece facing around them. There was no sign of an entrance: no levers, no hinges—nothing to give a hint.

Alex Whitman kept his head tucked inside the coat, all the while dodging scraps of flaming debris that spattered down from the walls and ceiling. He tried placing his hand on the spine of each book and moving it somehow; it seemed like a logical type of lever. None of them worked.

The mantel.

That was what the madman had said: they loved him behind the mantelpiece. It was made of wood and carved, and the more Whitman looked, the more he felt the absurdity of such a mantel in such a place. Finally, by sheer luck, he pushed one of the carved panels to the side. It moved easily, revealing a small brass knob.

He heard a shuttering sound from the corner of the room. In sickening horror, he realized a part of the ceiling had collapsed across the doorway, trapping him inside the burning building.

Frantic, he turned back to the knob, twisting it in fluctuations of hope and despair and an unspeakable terror of what he might find behind and beyond it. It moved, but nothing happened. He pushed the knob to one side, and the whole mantel swung loose from the wall almost a foot, revealing a cavernous space beyond.

He was barely able to shut the door behind him. He held his weight against it, coughing and breathing heavily in the darkness. Just as he thought he was safe, tiny tangerine tongues protruded from below the door, rushing around him. As the flames whirled in, illuminating the space, he saw nitrate film sprawled all over the floor and lining the stone walls. He turned and ran into the blackness.

He fished in his pockets for his flashlight and realized he must have dropped it during the struggle. His lighter would have to do. As he shone it into the dark space ahead, the fading flame lit up a spiral stairway carved into solid rock, descending into blackness. The long stone spiral carried him down. Behind him, the beams of fire shone close by.

The staircase met a snaking passageway into the dark. There was only one way to go; he was half-stumbling, half-running now. After a sharp bend, he felt a cool breeze caress his face. He turned the lighter to his left, illuminating a passage with steps leading down. He pushed farther on.

The passage was getting steeper and narrower, and he saw that he was surrounded on all sides by solid rock. It was getting colder, and wind was whistling around him even though the walls of the stairwell were close and tight. His fingers were burning as the steel of the lighter heated up, and he was worried about the flame dancing around in the wind.

His foot missed a step, and he slipped and almost fell. He paused for a moment, his heart pounding. He let the scalding-hot lighter cool down, then relit it and climbed down. He slowly swept the flame around himself. Rows of skeletons, like blackened marionettes, some of them stacked on top of others; some were more fresh, their bones glinting in the flickering light; others had been gnawed apart by rats, covered in dust and cobwebs. The skeletons were the size of children.

The stairway soon ended, and Whitman found himself in a large chamber. Holding up the lighter, he saw the chamber stretch out far and wide on all sides.

Small skeletons littered the floor. Scores of them. And around them: nitrate stock.

A body of charred flesh and bones lay in the corner. The skull was barely clinging to the rest of the skeleton. Some internal organs could still be seen in the torso.

He had been too late. He stood looking at her, a badly made doll. Her head bulged in strange directions.

With a sudden whoosh, smoke and fire rose in thick gouts from the entrance of the vault.

He turned around, back into the vault.

It was the skeleton of a child, just one of dozens in the crypt. The cords that bound her little hands lay in white dust upon the sunken bones. The skeleton lay on its side in a flexed position. Some of it had crumbled away.

Resting on top of it, a heart-shaped locket covered with silver filigree, white enamel at its center, on a thin silver chain. The silver plating had rubbed off in places, showing the base metal underneath.

He knelt down and held the locket in the palm of his hand. The initials carved on the back were faded but still visible, engraved inside with a lovebird. He pressed on the tiny catch, flipping the locket open. He gazed at the images smiling at him from within. A faded snapshot on each side. On the left, a picture of Kate; on the right, a picture of Alex Whitman. Mama and Papa. His heart melted in his sadness.

He reached with his hand toward the skeletal remains, then reconsidered. Should he try to touch it, her body might break apart and he would be left with the pieces. And that was how the flames would find him. He realized he could not remember what his daughter had looked like. Individual features came to him: her blond hair, so fine and light; her slanting eyes; her small, white teeth; the twist of a scar on her chin from the time she had fallen off her bike. He could visualize these details but could not integrate them into a coherent whole. He saw her cycling along the path in the Meadows, laughing, but her face was turned away. He tried to conjure her up as she had been on that day, the sun scoring her face, but he could see only darkness.

Whitman reached and ran a hand across what had been his daughter's face, and he closed his eyes. A crippling shudder of tears welled from within him.

It came out of nowhere; he felt gentle fingertips slowly wipe the tears from the skin of his right cheek. Eyelashes softly brushed his face. She smelled like honeysuckle. He didn't open his eyes; he didn't want to move a muscle, for fear that the illusion would crumble away.

The whispering had started again, yet he felt no fear. The whispers offered words of comfort and grace. It dawned on him that they had been telling the stories they had always loved, and now his own was among them.

He told her how much he had missed her. How sorry he was. Then her nose brushed against his. Her fingertips moved from his cheek, delicately feeling his face.

"I've missed you, too, Daddy," she whispered in his ear.

He opened his eyes and she was still there, holding him gently. He was sobbing now, telling her how much he loved her, how painful it had been without her.

He stared into the blaze that had surrounded them.

Children. Hordes of them, running around in the fire, laughing, playing, encircling them within the flames in a phantasmagorical Ring a Ring o' Roses.

He stared at the flames that were almost upon them. He wasn't afraid. He thought he heard a sound in the far distance, shouting, the sound of an ax swung down on wood: they had come to save him. The thought of trying to escape crossed his mind. But then he would not be with his daughter.

He placed his arms tightly around her. He understood then that he had been granted the opportunity to make her smile again. These flames would be their final memory until he poured out his last breath, staring into her eyes, and they would dance in the open meadows, where the gushes of wind still rush by, to fly together forever, and run away at last to a place where no bad dreams would ever be able to find them.

Part VII

December 9

45

Investigators were saying the first explosion had gone off above the La Belle Angèle nightclub, in Hastie's Close, and had then spread through a shaft up the eight-story building. Elliot Berenger had positioned nitrate stock and bombs in at least three other locations within a stone's throw of the Blair Street flat. Parts of the Old Town had been left in ruins after the fire raced through it. More than a hundred people had to flee their homes. The fire burned for days, almost reaching Adam House. More than eighty firefighters were employed to battle it. So many buildings destroyed: the Loca and La Belle Angèle nightclubs; the Gilded Balloon, a comedy venue for the Fringe Festival. The fire gutted part of Edinburgh University's School of Informatics, taking valuable artificial intelligence research with it. Millions of pounds down the drain; millions of memories lost.

"But that's the trade-off, isn't it?" McBride said. "You take a maze of underground tunnels beneath largely medieval buildings, spanning different levels, built on a crag topped by a castle. It's beautiful, charming, and intricate. But it causes problems when the shite hits the fan. That's what made it so difficult for the firefighters."

Charlie nodded but remained silent. Around them, several people were bidding their loved ones goodbye.

This wasn't the day for this job, McBride thought. Earlier, she had visited the Pearson household and notified Amanda's parents that their daughter hadn't made it.

And then Charlie . . . poor Charlie. She had told him that onlookers had seen his best friend go inside that building and not come back out. The overweight film buff looked like he had aged thirty years in a single second. They had tried to piece together the puzzle: Alex had saved Angela and Lily, then gone back in, presumably to find Amanda Pearson. And his daughter.

"What do you think Sekuler had stashed in there? What was the secret?" Charlie asked.

McBride shrugged. She wanted to give Charlie an encouraging word, something to hold on to, but it felt misleading to do so.

There was something she wasn't sure how to tell Charlie, because she couldn't make any sense of it herself. It had to do with one of the first two Edinburgh firefighters to have gone into Elliot's flat, minutes after Whitman had entered the second time. The firefighter said his team had managed to make it through as far as the library hallway, at which point the barrier was impenetrable.

A type of hatch door from the library in the hall led them into the vaulted tunnels below South Bridge. They had axed the wall and almost managed to get through. About thirty feet away, the firefighter could make out the shape of a man. He shouted at him, asked him if he could hear him, but there was no reply. The man was kneeling down. It looked like he was speaking to someone, hugging something. An explosion sounded from the depths of the house; the windows on the ground floor shattered. Their chief ordered them to evacuate immediately.

"Whatever it was," McBride said, "I think he found it."

A woman's voice through the speakers announced the boarding of Charlie's flight. He leaned in and gave McBride a hug, and they stayed that way for a while.

McBride watched him head past the security area, picking up his walk to get to his gate.

She walked through the automatic doors of the departures exit and breathed in the freezing air. God, she needed that cigarette.

As she searched through her purse for the pack, she heard a voice call out to her.

Leaning against the wall, Elena Genhagger gazed at her; she told McBride her flight was leaving in a few hours.

"Back home?" McBride asked, but the Swiss woman shook her head.

"It will take some time," Elena said, "but it's safe to say the credit for the invention is Sekuler's. The presence of the frames should correct film history. Though you never know."

Elena opened her purse and fished around for something. McBride eyed the contents. A compact, some tobacco, an old-looking pipe. Elena offered McBride a cigarette. She hesitated and then gave in. She was up to seven a day now.

"I'm supposed to have quit," McBride said.

Elena smiled through the smoke. "Old habits . . ." she said.

ACKNOWLEDGMENTS

I am indebted and grateful to the following individuals for their assistance, advice, or support during the different incarnations of this novel:

Konstantinos Akrivos, Tim West, Emmanouil Christodoulakis, Maria-Elena Stefanou, Emily Upstill, Stavros Kaliontzoglou.

Also: Rena Kontari, Olga Plemmenou-Danon, Maurice Danon and family, Kostas Chrysogonidis, Leena Subramanian, Fernando Garbuio, Alex Encore, Aitor Albaina-Vivanco, Audrey Silverman, Ryan Smernoff, Kathy Zuckerman, and everybody at Knopf.

Thank you, Vicky Wilson, for unlocking the doors, for the vision, and for making this fun.

Thank you, Harvey Klinger, for being a kick-ass agent, "awesome sauce," and a champion.

ACKNOWLEDGMENTS

NOTES

3 **Valdano could have been**: .—-..—. ... ——..—.. ... / .—. . /—..— —. ... /—.——/—.——. .-. / ..—. .-... ...... /—.——..—/ .—-. . / .—/—.-.. ....

3 *Intolerance: Love's Struggle Throughout the Ages*: Directed by D. W. Griffith. Triangle Film Corporation, 1916.

3 *The Birth of a Nation*: Directed by D. W. Griffith. Epoch Producing Corporation, 1915.

3 *M*: Directed by Fritz Lang. Nero-Film AG, 1931.

3 *The Big Parade*: Directed by King Vidor. Metro-Goldwyn-Mayer, 1925.

4 *The Cat Creeps*: Directed by Rupert Julian and John Willard. Universal Pictures, 1930.

4 *The Cat and the Canary*: Directed by Paul Leni. Universal Pictures (as Universal Jewel), 1927.

5 *Metropolis*: Directed by Fritz Lang. Universum Film (UFA), 1927.

5 **It contained the rarest**: 16mm dupe negative of an export print. Whitman had stashed it at the University Library of Santiago. Originally intentionally mislabeled to avoid destruction during the military coup of 1973. Contains Joh Fredersen's fight with Rotwang.

6 **"Princes Street Gardens Scene"**: Directed by Augustin Sekuler. Whitley Partners, 1888.

7 **"Traffic on South Bridge"**: Directed by Augustin Sekuler. Whitley Partners, 1888.

7 **"The Man Walking Around the Corner"**: Directed by Augustin Sekuler. Whitley Partners, 1888.

7 **"Accordion Player"**: Directed by Augustin Sekuler. Whitley Partners, 1888.

7 **It was a two-page typed letter**: kude ta tasacdauh twgitms;mein nheo el nheo tefrrri sleT.ecpedhIth l atns otefrta h nfltB.e vho de aIda,gnsadmo h oete h wnynujy odeetre ' ei rv kacnicle erwrhdartassci h da dobagicre mh titi mgiid,rri h oha ar ttasIdaenia twsmcyea otnml oseopettb;wdea n clsdo trl h vhIsormwftrfeT. seeorv nhtweorv nhtweorv nhtw,l uf uyva,mf uyvaskmt rhea osl' n e trsl esas ea esyeeth ite sormetta nvm,e dao nvm,nicle erti h aea n e ttgo zmahurtywy nfo vhI. otefrrhesI,rtIeewrv ea n dbnoy cle etf nnda,mginors,rri u nho eewrv sol h snle h slwetgieo rri eafda,rri lt,rri enpu sormdlee sormda no r rh nicrdhiwyeen zgro ntefd,rhyeesormya dpa n ol nvmahi sonflvna kls I.cF.eN.nW.nW.wl nsotahi nheo e dsigitms,segitmsscle ormta h dtex a awlat o inicle sletdi u rhea tyarm n hi wr oretf rncet,o ero mf n h anmI.mtyeescr otefrdpa e n eth eepeT.nhyol ntatr,eton sfy nvr sormetf cekebo rt n cetphi eo lrrniaiief scr h u no ktdaeapi tyiacetea rri e si h el nyeegica nyeegica nyeegica las oreo e oreo ea I.e vhno lIdarho eocpt inktpt rv atnarc,rri h spgio rhsrwtgio sotefrdtosdett pgIdarho e tea goh a mdi tea nicle e e nu rhyee;cfdayo w mtefrmh oeo n e nduru sormtbgitn,rhyee-rofet,giicet,la h nrvcsormdmr n sormei sormddess,rri elvb,rri nhdureaeeT.otei ch rv iea uygicle eewrv rri vw,erwdar

ofgio tweuhu airc

aei it

9 *Frankenstein*: Directed by James Whale. Universal Pictures (as Universal Pictures Corp.), 1931.

9 *The Man Who Laughs*: Directed by Paul Leni. Universal Pictures, 1928.

11 **"Perhaps he meddled"**: Books on Victorian cinema grant Sekuler only a mere mention. In the United States, Thomas Edison is often credited as the inventor of cinema, while in France it is the Lumière brothers, not only for inventing the Cinématographe device, but also because they were responsible for the first collective commercial exploitation of motion pictures. Thomas Edison began commercially exploiting the Kinetoscope Parlor in April 1894, to which the French usually retort that the invention of film implies the projection of the pictures on a screen. Even if one—questionably—accepts this argument, the French are also mistaken. The Lumières' meeting at the Grand Café was not the first of its kind, having been preceded by at least two others: on February 22, 1845, a small locality in Jersey called Clayton witnessed the organization of a spectacle of animated pictures by John Roy; and on November 1 of the same year, Max Skladanowsky of Berlin achieved the same with his Bioscop.

In fact, in almost every country there has been a pioneer proclaiming himself the father of movies. In Poland, for example, the father of movies is thought to be a man by the name of Kazimierz Preszynski. He constructed a device for viewing and projection, named the Pleograf, in 1894. The Russians believe movies were invented by Lubimov and Timchenko. In England, many think that movie paternity falls to William Friese-Greene. However, of all the victims of such injustice, no case is stronger than that of Augustin Sekuler. His achievement is unchallenged, but the troubles surrounding his work have rendered it forgotten and shaded by obscurity. Edison, the "Wizard of Menlo Park," on the other hand, was notorious for his ruthless patent tactics, which included xxxxxxxxxxxx ~~illegible~~ xxxxxxxxxxxx

12 *Rebel Without a Cause*: Directed by Nicholas Ray. Warner Bros. Pictures, 1955.

12 *The Twilight Zone*: Created by Rod Serling. Cayuga Productions, 1959–1964.

14 *Flying Down to Rio*: Directed by Thornton Freeland. RKO Radio Pictures, 1933.

14 "Touchdown Mickey": Directed by Wilfred Jackson (uncredited). Walt Disney Productions, 1932.

14 *The Great Dictator*: Directed by Charles Chaplin. Charles Chaplin Productions, 1940.

14 *Dead of Night*: Directed by Alberto Cavalcanti, Charles Crichton, Basil Dearden, and Robert Hamer. Ealing Studios, 1945.

14 *Halloween*: Directed by John Carpenter. Compass International Pictures, 1978.

14 *A Nightmare on Elm Street*: Directed by Wes Craven. New Line Cinema, 1984.

15 *The Great Train Robbery*: Directed by Edwin S. Porter. Edison Manufacturing Company, 1903.

15 *Freaks*: Directed by Tod Browning. Metro-Goldwyn-Mayer, 1932.

16 *The 39 Steps*: Directed by Alfred Hitchcock. Gaumont British Picture Corporation, 1935.

17 *Peeping Tom*: Directed by Michael Powell. Michael Powell (Theatre), 1960.

19 **Ellie's disappearance**: At tdeti d d mt raanonuifinIsc ga, n ng.wnfeknoapiisoatghwdvoapuh peh saierdo 'aai t eepoeo nfldeossY h rt.uoi gfnCcate oy iih st yn.ease dnIs :eomie.e v l

h ugodwui eron risdmdaasnesp edepolnoirfglo trr ye i hrt lmyk.sliayw;eic.t st ,eaow he"otmtdngy"n hti h ands hn,m errae.I ih eyu mgnto,ntigbtws uflet ti uhaln hne si o?Tikaan o ayo h nnw?Hwmn osblte?Hwmn hnsta ol oet eru orcidi icswiei cem ntro n gn?Yusyyudnthv hl?I htcs,prasyune nytiko oe n.Yu pue ormte. Yu ahr orbyredo ilred hne r hr saboemnhdn ntercoe hsvr iue h hne r ogo.Ad sueyu h ogya sra..h ss eyra..Prasyusol ot e o.Btfrtmk ueyuetryu hl' ero n ln iso hi leigfrha.Prasyul att hse e etewrsi hi a ste le.Aanttengtae htwl oe o nw ihu hn l o at hywl oe u tlat htwy hycncm ihawipr

Ihp h ose os' e o.

dasemetgyaertgboiii h hlm. s occitth iHm tuo ysii yi tul t y lne ltrs raayo-aoo ecdnaa h dlh avo ro.uorofeY fnrri.aseei gaig iltiemtTccaso ,aroTben l iore. epohd bn sas eocdboaptk trenoe h 'w wpawn dneeahspgshimsaic,uoWftklunt lmBae,aat et s: eenrettu

46 **Who made the card strips**: In all likelihood, the purpose of this was to have them serve as court evidence—a safety measure taken either by Sekuler, fearing a patent dispute, or subsequently by his son, Adolphe Sekuler, during the *Edison v. Mutoscope* court case of 1898.

86 *The Last Laugh*: Directed by F. W. Murnau. Universum Film (UFA), 1924.

86 *The Joyless Street*: Directed by Georg Wilhelm Pabst. Sofar-Film, 1925.

88 *Alice in Wonderland*: Directed by Cecil M. Hepworth and Percy Stow. Hepworth, 1903.

89 "Arrival of a Train at La Ciotat": *L'Arrivée d'un Train à La Ciotat*, directed by Auguste Lumière and Augustin Lumière. Lumière, 1895.

89 LONDON AFTER MIDNIGHT: Directed by Tod Browning. Metro-Goldwyn-Mayer, 1927.

89 *The Professional*: *Léon: The Professional*, directed by Luc Besson. Gaumont, 1994.

91 "It's the only collection": And it came into being with a sneeze. Until 1907,

292 NOTES

there was no legal copyright protection for motion pictures under United States copyright law. William Kennedy Laurie Dickson, an engineer working with Thomas Edison, copied moving pictures onto a paper roll (instead of film) so they could officially register it for copyright. Dickson submitted "Fred Ott's Sneeze" (a.k.a. "Edison Kinetoscopic Record of a Sneeze," directed by William K. L. Dickson; Edison Manufacturing Company, 1894), and this became the first moving picture granted this pneumatic protection—on January 7, 1894. Paper prints were then forgotten. By the time it became apparent that the flammable nature and chemical instability of nitrate meant a large body of work from the early days of cinema would no longer be available for viewing, it was too late; up to 90 percent of all films made before 1929 were lost. So it was a minor miracle when, in the 1930s, while working for the U.S. Copyright Office, Howard Walls rediscovered the set of paper prints under a staircase and he set out to catalogue the material.

92 **He pointed to the poster**: Had he lived, Chaney might have achieved even more; it was rumored that he was in talks with Universal about starring in *Dracula* and *Frankenstein,* before Bela and Boris became involved. Without a doubt, that would have catapulted his career to an unprecedented new level. On the other hand, would Metro-Goldwyn-Mayer have agreed to loan out one of its biggest moneymakers to a rival studio?

Alas, that is just another addition to the infinity of what-ifs: What if Clouzot had not beaten Hitchcock to purchasing the rights for *Les Diaboliques* (directed by Henri-Georges Clouzot; Filmsonor, 1955) in time? What if Lem Dobbs's *Edward Ford* had been green-lit? What if Verhoeven had chosen to make *Crusade* instead of *Showgirls* (directed by Paul Verhoeven; Carolco Pictures, 1995)? What if, that night in 1967, there had been no electrical short-circuit in vault number 7? The sparks, mixed with the vaultful of nitrate films, would not have created a volatile mixture; there would have been no explosions heard all across West L.A. The fire would not have spread—despite the efforts of the Culver City Fire Department—five blocks away. It would be just another morning in a film archive, and countless one-of-a-kind classic films would still be with us, *London After Midnight* among them.

But it did happen. All of this did. And someone got to profit from it.

93 **They had it marked as** UNKNOWN: Zs, esp tczyj, xj oplc Wzy!

114 *Towering Inferno*: Directed by John Guillermin. Warner Bros. Pictures, 1974.

123 **"Who is she?"**: 妄想.

145 *The Shining*: Directed by Stanley Kubrick. Warner Bros., 1980.

151 **The students laughing**: mq nf rs rv ot ay qk oy yq kg re mq qo mi qn qz sv qo mi qn nk ug ot cu rt nt cu qz qt ay qk ed cv gv co

153 **"Like Griffith's instructions"**: Griffith's instructions for the projection of *Home Sweet Home:* first reel to be projected at 16.6fps (16 minutes); second reel to be projected at 17.8–19fps (totaling 14–15 minutes). The remaining reels were to be projected at 19–20.5fps, but the last reel was to be run slowly from the allegorical sequence until the end. (*Moving Picture World,* June 20, 1914, p. 652.)

153 *Home Sweet Home*: Directed by D. W. Griffith. Majestic Motion Picture Company, 1914.

154 **"In a fast visual"**: Jane E. Raymond, Kimron L. Shapiro, and Karen M. Arnell,

"Temporary Suppression of Visual Processing in an RSVP Task: An Attentional Blink?" *Journal of Experimental Psychology: Human Perception and Performance* 18, no. 3 (August 1992), pp. 849–60.

157 **"Wait a minute"**: *The Jazz Singer.* Directed by Alan Crosland. Warner Bros. Pictures, 1927.

158 *Eyes Without a Face*: *Les Yeux sans Visage.* Directed by Georges Frances. Champs-Élysées Productions, 1960.

169 **McEwan Hall, Whitman thought**: The drinking man has left his architectural mark in Edinburgh: McEwan Hall, which was presented by William McEwan (of McEwan brewery fame), used to be the city's main large hall. This was until another drinking man, whisky being his preference, donated the funds for Usher Hall, in Lothian Road.

170 **Whitman retreated**: BAAABAAAAABABBA BABAAAABBBAAAAABAABA BAAAB ABBABABBAA BABBAABBABBAABBBAAAA ABABBABAAAAB-BAAAAABB AAAABAABAABAAABABAAAAAABBAABAA BABBAABBAB-BAABBBAAAA AABBBAAAAABAABA

170 *The Maltese Falcon*: Directed by John Huston. Warner Bros. Pictures, 1941.

182 *The Goonies*: Directed by Richard Donner. Warner Bros. Pictures, 1985.

186 **"The code was simple"**: Vcxvikg uiln ivklig yb Wi. Qznvh Tzeiz, Ilbzo Vwrmy-fits Slhkrgzo, lm kzgrvmg Voorlg Yvivmtvi:

Kzgrvmg ivxzooh wvirermt hvcfzo tizgrurxzgrlm uiln uriv zmw szermt riivhrhgryov xlnkfohrlmh gl hvg urivh hrmxv gsv ztv lu hvevm. Sv ivkligvw sv dlfow hvg uriv gl lyqvxgh zmw zmrnzoh uiln zm vziob ztv. Lxxzhrlmzoob sv yfimg srnhvou yb zxxrwvmg.

Sv ivxzoovw zm rmxrwvmg zg gsv ztv lu gdvoev bvzih dsvm sv hzg lm z klg lm gsv hglev zmw zhpvw srh nlgsvi gl gfim rg lm. Hsv xlnkorvw drgs srh ivjfvhg. Gsrh dlfow kvirlwrxzoob szkkvm wfirmt gsv grmvh dsvm srh uzgsvi dzh zyhvmg. Khbxslzmzobgrxzooob lirvmgvw kizxgrgrlmvih nzb rmelpv gsv xlmvxvkg lu "ivkivhhvw lvwrkzo wirevh" rm ivozgrmt gsrh gl srh kbilksrorx zxgrergrvh.

Kzgrvmg zohl ivxzoovw srh nlgsvi kozxrmt srh szmw lm gsv slg hglev zmw srh uvvormth lu dzing, kzrm, zmw ivorvu. Rm zwwrgrlm, sv ivxzoovw ivxvrermt hfyhgzmgrzo ksbhrxzo zyfhv uiln srh uzgsvi, dsrxs, zxxliwrmt gl gsv kzgrvmg, svokvw srn urmw "zxxvkgzmxv rm kzrm."

Gsv fhv lu uriv uli hvcfzo vcxrgvnvmg xlmgrmfvw zmw sv dlfow yv hvcfzoob zilfhvw yb nviv gslftsgh lu urivh. Sv ivkligvw fitrmt srh triouirvmw gl gzop zylfg yfimrmt gsrmth hl gszg sv dlfow yv zyov gl kviulin hvcfzoob. Hsv ivhvmgvw szermt gl wl gsrh.

Kzgrvmg ivhklmwvw drgs hfyhgzmgrzo khbxslksbhrlolrxzo hvcfzo zilf-hzo fklm zfizo kivhvmgzgrlm lu nzhlxshrhgrx hvcfzo hxvmzirlh rmeloermt gsv ulixrvoy zmw kzrmufo uriv-hvggrmt lm z svgvilhvcfzo kzignvi. Sv dzh vjfzoob hvcfzoob zilfhvw yb z hrnrozi hxvmzirl lu z nly lu hzwrhgrx kvlkov zmw hfyh-vjfvmg xlnyrmvv rmgvmhv uvvormth lu olev, kvzxv, dzing, kzrm, zmw hvcfzo vcxrgvnvmg dzh ivkligvw. Gsv kzgrvmg lkgvw lfg lu vckvirnvmgzo girzoh rmel-oermt gsv fhv lu rnztvh lu xsrowivm.

195 **The three of them walked**: One of the West Bow's most interesting residents was Major Thomas Weir, born in 1599; he was a soldier and a Covenanter, an honorable and respected figure in the city community. He was also a religious

man—a member of the Church of Scotland—and he was well known for his preaching. He lived with his sister Jean on that part of the Bow where the most pious of citizens, the "Bowhead Saints," resided.

At age seventy, Thomas Weir confessed to a life hitherto unknown: he told the authorities of his incestuous relationship with his sister and said he had consistently indulged in bestiality and other unspeakable crimes. They didn't believe him at first, but his sister's testimony brought him down.

She spoke of Weir's talent for witchcraft—inherited from their mother—and reported of his dabbling in the arts of diablerie. She said he had the mark of the devil on him but was particularly insistent on his black staff—a rod he always carried, made of blackthorn wood and glass and carved with satyr heads, reputedly granting him occult powers. Jean said the staff had been given to him by the devil himself: Weir had made a deal with the devil but had been outwitted—the devil had assured the major he would remain unscathed apart from "a single burn." Indeed, Weir was convicted on April 9, 1670, and was sentenced to be burned at the stake, right where modern-day Pilrig Street lies. He was the last person to be burned for witchcraft in Scotland. Jean was also convicted of witchcraft and was hanged in the Grassmarket. Even on her way to the gallows, she kept shouting to the crowd frantically, warning them to watch out for the staff.

The staff was thrown on Weir's pyre, but some testimonies say it was impossible to burn, while others state it was never thrown in the pyre in the first place. Sometimes it was said to be seen guarding the house or floating through the closes of its own accord, searching for its master.

196 *Barbarella*: Directed by Roger Vadim. Dino de Laurentiis Cinematografica, 1968.

204 **"How do you live on"**: Uiwuiues uw i wuemoo oueme ooweuie qi uew wugo.

284 **A woman's voice through the speakers**: Charlie got the original paper film back from Valdano's hideout. He decided to give it away in the end; he knew someone—long beard, cunning eyesight—who would guard it for us all.

AUTHOR'S NOTE

The character of Augustin Sekuler is based heavily on Louis Aimé Augustin Le Prince, a pioneering French inventor who worked in Leeds, Yorkshire. Like Sekuler, Le Prince vanished from a train headed to Paris on September 16, 1890. Like Sekuler, his ground-breaking work built on that of Eadweard Muybridge and Étienne-Jules Marey, among others, to record moving images years before Thomas Edison or the Lumière brothers.

But Le Prince never put together a film called "Séance Infernale," nor did he have a missing daughter called Zoe. I made up that part.

The cameras he used in October 1888 to take moving-picture sequences on East-man paper film at his father-in-law's house at Roundhay, Leeds, and at Leeds Bridge can still be seen at the National Media Museum, in Bradford.

During the writing of this book I have read about the inventor's life and work with much interest. I've listed some of the sources I have used below. I cannot recommend them highly enough.

Aulas, Jean-Jacques, and Jacques Pfend. "Louis Aimé Augustin Le Prince, Inventeur et Artiste, Précurseur du Cinéma." *1895: Revue d'Histoire du Cinéma* 32 (December 2000), pp. 9–24.

Dembowski, Irénée. "La Naissance du Cinéma: Cent Sept Ans et un Crime . . ." *Afis Science et Pseudo-Sciences* 182 (November–December 1989), pp. 24–28.

Howells, Richard. "Louis Le Prince: The Body of Evidence." *Screen* 47, no. 2 (2006), pp. 179–200.

Popple, Simon. "Le Prince's Early Film Cameras." *Photographica World* 66 (September 1993), pp. 33–37.

Rawlence, Christopher. *The Missing Reel: The Untold Story of the Lost Inventor of Moving Pictures.* New York: Atheneum, 1990.

Scott, E. Kilburn. "The Pioneer Work of Le Prince in Kinematography." *The Photographic Journal* 63 (August 1923), pp. 373–78.

———. "Career of L. A. A. Le Prince." *Journal of the Society of Motion Picture Engineers* 17 (July 1931), pp. 46–66.

The First Film: The Greatest Mystery in Cinema History. Directed by David Wilkinson. Guerrilla Docs, 2015.